Current Surgical Guidelines

Abdullah Jibawi

Specialist Registrar in Surgery
University Hospitals of Leicester;
Visiting Researcher to Oxford University

David Cade

Medical Director
Greater Manchester NHS CATS;
Previously Consultant General Surgeon
Mid Cheshire Hospitals NHS Foundation Trust

OXFORD
UNIVERSITY PRESS

OXFORD
UNIVERSITY PRESS

Great Clarendon Street, Oxford OX2 6DP

Oxford University Press is a department of the University of Oxford.
It furthers the University's objective of excellence in research, scholarship,
and education by publishing worldwide in

Oxford New York

Auckland Cape Town Dar es Salaam Hong Kong Karachi
Kuala Lumpur Madrid Melbourne Mexico City Nairobi
New Delhi Shanghai Taipei Toronto

With offices in

Argentina Austria Brazil Chile Czech Republic France Greece
Guatemala Hungary Italy Japan Poland Portugal Singapore
South Korea Switzerland Thailand Turkey Ukraine Vietnam

Oxford is a registered trade mark of Oxford University Press
in the UK and in certain other countries

Published in the United States
by Oxford University Press Inc., New York

British Library Cataloguing in Publication Data
Data available

Library of Congress Cataloging in Publication Data
Data available

Typeset by Cepha Imaging Private Ltd., Bangalore, India
Printed in Italy
on acid-free paper by
Lego Print S.p.A.

ISBN 978–0–19–955827–8

10 9 8 7 6 5 4 3 2 1

Foreword

It is with some trepidation that I began the task of reviewing the contents of this book. My trepidation was based on the fact that, having had a strong interest in guideline production and dissemination myself, I know just how insipid and monotonous guidelines can be. I need not have worried! Indeed, towards the end of my task, I was positively looking forward to reading the next chapter. The authors are to be commended on compiling such a comprehensive collection of contemporary surgical guidelines, and presenting them so clearly that the busy clinician will have no trouble whatsoever in reading and digesting their contents. The sensible use of simple tables makes it straightforward to identify the information relevant to a specific clinical problem.

I particularly enjoyed the first twenty chapters because they deal with everyday clinical issues that are relevant to surgeons practising in all branches of surgery. I have no doubt that junior doctors who base their day-to-day care of surgical patients on these guidelines will greatly improve the care that they offer. Experienced surgeons will not only find guidelines relevant to their specialist area but can rapidly access contemporary information from areas of surgical practice outside their immediate expertise. It is for these reasons that this book will be invaluable to all surgeons, be they Foundation year doctors or experienced consultants.

The guidelines are UK-based if they are available. Thereafter, the hierarchy is European guidelines followed by North American guidelines. This approach is sensible and pragmatic. In summary, the authors are to be congratulated on compiling and presenting contemporary surgical guidelines in such a way that they are interesting and immediately relevant to clinical practice. I am certain that I will be referring to my own copy on a very regular basis!

Professor Nick London
Professor of Surgery
University of Leicester

Preface

Documents written for guiding decisions in the diagnosis and management of specific diseases have been in use for many thousands of years. Unlike previous approaches that were often based on authority or tradition, modern guidelines reflect a consensus of expert opinion following a thorough and systematic review of currently available scientific evidence.

Clinical guidelines do not aim to replace the clinical judgement, but to support it. Guideline recommendations attempt to define practices that meet the requirement of most patients in most circumstances, but can give no guarantee of a successful outcome in every individual case. Clinical judgement and decision-making should consider the individual patient's condition, circumstances and wishes, as well as the quality and availability of expertise in the area where care is provided.

In recent years, the number of guidelines produced by national bodies, specialist associations, royal colleges, and others has increased enormously and it has become difficult for busy clinicians to keep up to date with rapidly changing fields. The focus of this handbook is to summarize currently available guidelines in general and vascular surgery in a concise, practical, and friendly way. Neither should it be considered that it includes all acceptable methods of management nor as a standard of clinical care. In short, 'we summarize the guidelines, you make the decision'.

We hope that this book will contribute to the implementation of high quality guidelines in surgical practice.

General outlines

The principles and rules throughout the book are limited in order to provide consistency in summarizing all the scattered guidelines.

We have used different search engines to find the most relevant and up-to-date guidelines for each topic. National Library for Guidelines (UK), National Guideline Clearinghouse (US), National Institute for Health and Clinical Excellence (NICE), Scottish Intercollegiate Guidelines Network (SIGN), Google™, and other online portals (e.g. the Association of Surgeons of Great Britain and Ireland, the Royal College of Surgeons of England, and BMJ Clinical Evidence) were accessed and systematically reviewed. Full text guidelines were retrieved, thoroughly evaluated, and summarized. Guidelines written on the same topic and published by different authorities were compared and referenced within the summary text as appropriate. Relevant chapters were reviewed independently by the authors and then by appropriate experts in each field.

We have integrated friendly statistics within different sections of each chapter to support a realistic decision-making process and allow informed decisions for patients at the point of care. These statistics can be used, for example, to understand the impact of a risk factor on a specific disease and allow for better understanding of any recommended screening programme (e.g. screening for abdominal aortic aneurysm at the age of 65, chapter 46); to realize the limitations of certain investigations in detecting (sensitivity) and confirming (specificity) certain pathology or disease severity (e.g. endoscopic ultrasound scan (EUS) in oesophageal cancer staging, chapter 21); and to provide the clinician with the latest figures on the efficiency and safety of different treatment options, and therefore, allow for better communication with patients and evidence-based supported decision-making (e.g. efficacy of local glyceryl trinitrate (GTN) for anal fissure healing, chapter 34).

Recommendations for a specific investigation, screening, or treatment have been graded as per the original guideline's grading system, which usually follows the main theme of grading as outlined in chapter 1.

Tables have been used extensively within the handbook for summarizing and easy access purposes. The recommended approach for each disease has been outlined using specially designed algorithms which formulate an integral part of each relevant chapter and have to be interpreted within this context. The recommended approach does not include all acceptable methods of diagnosis or management; sound clinical judgment is always required (chapter 1).

The audit process has become an integral part of the evaluation of an individual clinician's performance as well as the hospital internal activities. Audit requires appropriate tools to gather selected information (indicators) and compare to standards and guidelines in order to highlight the differences and make changes where appropriate. We have provided the reader with a distinct audit box under the title 'Know your results'. The audit ideas within the box are there to stimulate the reader's mind on the practicality of assessing and measuring guidelines in real life.

Some ideas have been derived from published audit work and are referenced where appropriate.

Finally, we used a quick reference script to allow for rapid and efficient access to information at the point of care. This style has been adopted based on some constructive feedback we have had during the development process; the handbook is not to replace the more traditional surgical textbooks or handbooks, but to provide the reader with consistent, up-to-date, and sound clinical information. We hope the book will stimulate the reader to read the original documents. Any comments or recommendations are welcomed (please visit our website at: www.surgicalguidelines.co.uk).

Acknowledgements

We would like to record our sincere thanks to our advisors on specific sections:

Prof. Nick London, Professor of Surgery, University of Leicester and Honorary Consultant Vascular and Endocrine Surgeon, University Hospitals of Leicester NHS Trust; **Ms. Linda De Cossart**, Vice President of the Royal College of Surgeons of England; **Prof Mohan de Silva**, University of Sri Jayawardenepura, Colombo, Sri Lanka; **Prof. A Ross Naylor**, Professor of Vascular Surgery, University Hospitals of Leicester NHS Trust; **Prof. Robert Sayers**, Professor of Vascular Surgery, University Hospitals of Leicester NHS Trust; **Mr. Mark McCarthy**, Consultant Vascular Surgeon and Honorary Senior Lecturer, University Hospitals of Leicester NHS Trust; **Mr. Martin Dennis**, Consultant Vascular Surgeon, University Hospitals of Leicester NHS Trust; **Mr. Akhtar Nasim**, Consultant Vascular Surgeon, University Hospitals of Leicester NHS Trust; **Mr. Sukhbir Ubhi**, Consultant Surgeon, University Hospitals of Leicester NHS Trust; **Mr. Chris Sutton**, Consultant Surgeon, University Hospitals of Leicester NHS Trust; **Mr. Roddy Nash**, Consultant Surgeon, Derbyshire Royal Infirmary; **Dr Douglas A B Turner**, Consultant Anaesthetist and Critical Care, University Hospitals of Leicester NHS Trust; **Dr. Sue Povard**, Consultant Haematologist and Lecturer at the University of Leicester; **Dr. Andrew Swann**, Consultant Microbiologist, University Hospitals of Leicester NHS Trust; **Ms. Michelle Lapworth**, Vascular and Wound Specialist Practice Nurse, University Hospitals of Leicester; **Mr. John Jameson**, Consultant Surgeon, University Hospitals of Leicester NHS Trust; **Mr. Ashley Dennison**, Consultant Surgeon, University Hospitals of Leicester NHS Trust; **Mr. David Berry**, Consultant Surgeon, University Hospitals of Leicester NHS Trust; **Mr. David Corless**, Consultant Surgeon, the Mid Cheshire Hospitals NHS Trust; **Mr. Magdi Hanafy**, Consultant Surgeon, the Mid Cheshire Hospitals NHS Trust; **Mr. Sulaiman Shoaib,** Consultant Surgeon, The North West Wales NHS Trust; **Mr. Lloyd Jenkinson**, Consultant Surgeon, The North West Wales NHS Trust.

We would like also to heartedly appreciate the constructive feedback we had from **Prof. Nick London**, Professor of Surgery at the University of Leicester (UK), **Prof. Murray Brennan**, Professor of Surgery at the Memorial Sloan Kettering Cancer Centre (USA), and **Prof. Jonathan Meakins**, Professor of Surgery at the Nuffield Department of Surgery, University of Oxford (UK).

Finally, we would like to thank our families, without their support this work would not have been completed ever, and our colleagues for their contributions and feedback: Mohammed Ballal (UK), Chris Mann (UK), Caroline Gjorup (Denmark), Baraa Zuhaili (US), Khalid Osman (UK), and Kee Wong (UK).

Symbols and abbreviations

+ve	positive
−ve	negative
°C	degree centigrade
%	percentage
~	approximately
±	with or without
>	greater than
<	less than
▶	important
📖	cross reference
≥	equal to or greater than
≤	equal to or less than
α	alpha
β	beta
µ	micro
®	registered
™	trademark
AAA	abdominal aortic aneurysm
ABG	arterial blood gases
ABPI	ankle brachial pressure index
A&E	Accident and Emergency
ACA	adenocarcinoma
ACE	angiotensin-converting enzyme
ACTH	adrenocorticotropic hormone
AF	atrial fibrillation
AFP	alpha-fetoprotein
AGA	American Gastroenterological Association
AI	aromatase inhibitor
AK	above knee
ALT	alanine transaminase
am	*ante meridiem* (before noon)
ANC	axillary node clearance
ANS	axillary node sampling
APACHE	acute physiology and chronic health evaluation

APC	argon plasma coagulation
APR	abdominal perineal resection
aPTT	activated prothromboplastin time
ARF	acute renal failure
ARR	absolute risk reduction
ASA	American Society for Anaesthesiologists
AST	aspartate aminotransferase
ATN	acute tubular necrosis
AXR	abdominal X-ray
BADS	British Association of Day Surgery
BAPEN	British Association for Parenteral and Enteral Nutrition
BCS	breast-conserving surgery
bd	*bis die* (twice daily)
BK	below knee
BMI	body mass index
BP	blood pressure
bpm	beats per minute
BUN	blood urea nitrogen
Ca	calcium
CA	carbohydrate antigen
CBD	common bile duct
CBDS	common bile duct stones
CDR	clinical decision rule
CEA	carcinoembryonic antigen; carotid endarterectomy
CER	control event rate
CFTR	cystic fibrosis transmembrane regulator
CgA	chromogranin A
Ch	chapter
CI	contraindicated, confidence interval
CJD	Creutzfeldt–Jakob disease
CLI	critical limb ischaemia
CLO	columnar-lined oesophagus
cm	centimetre
CMM	conventional medical management
CMV	cytomegalovirus
CO_2	carbon dioxide
COPD	chronic obstructive pulmonary disease
CPAP	continuous positive airways pressure
CPD	continuing professional development
CRC	colorectal cancer

CRP	C-reactive protein
CT	computed tomography
CVA	cerebrovascular accident
CVI	chronic venous insufficiency
CVP	central venous pressure
CXR	chest X-ray
D&F	diet and fluid
d	day
DCIS	ductal carcinoma *in situ*
DEXA	dual energy X-ray absorptiometry
DIC	disseminated intravascular coagulation
dL	deciliter
DSA	digital subtraction arteriography
DVT	deep vein thrombosis
EBM	evidence-based medicine
ECG	electrocardiogram
EDV	end diastolic velocity
EER	experimental event rate
e.g.	*exempli gratia* (for example)
ELISA	enzyme-linked immunosorbent assay
EMS	endoscopic mucosal resection
EPO	evening primrose oil
ER	oestrogen receptor
ERCP	endoscopic retrograde cholangiopancreatography
ERP	enhanced recovery programme
ESRD	end-stage renal disease
EU	European Union
EUA	examination under anaesthesia
EUS	endoscopic ultrasound scan/ultrasonography
EVAR	endovascular aneurysm repair
EVL	endoscopic variceal ligation
EVLT	endovenous laser therapy
EWMA	European Wound Management Association
FBC	full blood count
18-FDG	18-fluoro-2-deoxyglucose
FA	folinic acid
FAP	familial adenomatous polyposis
FENa	fractional excretion of sodium
FEV(1)	forced expiratory volume in 1 minute
FFP	fresh frozen plasma

FIO_2	fraction of inspired oxygen
FNA	fine needle aspiration
FNAc	fine needle aspiration cytology
FOB	faecal occult blood
FP	focused parathyroidectomy
FRC	functional residual capacity
5-FU	5-fluorouracil
FVC	forced vital capacity
g	gram
GA	general anaesthesia
GBS	gastric bypass surgery
GCS	graduated compression stocking
GFR	glomerular filtration rate
GI	gastrointestinal
GMC	General Medical Council
GOJ	gastro-oesophageal junction
GORD	gastro-oesophageal reflux disease
GP	general practitioner
GTN	glyceryl trinitrate
Gy	gray
h	hour
H2	histamine-2
Hb	haemoglobin
HBV	hepatitis B virus
HCAI	health care-associated infection
HCC	hepatocellular carcinoma
HCV	hepatitis C virus
HDU	high dependency unit
HER-2	human epidermal growth factor receptor-2
5-HIAA	5-hydroxyindoleacetic acid
HIV	human immunodeficiency virus
HNPCC	hereditary non-polyposis colorectal carcinoma
H_2O	water
HPC	history of presenting complaint
HPT	hyperparathyroidism
HPV	human papillomavirus
HRT	hormone replacement therapy
ICA	internal carotid artery
ICP	Integrated Care Pathway
ICU	intensive care unit

IDDM	insulin-dependent diabetes mellitus
i.e.	*id est* (that is)
IE	infective endocarditis
Ig	immunoglobulin
IJCP	idiopathic juvenile chronic pancreatitis
IL	interleukin
IM	intramuscular
INR	international normalized ratio
IOC	intra-operative cholangiography
IONM	intra-operative nerve monitoring
IPC	intermittent pneumatic compression
iPTH	intra-operative parathyroid hormone
ISCP	idiopathic senile chronic pancreatitis
ITU	intensive treatment unit
IU	international unit
IV	intravenous
K^+	potassium
kcal	kilocalorie
kg	kilogram
kPa	kilopascal
KUB	kidney-ureter-bladder
L	litre
LA	local anaesthesia
LACI	lacunar infarction
LAGB	laparoscopic adjustable gastric banding
LA-VBG	laparoscopic-adjusted vertical banded gastroscopy
LCBDE	laparoscopic common bile duct exploration
LCIS	lobular carcinoma *in situ*
LFT	liver function test
LIF	left iliac fossa
LMWH	low molecular weight heparin
LOS	lower oesophageal sphincter
LT4	levothyroxine
m	metre
MAOI	monoamine oxidase inhibitor
MAP	mean arterial pressure
MDT	multidisciplinary team
MEN	multiple endocrine neoplasia
μg	microgram
mg	milligram

Mg	magnesium
μg	microgram
MI	myocardial infarction
min	minute
mL	millilitre
mmHg	millimetre mercury
mmol	millimole
mo	month
MR	magnetic resonance
MRA	magnetic resonance angiography
MRCP	magnetic resonance cholangiopancreatography
MRI	magnetic resonance imaging
MRSA	methicillin-resistant *Staphylococcus aureus*
MTC	medullary thyroid cancer
MUST	Malnutrition Universal Screening Tool
NBM	nil by mouth
NET	neuroendocrine tumours
NF	neurofibromatosis
ng	nanogram
NGT	nasogastric tube
NHS	National Health Service
NICE	National Institute for Health and Clinical Excellence
NNT	number needed to treat
NPI	Nottingham prognostic index
NSAID	non-steroidal anti-inflammatory drug
od	*omni die* (once daily)
OGD	oesophagogastroduodenoscopy
OHCM	Oxford Handbook of Clinical Medicine 7th edition, OUP
OHCS	Oxford Handbook of Clinical Surgery 3rd edition, OUP
OR	odds ratio
p	probability
PACI	partial anterior circulation infarction
$PaCO_2$	partial pressure of carbon dioxide in arterial blood
PAD	peripheral arterial disease
PC	presenting complaint
PCA	patient-controlled analgesia
PCO_2	partial pressure of carbon dioxide
PDT	photodynamic therapy
PE	pulmonary embolism
PEF	peak expiratory flow

PEG	polyethylene glycol
PEI	percutaneous ethanol injection
PET	positron emission tomography
PFT	pulmonary function tests
PHP	primary hyperparathyroidism
PMI	perioperative myocardial infarction
PO	*per os* (by mouth)
PO_2	partial pressure of oxygen
PO_4	phosphate
POCI	posterior circulation infarction
PPI	proton pump inhibitor
PR	*per rectum* (by the rectum) / progesterone receptors
PRN	*pro re nata* (when necessary)
PSS	post-splenectomy sepsis
PSV	peak systolic velocity
PT	prothrombin time
PTH	parathyroid hormone
QALY	quality adjusted life year
qds	*quater die sumendus* (to be taken 4 times daily)
RBC	red blood cell
RBL	rubber band ligation
RCT	randomized controlled trial
RF	radiofrequency
Rh	rhesus
RhAPC	recombinant human activated protein C
RIF	right iliac fossa
rpm	respirations per minute
RR	relative risk
RRR	relative risk reduction
SAPS	simplified acute physiology score
SCC	squamous cell carcinoma
SCS	spinal cord stimulation
SD	standard deviation
SECU	surgical extended care unit
SF	stress factor
SFJ	saphenofemoral junction
SPJ	saphenopopliteal junction
SIGN	Scottish Intercollegiate Guidelines Network
SIRS	systemic inflammatory response syndrome
SLNB	sentinel lymph node biopsy

Detailed contents

Part 1

Principles of evidence-based medicine

Chapter 1

Principles of evidence-based medicine

Principles of evidence-based medicine

Key guidelines

- Oxford's Centre for Evidence-Based Medicine.
- The Cochrane collaboration.
- Sackett *et al.* (2000). *Evidence-based medicine*, 2nd ed. Churchill Livingstone.

Basic facts

- **Definition**—Evidence-based medicine (EBM) is a process of systematically reviewing, appraising, and applying clinical research findings to support the optimum delivery of clinical care to patients.[1,2,3]
- **Challenges**—The overwhelming number of published scientific papers everyday (>2,000,000 each year), the busy clinical life to fulfil the knowledge gaps (if identified!), the shortage of time required to keep up to date with existing information, and the weak continuing professional development (CPD) strategies to address the problem of declining knowledge require a different approach to clinical learning. EBM has been identified to address all these issues and to keep physicians up to date at the point of care for their patients.[3,4,5]
- **EBM process**—requires the identification of one's own knowledge gaps (where there is a lack of any justifying evidence of the practice), formulation of appropriate 'answerable' questions (**PICO**: what is the clinical **P**roblem, what is the **I**ntervention under question, what is the **C**omparison group, and what is the **O**utcome to measure), searching for the best scientific evidence (using clinical guidelines, systematic reviews, clinical evidence sources, and even individual quality research), critically appraising the selected evidence (using valid tools), and application of the best acceptable conclusions into one's practice.
- **How important**—EBM has become an essential part of modern surgical practice.[7] Surgeons should be aware of current clinical guidelines in their field of practice and the advice they contain [Good Surgical Practice 2008].[7] The unique features of the individual patient in terms of biology, needs, and special circumstances, often have the ultimate effect on decisions and outcome; the evidence is but one part of a rather versatile question.[6]

EBM useful terms and techniques

- **Understanding EBM**—requires familiarity with certain terms and definitions. For example, studying the effect of a *risk factor* requires a good understanding of incidence and prevalence, relative risk, and odds ratios. Studying the effectiveness of a *diagnostic test* requires familiarity with certain concepts such as sensitivity and specificity. Finally, studying the effect of a *treatment* requires deep understanding of odds ratios and number needed to treat, among other things. Supporting examples are used herein for better understanding.
- **Prevalence and incidence.**
  - *Prevalence*—is the total number of existing cases of the disease in the total population at one time.

- *Incidence*—is a measure of the risk of developing some new condition within a specified period of time.[4] Incidence is calculated by measuring the number of new cases within a specified time period divided by the size of the population initially at risk. For example, if a population initially contains 10,000 non-diseased persons and 580 develop a condition over 2y of observation, the incidence proportion is 58 cases per 1,000 persons, i.e. 5.8%.
- **Relative risk (RR)**—is the risk of an event (or of developing a disease) relative to exposure. For example, if the probability of developing oesophageal cancer among smokers was 10% and among non-smokers 1%, then the relative risk of cancer associated with smoking would be 10. Smokers would be ten times as likely as non-smokers to develop oesophageal cancer. We express such relative risk as RR×10.[6]
  - *Relative risk can also be defined*—as the rate of an event in a treatment group (experimental event rate or EER) divided by the rate of this event in the control group (control event rate or CER), expressed mathematically as EER/CER.
  - *Absolute risk reduction (ARR) (or increase)*—is used to express the effect of the treatment without that from placebo. For example, if 55% of patients achieved a satisfactory pain relief on using ibuprofen, compared to 18% on placebo, then ARR is 37% (55–18).
  - *Relative risk reduction (or increase)*—is used to express in percentage the absolute risk reduction (or increase) in relation to the control group. This is calculated using the formula: (EER–CER)/CER. For example, if 55% of patients achieved a satisfactory pain relief on using ibuprofen, compared to 18% on placebo, then the relative risk (RR) would be 3.1 (0.55/0.18). Ibuprofen is theoretically three times more effective than control. The absolute effect of ibuprofen (excluding that from placebo) can be estimated by calculating the relative risk reduction (55–18)/18, expressed in percentage (206%).[6]
- **Number needed to treat (NNT)**—is an epidemiological measure used to assess the effectiveness of an intervention by calculating the number of patients who need to be treated in order to achieve one positive effect or to prevent one additional bad outcome. For example, if 55% of patients achieved a satisfactory pain relief on using ibuprofen, compared to 18% on placebo, then the number needed to treat to achieve this 'satisfactory' pain relief is 2.7 (1/0.55–0.18), i.e. we have to treat 2.7 patients with ibuprofen for one to benefit 'satisfactorily' from the ibuprofen.
  - NNT is calculated using the inverse of ARR (NNT=1/ARR).
  - The ideal NNT is 1, whereby everyone would improve with treatment and no one would do in the control group. The higher the NNT, the less effective the treatment is expected to be.

Table 1.1 Types of research studies[1,4]

- *Systematic review of randomized controlled trials*—focused on a single question, systematic reviews are a literature review with the aim of identifying, appraising, selecting, and synthesizing a high quality research evidence relevant to that question.

- *Randomized controlled trials (RCTs)*—involve the random allocation of different types of interventions to subjects. This ensures that confounding factors are evenly distributed between treatment groups, provided that the number of subjects is sufficient enough to obtain valid randomization.

- *Cohort studies*—studies involving a group of people who share common features or exposure within a defined period and compare their outcome to a comparison group (from the general population from which the cohort is drawn, or from another cohort of people thought to have had little or no exposure to the investigated intervention).

- *Case-control studies*—compare subjects who have a condition (the 'cases') with subjects who do not have the condition, but are otherwise similar (the 'controls').

- *Case series*—are observational studies that track a series of patients who had similar exposure (same operation) or similar disease prospectively or retrospectively.

Table 1.2 Level of evidence[4,8]

Level 1	Evidence obtained from meta-analyses, systematic reviews of RCTs, or at least one properly designed RCT. Evidence can be labelled as (++) for high quality studies and low risk of bias, (+) for well-conducted studies, and (−) for studies with high risk of bias.
Level 2	Cohort or case-control studies. This can be labelled as (++) for high quality systematic reviews and low risk of bias, (+) for well-conducted studies, and (−) for studies with high risk of confounding or bias.
Level 3	Evidence obtained from respected authorities, clinical experience, or descriptive studies (case series or case report studies).
Level 4	Expert opinion or formal consensus decisions.

- *Odds ratios (OR)*—are another way of calculating the risk of an event (or of developing a disease) with some difference.
  - The odds of an event are calculated as the number of events divided by the number of non-events. For example, if 22 out of 40 patients achieved a satisfactory pain relief on using ibuprofen, compared to 7 out of 40 patients (18%) on placebo, then the odds ratio would be 5.7 ((22/18)/(7/33)).
  - The main difference between OR and RR is that the range that RR can take depends on the baseline event rate; OR does not need a baseline: it gives the risk of the cases relative to the controls, not relative to the baseline absolute value.[6]
  - In many situations in medicine, we can understand and interpret the odds ratios by pretending that they are relative risks: when events are rare, risks and odds are very similar; otherwise, odds ratios will be different.

- **Sensitivity and specificity**—are statistical measures of the performance of a test.
  - *Sensitivity*—measures the proportion of people with the target disorder who have a positive test. For example, a test with high sensitivity is usually positive for real sick people who have the condition, and negative for non-sick people. As a rule, a negative result of a high sensitive test rules out the diagnosis; a positive result CANNOT prove the existence of this specific disease.[6]
  - *Specificity*—measures the proportion of people without the target disease who have a negative test.[6] As a rule, a positive test result of high specificity confirms the diagnosis of this disease type.
  - *Accuracy*—is used to refer to both specificity and sensitivity. Accuracy is closely related to precision, reproducibility, or repeatability, whereby further measurements or calculations are expected to show the same or similar results.[4,6] Accuracy can be determined from sensitivity and specificity if the prevalence is known, using the following equation:[4]

    $$Accuracy = (sensitivity)(prevalence) + (specificity)(1 - prevalence)$$

- **Types of research studies**—the hierarchy of studies used for obtaining evidence is listed in Table 1.1.
- **Types of research questions.**[1,3]
  - *Questions on symptom prevalence or differential diagnosis*—are best answered using non-comparative studies (cohort studies, ecological studies, and case series).
  - *Questions on confirming diagnosis*—are best answered by using diagnostic studies (studies that test the quality of a specific diagnostic test (validation studies) or studies that model the data to obtain relevant diagnostic factors (exploratory studies)). Other useful types of studies to answer this type of questions include: Clinical decision rule (CDR) studies (scoring systems which lead to diagnostic pathways or prognostic estimations), absolute **SpPin** studies (studies with diagnostic finding whose **Sp**ecificity is high enough that a **P**ositive result rules **in** the diagnosis)[1], and absolute **SnNout** studies (studies with diagnostic finding whose **Sen**sitivity is high enough that a **N**egative result rules **out** the diagnosis).[1]
  - *Questions on prognosis*—best answer can be obtained from cohort studies or CDR studies. Untreated control group in randomized controlled trial (RCT) studies can be used for answering this question. Other types of studies include 'outcome' research and case series studies.[1,3]
  - *Questions on treatment, prevention, aetiology, and harm*—best answer can be obtained from RCTs and their systematic reviews. Other lower types of studies include cohort, outcome, and case-control studies.[1,3]
- **Level of evidence**—a ranking system developed to stratify evidence by quality and ability to answer a specific research question. Different systems have been developed (NICE, SIGN, US Preventive Services Task Force, etc.) with a generally similar concept (Table 1.2).

- *Grading of recommendations*—recommendations for using certain approach/intervention can be classified by grading systems that balance the risks and benefits of the intervention and the level of evidence on which this decision is based.[4] This takes into account more dimensions than just the quality of the research evidence.[4]
  - The grading of recommendations outlined by many guideline development groups (NICE, SIGN, American College of Chest Physicians, etc.) follows a similar approach. Table 1.3 outlines a generic recommendation system.
  - The Grading of Recommendations Assessment, Development and Evaluation (GRADE) approach is increasingly being adopted by organizations worldwide to provide a more pragmatic and transparent system for rating quality of evidence and strength of recommendations.[10]

Table 1.3 Generic grading of recommendations[1,4*]

Grade A	Research evidence is strong enough to suggest that the benefits of the clinical service/intervention substantially outweigh the potential risks.
Grade B	Research evidence is fairly convincing to suggest that the benefits of the clinical service/intervention outweigh the potential risks.
Grade C	Research evidence suggests that there are clear benefits provided by the clinical service/intervention. Nevertheless, the balance between benefits and risks are too close for making general recommendations.
Grade D	Recommendations with evidence level 3 or 4 or those based on a formal consensus approach.

*Good practice (G) has also been used occasionally in a few guidelines to reflect lower level, but convincing supporting evidence to the specific recommendation.

Further reading

1. Oxford's Centre for Evidence-Based Medicine (Bandolier). Available from: http://www.medicine.ox.ac.uk/bandolier/aboutus.html.
2. The Cochrane collaboration. Available from: http://www.cochrane.co.uk/en/colloboration.html
3. Sackett DL, Straus S, Richardson S, Rosenberg W, Haynes B (2000). *Evidence-based medicine: how to practise and teach EBM*, 2nd ed. Churchill Livingstone, London.
4. Wikipedia. Evidence-based medicine. Available from: http://en.wikipedia.org/wiki/Evidence-based_medicine.
5. Sackett DL, Rosenberg WM, Gray JA, Haynes RB, Richardson WS (1996). Evidence-based medicine: what it is and what it isn't. *BMJ* 312, 71–2.
6. Bandolier. Evidence-based thinking about health care. URL: http://www.medicine.ox.ac.uk/bandolier. Accessed May 2009.
7. The Royal College of Surgeons of England (2008). Good surgical practice. URL: http://www.jchst.org/publications/docs/good-surgical-practice-1/attachment_download/pdffile.
8. National Institute for Health and Clinical Excellence (2005). Reviewing and grading the evidence. Available from: http://www.nice.org.uk/niceMedia/pdf/GDM_Chapter7_0305.pdf.
9. EBM glossary (2008). Available from: http://ebm.bmj.com/cgi/reprint/13/4/128.
10. Goyatt G, Oxman A, Vist GE, Konz R, Falck-Ytter, Alonso-Coello P, Schünemann HJ. GRADE: an emerging consensus on rating quality of evidence and strength of recommendations. *BMJ* 2008; 336:924–926 (26 April).

Part 2

General care of the surgical patient

Principles of good surgical practice

Principles of good surgical practice

- The Royal College of Surgeons of England (2008). Good surgical practice.
- GMC (2006). Good medical practice.

Background

- All doctors are expected to provide a good standard of surgical practice and care. Patients must be able to trust doctors and doctors have to justify that trust.[1] Dignity and confidentiality must be respected.[1] Appraisal of surgeons is based on the seven core headings presented in *Good Medical Practice* (2006),[2] which sets out the standards required by all doctors (Table 2.1).
- *Good surgical standards* outline the accepted level of surgical practice, provide quality guidance for appraisal and revalidation processes, and set a framework for authorities to make judgements about surgeons' practice.[1] It is for surgeons to reflect on their practice and work to the set standards.[1] Serious or persistent failure to follow the GMC guidance will put one's registration at risk.[1] We highly recommend reviewing the sample and highly informative cases provided on the GMC website (case no. 215 for example).[4]

Terminology

In *Good Medical Practice*, the terms 'you must' and 'you should' are used in the following ways:[2]

- 'You must' is used for an overriding duty or principle.
- 'You should' is used when the General Medical Council (GMC) is providing an explanation of how that overriding duty is to be met.
- 'You should' is also used where the duty or principle will not apply in all situations or circumstances or where there are factors outside your control that affect whether or how you can comply with the guidance.
- 'Ensure' is used where surgeons must do all that is within their control to make sure that the event takes place.[2]

Good Medical Practice came into effect on 13 November, 2006. The terms used have major medico-legal implications. The majority of recommendations are 'you must'.

By the bedside[1]

- **Ensure appropriate and safe environment**—accommodate for any special needs requirements.
- **Maintain compassionate and clear communication**—with patients, supporters and, in case of children, parents or responsible adults.
- **Respect privacy**—this is a natural requirement for patients to disclose problems and concerns.
- **Provide enough time**—discuss with patients and their supporters any proposed procedure and other concerns.

Table 2.1 Standards required by all doctors[2]

1	Good clinical care
2	Maintaining good medical practice
3	Relationships with patients
4	Working with colleagues
5	Teaching and training
6	Health
7	Probity

Table 2.2 Sample of standard operative notes

Patient name: **Hospital ID:**   **DOB:**
Date and time:

NAME OF OPERATION PERFORMED

- *Type of procedure:* elective/emergency.
- *Name of:* supervising surgeon/operating surgeon/assistant(s)/scrub nurse/anaesthetist.
- *Type of anaesthesia, antibiotics, etc.:* **GA/LA/spinal.**

- *Incision:* midline, subcostal, 4 key holes, etc.
- *Findings:* perforated appendix, liver metastasis, etc.
    - Any problems/complications.
- *Procedure:* in concise details.
    - Extra procedures performed with reasons.
    - Details of tissue removed, added or altered.
    - Identification of any prosthesis used, including serial numbers of prostheses and other implanted materials.
- *Closure:* sutures, layers, etc.

- *Post-operative care instructions:*
    - Monitoring: specific signs and schedule.
    - Level of allowed activity: bed rest for 4h, etc.
    - Diet and fluid: NBM for 24h, allow D&F, etc.
    - Physiotherapy.
    - Prophylactic: antibiotics, DVT, PPIs, etc.
    - Suture removal.
    - Follow-up.

Signature.

Clinical assessment

- *Adequately assess your patient's condition*—ensure good history taking (including symptoms, psychological, and social factors) and physical examination where appropriate.[1]
- *Standard history taking and physical examination.* See 📖 OHCM Ch. 3.
- *Providing information*—patients, including children, should be given information about treatment options and any alternatives, main risks, side effects, and possible complications.[1]
- *Prioritization*—ensure that patients are prioritized and treated according to their clinical need.[1]
- *Informed decision*—patients need the opportunity to make a fully informed and unharassed decision. Patients must agree to treatment suggested before proceeding. Where appropriate, they may indicate by signature their willingness to proceed (see 📖 Chapter 5, pp.27–30).[1]

Record keeping

- *Ensure accurate records*—all records should be timed and dated, legible, complete, signed, and contemporaneous. Any changes in treatment plans should be recorded.[1,2]
- *Ensure labelled records*—always use patient's identification details on relevant records. The name of the most senior surgeon should be used to label the visit and ward round.[1,2]

Performing procedures

- *Know your limits*
  - Always carry out surgical procedures within the limits of your competence and in a timely and safe manner.[1]
  - Ensure that unfamiliar operative procedures are performed only if there is no clinical alternative, if there is no more experienced colleague available or if transfer to a specialist unit is considered a greater risk.[1]
- *Know your results*
  - You should always be aware of your immediate results, results obtained by peer groups, and where possible, personal and published audits of long-term outcomes.[1]
  - Ensure that patients receive satisfactory post-operative care and that relevant information is promptly recorded and shared with the caring team, the patient, and their supporter(s).[1]
- *Write legible operative notes*—typed if possible (see Table 2.2)
  - Notes should accompany the patient into recovery and then to the ward, and should be in sufficient detail to enable the effective continuity of care by the team.[1]

Discharge patients and handover practice

- *Safe discharge*—provide appropriate information to the patient and/or their carer(s) on discharge.[1] Follow-up notes should be sufficiently detailed to allow another doctor to continue the care of the patient at any time.[1]
- *Safe handover*—ensure a proper formal handover of patient's condition to the appropriate colleagues following your period on duty.[1,3]

Table 3.1 Admission instructions[1]

1. Level of admission unit
2. Clinician in charge with his/her bleep/contact number
3. Admission diagnosis
4. Level of allowed activity
5. Diet, nursing, monitoring schedule
6. IV fluid requirements, medications
7. Laboratory tests and imaging required

Table 3.2 Discharging criteria[1]

- *Stable medical condition*—stable vital signs (for at least 1h in the case of day surgery), full orientation to persons, place and time, good pain control (including enough supply of oral analgesics), minimum complaint of nausea, vomiting or dizziness, minimum bleeding from the operative site, and ability to take oral fluid in case of day surgery.

- *Appropriate social condition*—availability of appropriate carer at home, full understanding and written instructions of post-operative care and contact numbers, and clear scheduled plan for follow-up.

Table 3.3 Information on discharge[1,3]

- *Discharge medications*—clear instructions on prescribed analgesia, antiemetics, or antibiotics.

- *Care of wound*—e.g. change of dressing and suture removal.

- *Suitable timing*—for bath or shower.

- *Appropriate time*—to resume normal activities and work.

- *Expected symptoms after discharge*—and how to manage or call for help. All contact telephone numbers for any further enquiries or emergency situations must be written out for the patient and/or carers.

Effective admission management—audit areas

Is the discharge practice of acceptable quality?

- Sufficient information, contact numbers, forward planning, need for overnight admission.
  - *Standard*—adherence to discharge criteria, sufficient information on discharge.
  - *Indicators*—% of patients receiving information on operation (preoperatively), wound care, time for bath or shower, expected symptoms post-discharge, etc.).

Other audit suggestions

- Is admission information received from GP/clinic of sufficient quantity/quality to allow a smooth admission process?

Further reading

1. Healthcare Commission. Guide to admissions management. (2006) (UK) URL: http://www.cqc.org.uk/_db/_documents/Admissions_Management_Topic_Guide.pdf. Accessed May 2009.
2. Joint Commission Mission. Hospital Accreditation. (2006) (US) URL: http://www.gao.gov/new.items/d0779.pdf. Accessed May 2009.
3. British Association of Day Surgery. Guidelines about the discharge process and the assessment of fitness for discharge. URL: http://www.nodelaysscotland.scot.nhs.uk/SiteCollectionDocuments/NoDelays/Documents/Adobe%20PDFs/RG0029%20BADS%20Discharge%20Criteria.pdf. Accessed May 2009.
4. The Royal Pharmaceutical Society of Great Britain (2006). Guidance on discharge and transfer planning. Available from: http://www.rpsgb.org.uk/pdfs/dischtransfplanguid.pdf.

Day case surgery

Day case surgery

Key guidelines

- Department of Health (2002). Day surgery: operational guide.
- British Association of Day Surgery (2004). Integrated care pathways for day surgery patients.
- Association of Anaesthetists of Great Britain and Ireland (2005). Day surgery.

Background

- *Definition*—the admission of selected patients to hospital for a planned surgical procedure, returning home on the same day.[1] Procedures not requiring full operating theatre facilities and/or general anaesthesia (like endoscopy or outpatient procedures) are not classified as a 'true' day surgery.
- *Benefits*—include patients, clinicians, staff, and trusts.
  - *Patients*—reduced disruption to normal daily life, avoidance of prolonged waiting lists and hospital stay, decreased hospital acquired infection rate, and avoidance of unexpected cancellation due to emergency cases.[1] This mode of treatment is the preferred choice for most patients.[1,2]
  - *Clinicians*—better organized and relaxing working environment, and ability to release inpatient beds for major cases.
  - *Staff*—better quality of work facilities and rewarding working environment.
  - *Trusts*—improved Integrated Care Pathway (ICP) setting, reduced waiting times, and facilitated 'choose and book' process.[1]

Selection criteria

- *Which procedure*—any operation of relatively short duration, low incidence of post-operative complications, and minimum or no requirement for major perioperative interventions (blood transfusion, major analgesia, catheters, etc).[2] These include all intermediate and selected major operations where no specific contraindications exist.[1]
  - Selection criteria should be collaboratively agreed by surgeons, anaesthetists, and nurses involved.[3]
  - The Audit Commission's revised 'basket' of 25 procedures (2001) was later changed to a 'trolley'.[5] New procedures, especially laparoscopic, and older established operations, such as thyroid lobectomy and axillary clearances, are being increasingly added to the list of procedures to be considered for day surgery.
- *Which patient*—selection requires a balance between the extent of procedure, the fitness of patient, the use of general, regional, or local anaesthesia, the experience and particular skills of the clinicians, and the home conditions (Table 4.1).

Table 4.1 Patient selection for day case surgery

Social circumstances
- *Accompanying responsible carer*—to stay with patient for 24–48 hours post-discharge.
- *Suitable transport method*—to be available on going home.
- *Private telephone*—to be accessible for emergency and unexpected situations.
- *Distance to home*—not to exceed 1–1.5h.

Age limits
- Arbitrary limits for age (65 or 70) are increasingly considered inappropriate. Associated medical conditions (hypertension, obesity, smoking, asthma, and gastro-oesophageal reflux) are the most important factors, not the age per se.[1,5,6]

Body mass index (BMI) limits
- Upper BMI ceiling limits for safe and effective day surgery differs between units. A BMI of 30 to 40 was later challenged with super obese patients' series up to 62.7kg/m^2 with no weight-related complications.[8] Obesity is not an absolute contraindication to day care in expert hands and with appropriate resources and agreements.[3]

Associated medical conditions
- Type 1 diabetes mellitus, depending on its control and the extent of the procedure, can be managed as a day case if they are fit to eat and drink post-operatively. Asthma should be well controlled.

Other factors
- Times of operating, e.g. easier to get patients home if their operation is on a morning list. Where possible, configure morning lists with the more complex surgical and/or anaesthetic problems.

Discharging patients

Medical care
- Patients must have good analgesic control—local anaesthetic (LA) infiltration or block; oral or suppository medication (e.g. NSAID/paracetamol/codeine); and sufficient medications to maintain this state with clear instructions.
- Post-operative nausea and vomiting must be avoided where possible and controlled adequately before discharge. Anaesthetists will advise if they think prophylactic antiemetics should be prescribed (e.g. after a laparoscopic cholecystectomy).[3]
- Constipation should be anticipated and aperients supplied if thought necessary.

Instructions
- Verbal and written instructions must be given. The patient should be advised not to drink alcohol, operate machinery, or cook until the following day.[3] Advice should be given on the levels of activity and when to commence driving depending on the surgical procedure. Clear information must be given about dressings, suture removal, and district nurse or general practice attendance as well as appointments back at the hospital if necessary.
- Discharge summaries to be available when the patient leaves the unit. See 📖 Chapter 2, pp. 11–16.
- Sick note provided if necessary.

Follow-up
- Generally post-operative support and follow-up of patients occurs by telephone and is provided by day surgery nurses. Patients are given emergency contact numbers for expert nursing advice.[1]
- Generic discharge criteria are difficult to draw, and common sense with sensible judgment should be used at all times.

Know your results

How good your day surgery practice is—audit areas[9]

- Are information given to patients before planned day surgery sufficient, comprehensible, and on time to reduce patients' anxiety and increase their satisfaction?
  - *Standard*—quality and quantity of information and their effect on patients.
  - *Indicators*—% of procedures and information leaflets meeting the criteria; % of satisfied patients.
- Is the pre-admission assessment effective enough in choosing appropriate patients for day surgery to improve their experience and reduce cancellation rate?
  - *Standard*—agreed selection criteria by the unit.
  - *Indicators*–% of patients been assessed using protocols; % been refused day surgery; % cancelled within 2d of operation.

Other audit suggestions
- How effective the pain management plan in controlling post-operative pain and increasing patient satisfaction.
- Is theatre utilization efficient enough to meet the government targets of doing 75% of elective surgery as a day case?
- How efficient the discharge protocols in achieving safe and effective discharge process?

Beyond the guidelines and the future

Clinicians who recognize the quality benefits of day surgery are surprised and exasperated by the failure of so many to exploit the advantages it brings to patients and their health communities. The NHS Modernisation Agency final report on the ten changes in the NHS that would have the greatest impact listed treating day surgery as the norm at the top of the list. Day surgery will increase, but as is so often the case, predicting the catalyst and speed of change is difficult. Day surgery enthusiasts, surgeons, anaesthetists, and nurses working together will continue to broaden the scope of procedures suitable for the day surgery environment. The British Association of Day Surgery (BADS) Directory of Procedures gives an idea of what is achievable in dedicated facilities with appropriate equipment and trained staff. To many, day surgery is the simple and less fulfilling end of the surgical spectrum of procedures. This Directory shows that is not the case.

Surgery will continue to become less and less invasive with the help of new technology and surgical skills. In parallel, day surgery anaesthetic practice will exploit the value of regional and local anaesthetics to avoid systemic upset caused by strong analgesia, reduced surgical trauma aiding this change of practice. Mortality is an easily recognized measure of failure. Although obviously important, it is infrequent and not a good measure of the surgical experience. Quality of recovery affects all and is the standard by which the surgical experience should be judged. The ultimate is minimal upset by either drugs or trauma of an ever increasing range and complexity of surgical procedures such that patients need only leave home for their time in the operating theatre. In the years to come, this will be the norm. The likely catalyst will be the expansion of dedicated day surgical units led by clinicians and managers who have day surgery as their priority. *Mr. Roddy Nash, Council Member, British Association of Day Surgery (BADS).*

Further reading

1. Department of Health. Day Surgery: Operational Guide. (UK) 2002. URL: http://www.dh.gov. uk/en/Publicationsandstatistics/Publications/PublicationsPolicyAndGuidance/DH_4005487. Accessed May 2009.

2. British Association of Day Surgery. Integrated Care Pathways for Day Surgery Patients. (UK) 2004 URL: http://www.daysurgeryuk.net/bads/joomla/files/Handbooks/ IntegratedCarePathways.pdf. Accessed by May 2009.

3. Association of Anaesthetists of Great Britain and Ireland. Day Surgery. Revised edition. London: 2005 URL: http://www.aagbi.org/publications/guidelines/docs/daysurgery05.pdf. Accessed May 2009.

4. Royal College of Nursing. Selection Criteria and suitable procedures. Royal College of Nursing Publications. 2004 URL: http://www.rcn.org.uk/__data/assets/pdf_file/0004/78511/001436.pdf. Accessed by May 2009.

5. Osborne GA, Rudkin GE (1993). Outcome after day-care surgery in a major teaching hospital. *Anaesth Intensive Care* 21, 822–7.

6. Watkins BM, Montgomery KF, Ahroni JH, Erlitz MD, Abrams RE, Scurlock JE (2005). Adjustable gastric banding in an ambulatory surgery centre. *Obes Surg* 15, 1045–9.

7. British Association of Day Surgery: Discharge Criteria. URL: http://www.nodelaysscotland.scot. nhs.uk/SiteCollectionDocuments/NoDelays/Documents/Adobe%20PDFs/RG0029%20BADS% 20Discharge%20Criteria.pdf. Accessed May 2009.

8. The Royal College of Anaesthetists. Raising the standard: a compendium of audit recipes. Available from: http://www.rcoa.ac.uk/docs/ARB-section5.pdf.

Good consent practice*

* The guidelines on this chapter have been sourced and summarized from different UK, Europe, and international government sources, professional organizations, and medical specialty societies. Leading guidelines have been listed in the Key guidelines box.

Good consent practice

Key guidelines

- General Medical Council (2008). Consent: patients and doctors making decisions together.
- The Royal College of Surgeons of England (2008). Good surgical practice.

Background

- By definition, a person can give consent when he/she can appreciate and understand the facts and implications of an action.[1] Consent principles apply to any interaction with patients.
- 'You must' is an imperative in much of the advice rather than 'you should'. This must be borne in mind when gaining consent. Good documentation is advisable at all times.

Providing sufficient information

- *How sufficient*—information should be understandable enough to enable for weighing risks and benefits of any procedure and for making appropriate informed decisions about care.[1,2] Sufficient information is a right for patients and is protected by law.[1,2]
- *How much information*—varies between individual patients. Factors affecting this include the type and complexity of treatment, possible side effects and risks, patients' beliefs, culture, occupation, level of education, and patients' wishes. Decision should be based on an individual basis and the patients' views respected. Patients must be told if there is a potential serious outcome even if the likelihood is very small (Chester vs Afshar).
- *Consent scope and limits*—if treatment has to be delivered in stages, for example, or has to involve more than one specialty, then information about whether or when to move from one form of treatment to another should be fully discussed with patient and documented. The need to seek further consent at a later stage should be clarified.[1]

Who should obtain consent?

- *Best person*—the clinician doing the investigation and providing the treatment.[1]
- *Delegation*—is only acceptable for appropriately trained and qualified staff with sufficient knowledge of delivery method of the procedure/investigation, main techniques, benefits, and risks. They do not have to be able to do the procedure themselves.[1]

Good consent practice[1,2]

- *Work always in partnership with your patient*—no one else can make a decision on behalf of an adult who has capacity.
- *Review*—all available information before interviewing the patient.
- *Find appropriate time and setting*—where patients are able to understand and retain information.

- *Present information*—using up-to-date written and visual material, arrange for language and communication requirements as well as the presence of relatives or friends if requested by patient (offer the option), and give distressing information in a considerate way.
- *Discuss expected diagnosis*—what is the most likely diagnosis (if available) and possible outcome if disease left untreated. If the diagnosis is still uncertain, what further investigations prior to treatment are required?
- *Discuss options*—all available options for treating the condition, including the 'not to treat' option.
- *Discuss benefits and risks*
  - Main purpose and likely benefits of different options (diagnostic, curative, palliative, approved trial, etc.).
  - The common and serious possible side effects.
- *Discuss main details*
  - Technical details (that can be understood by patient).
  - Perioperative experience.
- *Overall responsible doctor for the treatment*—and extent of doctor in training or medical students' involvement.
- *Reflection*—allow patients enough time to reflect on the appropriate decision, and involve nurses and other health care members in discussions.
- *Final reminder*—that patients can change their minds about their decision at any time and can seek a second opinion.
- *Questions*—should be answered fully, accurately, and honestly. Some questions might be difficult to answer. Seeking further advice from others is helpful.

Withholding information

- *Sharing information*—all relevant information necessary for decision making should be shared with the patient.
- *Exceptional circumstances*—include those where disclosing information may cause serious harm to the patient (serious harm does not just mean that the patient would become upset and refuse treatment); in special circumstances, withholding the selected information can be considered appropriate. Seeking help and advice in such cases is recommended. Keeping good records is essential.[1]

Patients lacking capacity

- To facilitate decision making, the views of the patient's legal representative and the people close to the patient should be sought. Help should be requested when necessary. The care of the patient is the primary concern.

Know your results

Good consent practice—audit areas

Is consenting practice of acceptable quality?

- Quantity and quality of information, documentation, level of experience of consenting physician, etc.
  - *Standard*—quality and quantity of information.
  - *Indicators*—% of specific documented procedure, % of forms holding identifiable patient information, % of forms with documented site/side of operation, % of documented general/specific possible side effects, level of consenting physicians, etc.)

Other audit suggestions

- Patients' satisfaction/views on the consenting practice for specific operations/procedures.

Further reading

1. General Medical Council (2008). Consent: patients and doctors making decisions together. Available from: http://www.gmc-uk.org/guidance/ethical_guidance/consent_guidance/Consent_guidance.pdf.
2. The Royal College of Surgeons of England (2008). Good surgical practice. Available from: http://www.jchst.org/publications/docs/good-surgical-practice-1/attachment_download/pdffile (with kind permission).
3. Wikipedia. Informed consent. Available from: http://en.wikipedia.org/wiki/Informed_consent.

See also:
📖 OHCS pp12–3.
📖 OHCM p554.

Preoperative assessment

Preoperative assessment

Background
- Patients undergoing operations should, wherever possible, have a preoperative assessment (face-to-face, telephone, or questionnaire) by a suitably trained individual.[6]
- *Objectives*—to improve the surgical outcome by identifying any coexisting medical disorder, confirming its presence and severity with appropriate tests, treating conditions that may adversely influence the outcome, avoiding late cancellations, and/or deferring surgery if deemed necessary. Preoperative assessment can also be used to ensure that the patient has fully understood the proposed operation and is ready to proceed.[6]

General evaluation
Apply the same principles of taking (or receiving) history and performing physical examination with special attention to risk factors.
- *Clinical history*
  - *Proposed procedure*—indications and any unexpected changes since been booked, urgency of surgery, previous anaesthetic records, and grade of surgery.
  - *Systems review*—as applied to the specific surgery (Fig. 6.1). Be familiar with the documentation being used in your own hospital.
  - *Drug history*—complete list of medications including over-the-counter and herbal products, and drug allergies, including previous reactions.
  - *Social history*—smoking, alcohol, drugs, other personal behaviour of importance.
- *Physical examination*—thorough and guided by clinical history.
- *General impression*—regardless of age, patients who live independently, do their shopping and gardening, and can climb up several steps of stairs to go to their bedroom, are unlikely to have major serious medical disorders that would affect significantly the operative outcome in moderate surgical procedures.[7]
- *ASA grade*—the American Society for Anaesthesiologists (ASA) grading system is commonly used (Table 6.1).

Vascular preoperative assessment checklist

Operation details:	Investigations / results
Proposed operation:	one-sentence summary
	☐ ECG
	☐ CXR
	☐ Spirometry
Proposed date:	☐ Duplex:
Indications:	☐ Angio:
	☐ Vein scan:

Comorbidities ☐ Fairly fit & well	
Stable or active. e.g.	☐ Echo:
MI 5y (stable) – AF (active) –	
IDDM (stable) – MRSA (+ve) –	☐ Others:
High risk for HIV, etc.	

QoL	Prophylaxis
☐ Independent / bed-bound / etc.	LMWH
☐ Lives in own house / bungalow /	Clopidogrel
residential house / nursing home / etc.	Antibiotics
☐ Own shopping / carer 3 times / etc.	PPIs
	IV fluid

Bloods	Final check
Date: (acute or chronic)	☐ On list
WCC Hg	☐ Consent
PT PTT INR	☐ Family informed
Urea Cr Na K	☐ Marked
ABGs:	☐ HDU – ITU bed
	☐ Anaesthetic review
	☐ Special arrangements: Vascular
	study unit (VSU), angio team, stents
	☐ Others

Medications
Aspirin   Clopidogrel   LMWH
PPI   Antibiotics
Statin
Insulin   Metformin
Allergies

Fig. 6.1 Example of preoperative assessment checklist

Preoperative investigations

- *Rationale*—tests should make an important contribution to the process of perioperative assessment and management without causing unnecessary disadvantage/harm.
- *Possible disadvantages*—unnecessary delay of surgery, false positive findings leading to costly and risky investigations, and diversion of hospital resources into unnecessary costly service.[1]
- *Choosing the appropriate preoperative tests in elective operations*—have been recommended by NICE based on expert opinion using a consensus development process (level of recommendations: D).[1]

A derived practical algorithm is provided in Figs. 6.2 and 6.3, based on the three main factors recommended by NICE: patient age, surgery grade, and ASA grade.

Table 6.1 ASA grades (See also 📖 OHCM p553)

Grade 1	Normal healthy patient (no clinically significant 'comorbid' disorder)
Grade 2	Mild systemic disease (significant 'comorbid' disease that does NOT limit the patient activities)
Grade 3	Severe systematic disease (significant 'comorbid' disease that DOES limit the patient activities)
Grade 4	Severe life-threatening 'comorbid' disease

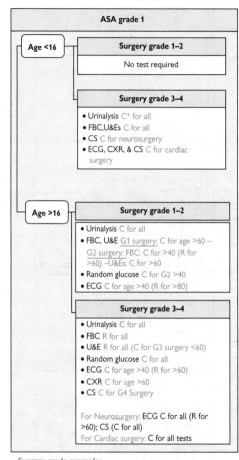

ASA grade 1

Age <16

Surgery grade 1–2

No test required

Surgery grade 3–4

- Urinalysis C* for all
- FBC,U&Es C for all
- CS C for neurosurgery
- ECG, CXR, & CS C for cardiac surgery

Age >16

Surgery grade 1–2

- Urinalysis C for all
- FBC, U&E G1 surgery: C for age >60 – G2 surgery: FBC: C for >40 (R for >60) –U&Es: C for >60
- Random glucose C for G2 >40
- ECG C for age >40 (R for >80)

Surgery grade 3–4

- Urinalysis C for all
- FBC R for all
- U&E R for all (C for G3 surgery <60)
- Random glucose C for all
- ECG C for age >40 (R for >60)
- CXR C for age >60
- CS C for G4 Surgery

For Neurosurgery: ECG C for all (R for >60); CS (C for all)
For Cardiac surgery: C for all tests

Surgery grade examples
Grade 1 (minor) Incision and drainage of breast abscess; excision of skin lesions.
Grade 2 (intermediate) Inguinal hernia repair; varicose vein surgery.
Grade 3 (major) Thyroidectomy; total abdominal hysterectomy (TAH).
Grade 4 (major+) Colonic resections; lung operations; neurosurgery; cardiovascular surgery.

Fig. 6.2 Recommendations: *C=consider the test, R=test recommended/required for the specific group

ASA grade 2–3

Cardiovascular comorbidities

Surgery grade 1–2

- **Urinalysis** C for all
- **FBC** C for all
- **U&E** C for all (R >60 & G2 surgery/R for all ASA G3)
- **Random glucose** not recommended
- **ECG** R for all
- **CXR** C for all (not for age <40 with surgery G1)
- **ABGs** R for ASA G3

Surgery grade 3–4

- **Urinalysis** C for all
- **FBC** R for all
- **U&E** R for all
- **Random glucose** not recommended
- **ECG** R for all
- **CXR** C for all (R for age >60 with ASA G3)
- **ABGs** C for all
- **CS** C for all (Not for ASA2 with surgery G2)

Respiratory comorbidities

Surgery grade 1–2

- **Urinalysis** C for all
- **FBC** C for all (R for >80 for ASA G3)
- **U&EC** for all ASA G3, C for age >40 with surgery G2, C for age >60 and surgery G1
- **ECG** C for age >40 (C for all if ASA G3, R for age >60)
- **CXR** C for all (only for >40 with surgery G1)
- **ABGs** C for all - **Lung functions** not recommended

Surgery grade 3–4

- **Urinalysis** C for all
- **FBC** R for all
- **U&E** R for all (C for age <60 and ASA G2)
- **[Glucose]**
- **ECG** R for all (C for age <60 and ASA G2)
- **CXR** C for all
- **Pulm Func tests** C for all (not for age <40 with ASA G2)
- **CS** C for all if surgery G4

Surgery grades examples

Grade 1 (minor) Incision and drainage of breast abscess; Excision of skin lesions.
Grade 2 (intermediate) Inguinal hernia repair; varicose vein surgery.
Grade 3 (major) Thyroidectomy; total abdominal hysterectomy (TAH).
Grade 4 (major+) Colonic resections; lung operations; neurosurgery; cardiovascular surgery.

Fig. 6.3 Recommendations: C=consider the test, R=test recommended/required for the specific group

Further reading

1. NICE (2003). The use of preoperative tests in elective surgery. (UK) available from: www.nice. org.uk/nicemedia/pdf/Preop-fullguideline.pdf
2. NHS Scotland (2003). Care before, during and after anaesthesia. (UK) available from: www. nhshealthquality.org/nhsqis/files/Anaesthesia National Overview - Sep2005.pdf
3. ICSI (2008). Preoperative evaluation. (US) available from: www.issi.org/preoperative_evaluation/ preoperative_evaluation_2328.html
4. ACC/AHA Guideline (2007). Perioperative Guidelines. (US) available from: http://anesthesiology. med.miami.edu/documents.mm_articles/105.pdf
5. AAGBI (2001). Pre-operative Assessment. The role of the Anaesthetist. (UK) available from: www.aagbi.org/publications/guidelines/docs/preoperativeass01.pdf
6. Modernisation Agency NHS National Good Practice Guidance on Preoperative assessment for day surgery. available from: www.cancerimprovement.nhs.uk\documents\publications from NHS modernisation Agency/Pre-operative guidance for daycase surgery.pdf
7. Charles R, Smith R (1998) *Atlas of general surgery*, 3rd ed, Hodder Arnold. p. 124

Know your results

Compliance with preoperative NICE guidelines—audit areas[1]

How compliant is preoperative testing practice with NICE guidelines?

- *Standards*—patients who require testing should be tested, and those who are not recommended to be tested should not be tested. Patient's age, ASA grade, and surgery grade should be used for adjustment.
- *Data required*—patient details, age, main diagnosis/operation, main comorbidities, ASA grade, and blood, urine and other tests ordered.
- *Indicators*[1]—% of patients who are **not** tested, in compliance with the guideline; % of patients who **are** tested, in compliance with the guideline; % of patients who are **not** tested, against the recommendations of the guideline; of patients who **are** tested, against the recommendations of the guideline, % of patients who are tested and for whom one or more reasons for testing are documented.
- Compare results with NICE recommendations.

Assessment of cardiovascular system

Key guidelines

- NHS Scotland. Care before, during and after anaesthesia. (UK) 2003
- ICSI. Preoperative evaluation. (US) 2008
- ACC/AHA Guideline. Update on Perioperative Cardiovascular Evaluation for Noncardiac Surgery. (US) 2007

Background

- Post-operative cardiac death or major cardiac complications occur in ~1–7% of patients undergoing major non-cardiac surgery.[4,5]
- Over 50% of perioperative deaths are caused by cardiac events. Most occur within 72h of operation (peak at 48h). Perioperative infarction has a 50% risk of death.[3,4] Detection and treatment of cardiac disorders in patients undergoing operative procedures can have significant impact on the surgical outcome.

Cardiac risk factors

Age

- In general, cardiac risk is higher in patients over the age of 70 (RR × 1.9). Age is a minor independent factor.

Ischaemic heart disease

- The risk is major with unstable coronary syndrome (acute or recent (<30d) MI or unstable angina), and *intermediate* with stable coronary syndrome (stable angina, or previous MI by history or pathologic Q waves).

Congestive heart failure

- *The risk is major* with decompensated heart failure, and *intermediate* with compensated or prior heart failure.[3]

Arrhythmias

- *Cardiac risk is major* in patients with significant arrhythmias (high-grade AV block, symptomatic ventricular arrhythmias in the presence of underlying heart disease, or supraventricular arrhythmias with uncontrolled ventricular rate) and *minor* in patients with minimal ECG changes (left ventricular hypertrophy, left bundle branch block, ST–T abnormalities) or if the rhythm was not sinus (e.g. atrial fibrillation).[3]

Valvular heart disease

- *In general*, cardiac risk is higher when clinical findings suggest a significant valvular heart disease and *major* if valvular disease was severe.[3]

Type of surgery

- *High-risk surgery*—include emergency major operations, aortic and other major vascular surgery, peripheral vascular surgery, and prolonged surgical procedures with associated large fluid shifts and/or blood loss. Estimated cardiac complication rate is >5%.
- *Intermediate risk surgery*—include carotid endarterectomy, head and neck surgery, intraperitoneal and intrathoracic surgery, orthopaedic

surgery, and prostate surgery. Estimated cardiac complication rate is 1–5%.

- *Low-risk surgery*—include endoscopic procedures, superficial procedure, cataract surgery, and breast surgery. Estimated cardiac complication rate is <1%.

Other factors

- *In general,* cardiac risk is higher in the presence of cerebrovascular ischaemia (RR × 2.9–4.7), IDDM (RR × 3.5), renal failure with serum creatinine above 2mg/dL (RR × 5.2), and in poor general condition (RR × 1.8).[4,5]
- *The risk is intermediate* in diabetes mellitus and renal insufficiency, and *minor* in the history of stroke and in controlled systemic hypertension.[3]

Cumulative cardiac risk index

- The risk of cardiac death, non-fatal myocardial infarction, and non-fatal cardiac arrest can be estimated using the modified Goldman's Scoring System based on six factors (Table 6.2).[6,7]

Action plan

- *Major risk factors*—require intensive investigations and management as appropriate, which may result in delay or cancellation of non-emergency surgery. Waiting 4–6wk after a myocardial infarction (MI) to perform elective surgery is recommended.[3]
- *Intermediate risk factors*—are well-validated markers of enhanced risk of perioperative cardiac complications and justify careful assessment of the patient's current status.

Table 6.2 Estimation of cardiac risk[6,7]

Cardiac risk factors
1. *Ischaemic heart disease*—history of MI, current complaint of ischaemic chest pain or use of nitrate therapy, positive exercise test, or ECG with Q waves.
2. *Heart failure*—history of congestive heart failure, pulmonary oedema, paroxysmal nocturnal dyspnoea, presence of bilateral crepitations or S3 gallop, or the presence of pulmonary vascular redistribution.
3. High-risk surgery—see text.
4. Cerebrovascular ischaemia.
5. IDDM.
6. Serum creatinine >2mg/dL.

Risk estimation
1. No risk factors—0.4%.
2. One risk factor—1.0%.
3. Two risk factors—2.4%.
4. Three or more risk factors—5.4%.

Further reading

1. NICE (2003). The use of preoperative tests in elective surgery. (UK) available from: www.nice. org.uk/nicemedial/pdf/Preop-fullguideline.pdf
2. NHS Scotland (2003). Care before, during and after anaesthesia. (UK) available from: www. nhshealthquality.org/nhsqis/files/Anaesthesia National Overview - Sep2005.pdf
3. ICSI (2008). Preoperative evaluation. (US) available from: www.issi.org/preoperative_evaluation/ preoperative_evaluation_2328.html
4. ACC/AHA Guideline (2002). Update on Perioperative Cardiovascular Evaluation for Noncardiac Surgery. (US) 2007 available from: http://anesthesiology.med.miami.edu/documents/ mm_articles/105.pdf
5. Mangano DT, Goldman L (1995). Preoperative assessment of patients with known or suspected coronary disease. *N Engl J Med* 333, 1750–6.
6. Devereaux, PJ, Goldman, L, Cook, DJ, Gilbert K, Leslie K, Guyatt GH (2005). Perioperative cardiac events in patients undergoing non-cardiac surgery: a review of the magnitude of the problem, the pathophysiology of the events, and methods to estimate and communicate risk. *CMAJ* 173, 627–34.
7. Morris PJ, Wood WC (2001). *Oxford Textbook of Surgery*. Oxford, Oxford University Press.

Assessment of respiratory system

Key guidelines

- NHS QIS Scotland. Care before, during and after anaesthesia. (UK) 2003
- ICSI. Preoperative evaluation. (US) 2008

Background

- Post-operative respiratory complications occur in 5–10% of major non-cardiac procedures and are more common than cardiac complications.[3]
- Respiratory complications are significant if resulted in prolonged hospital stay or increased morbidity and mortality.[4]
- *Common significant respiratory complications*—include bronchospasm, atelectasis, pneumonia, respiratory failure with prolonged mechanical ventilation, and exacerbation of underlying chronic lung disease.

Risk factors

- *Advanced age*—increases pulmonary risks significantly (RR × 1.9–2.4)[4] The correlation is mostly related to coexisting conditions, not to chronologic age.
- *Obesity*—slight non-significant increase in pulmonary complications (RR × 1.3), contrary to common beliefs.
- *Smoking*—significant risk factor (RR × 1.4–4.3). Stopping smoking >8wk preoperatively reduces the risk significantly (by 50%); stopping in <8wk may increase the risk.[4]
- *General health status*—strong predictor, especially in patients with ASA grade above two (RR × 1.5–3.2).[4]
- *COPD patients*—significantly at risk (RR × 2.7–4.7).[4]
- *Controlled asthma*—no effect on risk.
- *Type of surgery*
  - *Site of surgery*—risk of complications is higher in upper abdominal and thoracic surgery (10–40%) compared to lower abdominal surgery (0–15%). Risk is minimum in laparoscopic cholecystectomy (0.3–0.4%) as compared to open cholecystectomy (13–33%).[4]
  - *Duration of surgery*—higher risk if surgery duration exceeds 3 hours (RR × 1.6–5.2), and in surgery under GA (RR × 1.2).[4]

Predicting pulmonary risk

- *Epstein and colleagues model*—uses a sum of modified Goldman cardiac index plus main pulmonary risk factors.[5] Factors include smoking, obesity, productive cough, diffuse wheezing, rhonchi, FEV(1): FVC ratio <70%, and $PaCO_2$ >45mmHg.[5] Most useful in lung resection operations.
- *Risk estimation in abdominal operations*[5]
  - With abnormal findings on chest examination: risk increase by 5.8 folds.
  - With concomitant abnormal CXR findings: risk increases by 3.2.
  - Each extra point on the Goldman cardiac risk index: risk increases by 2.04.

Risk reduction strategies

Preoperatively
- Encourage cigarette cessation for >8wk before surgery.
- Treat COPD as appropriate.
- Use antibiotics and possibly delay surgery in respiratory infections.
- Educate patient on lung expansion manoeuvres (able to reduce respiratory complications from 60 to 19%).

Intraoperatively
- Use spinal or epidural anaesthesia.
- Use laparoscopic approach if possible.
- Aim at operative duration of <3h.

Post-operatively
- Use epidural analgesia.
- Use nerve block.
- Use deep breathing exercises.
- Use CPAP if necessary.

Other preoperative issues—specific advice and organization

- Fasting, the pill, and prophylactic prevention of DVTs are dealt with in later chapters (see ☐ Chapter 7, pp.45–48; ☐ Chapter 12, pp.87–90).
- Diabetes mellitus—general principles: no oral hypoglycaemics on the day of surgery; usually one third to half of the patient's morning insulin dosage may be administered (see ☐ Chapter 8, pp.49–64).
- Smoking—although in general, smoking cessation should be advised, there is no strong evidence to recommend smoking cessation in the immediate short term prior to surgery as a means to achieve improved outcomes and reduce post-operative complications.[5]
- Patients advised to take their normal medications (excluding anticoagulants, see ☐ Chapter 12, pp.87–90), and particularly important to continue with β-blockers. Aspirin for the prevention of MI or CVA should be continued unless instructed by local protocol.
- Procedure and anaesthetic leaflets provided to aid informed consent.
- The patient should have telephone contact if a day patient.
- A responsible adult and home support must be available.
- Home circumstances, e.g. stairs and transport, need to be enquired about.
- Advice given about getting back to normal activities and work.
- A contact point at the hospital if needed in the post-operative period at home.

Further reading

1. NHS QIS Scotland (2003). Care before, during and after anaesthesia. NHS Scotland.
2. ICSI (2008). Preoperative evaluation (guideline). ICSI, Bloomington, USA.
3. Hata TM, Moyers JR (2006). Preoperative evaluation and management. In: Barash PG, Cullen BF, Stoelting RK, eds. *Clinical Anaesthesia.* 5th edition. Lippincott Williams & Wilkins, Philadelphia.
4. Smetana GW (1999). Preoperative pulmonary evaluation. *N Engl J Med* 340,937–944.
5. Epstein SK, Faling LJ, Daly BD, Celli BR (1993). Predicting complications after pulmonary resection. Preoperative exercise testing vs a multifactorial cardiopulmonary risk index. *Chest* 104, 694–700.

Table 7.1 Fasting recommendations in healthy adults

Diet type	Recommendations	Grade
Water	Safe and beneficial to drink with unlimited amounts up to 2h before induction	A
Clear fluids	Clear tea, black coffee, etc.—safe to drink with unlimited amounts up to 2h before induction	A
Free fluid	Milk, tea with milk, coffee with milk—safe to drink up to 6h before induction	B
Solid food and sweets	Safe to take up to 6h before induction	D
Chewing gum	Unsafe to use on the day of operation and should not be permitted	B

Table 7.2 Fasting recommendations for healthy children

Diet type	Recommendations	Level
Water	Safe and beneficial to drink with unlimited amounts up to 2h before induction	A*
Milk	Breast milk—safe up to 4h before induction	D
	Formula milk/cow's milk—safe up to 6h before induction	
Solid food and sweets	Safe to take up to 6h before induction	D
Chewing gum	Unsafe to use on the day of operation and should not be permitted	D

* Level of recommendation is **A** for ≥1y and **D** for <1y

Table 7.3 Medication check preoperatively

Steroids, anticoagulant, oral contraceptives, antiplatelets, etc.

- *Fasting guidelines*—follow the one for healthy adults or children, unless contraindicated [D].
- *Special manoeuvres*—may be considered in high-risk patients for safety issues [D]:
  - H2-receptor antagonists and proton pump inhibitors.
  - Sodium citrate and gastrokinetic agents.
  - Rapid sequence induction.
  - Tracheal intubation.
  - Nasogastric tube.
- *Emergency cases*—treat as full stomach and apply manoeuvres to reduce aspiration [D].

Post-operative oral intake in elective surgery

- *Adults*—encourage drinking when patients feel ready for it, providing there are no contraindications [A].
- *Children*—offer oral fluids when fully awake from anaesthesia, providing there are no contraindications [A]. Clear fluids or breast milk should be considered first [D].

Exceptions from the guidelines

Patients having a procedure under sedation should follow the unit protocols. Instructions on post-operative fasting in major abdominal surgery or gastrointestinal tract should be planned individually with the surgeon in charge.

Further reading

1. The Royal College of Nursing (2005). Perioperative fasting in adults and children. Available from: http://www.rcn.org.uk/__data/assets/pdf_file/0009/78678/002800.pdf.

Perioperative medical complications*

* The guidelines on this chapter have been sourced and summarized from different UK, Europe, and international government sources, professional organizations, and medical specialty societies. Leading guidelines have been listed in the Key guidelines box.

Cardiovascular complications

Key guidelines

- Scottish Intercollegiate Guidelines Network (2004). Postoperative management in adults.
- Scottish Intercollegiate Guidelines Network (2007). Acute coronary syndromes.
- National Institute for Health and Clinical Excellence (2006). Atrial fibrillation.
- ACC/AHA/ESC (2006). Guidelines for the management of patients with atrial fibrillation.
- National Institute for Health and Clinical Excellence (2009). Thoracoscopic epicardial radiofrequency ablation for atrial fibrillation.

Perioperative myocardial infarction (PMI)

- *Incidence*—affects about 2–3% of patients perioperatively after major non-cardiac surgery.[1] Minimal risk in patients with no clinical atherosclerotic disease, and highest incidence (4–7%) in patients with known coronary disease.[2]
- *Presentation*—many (~50%) have no specific complaints. Few (~15%) complain of chest pain.[5] Presents occasionally with signs of congestive heart failure (e.g. short of breath).
- *Diagnosis*—maintain a high index of suspicion in high-risk patients, males, and elderly (See also 📖 OHCM Ch. 5).
  - Review patients' risk factors.
  - Seek specialist medical advice—early on clinical suspicion [CS]*[4]
  - Obtain 12-lead electrocardiogram (ECG)—immediately [D].[5] High-risk asymptomatic patients should always have ECG performed on admission (baseline), immediately after surgery, and daily for two days post-operatively [CS].
  - Check troponin levels (I or T)—raised levels can be detected in almost all patients within 6–9h after PMI onset (earlier using sensitive assays and low cut-off values). Sensitivity, specificity, positive and negative predictive values are remarkably high (>90%).[1] High-risk asymptomatic patients should routinely have troponin levels measured 24h after surgery [B].[4]
  - Confirm diagnosis—this can be established (within appropriate clinical and ECG findings) on finding raised (or fall from raised) troponin levels in 12h from onset of symptoms, with no other explanation (e.g. PE, AF) [B].[5]
- *Treatment*—see Table 8.1 (see also 📖 OHCM p783).

Atrial fibrillation (AF)

- *Incidence*—affects ~4 and 35% of patients undergoing major non-cardiac and cardiac surgery, respectively.[4,6] Morbidity, mortality, and length of hospital stay increases significantly in complicated cases.

---

* CS = consensus statement used by Scottish Intercollegiate Guidelines Network to refer to statements developed from structured discussion and validated using a formal scoring system.[4]
G = good practice recommendation

Table 8.1 Post-operative MI—treatment

- *Level of care*—admit to a specialist cardiology unit [C].[5] Use continuous ECG monitoring to detect the potentially lethal but treatable arrhythmias (ventricular fibrillation and pulseless ventricular tachycardia) [D].[5]

- *High-flow oxygen*—apply mainly for patients with hypoxia, pulmonary oedema, and PMI [D].[5]

- *Secure IV access, draw blood samples.*

- *Aspirin*—300mg immediately [A].[5] Aspirin reduces the rate of further vascular event (death, stroke, MI) by 30 and 50% in unstable angina and MI, respectively.

- *Nitrates*—GTN 2 puffs (or sublingual tablet) to relieve pain and support acute heart failure management [G].[5]

- *Morphine 5–10mg IV (± metoclopramide)*—as appropriate if nitrates failed to control pain.

- *Other types of treatment*—intensive blood glucose control in hyperglycaemic or diabetic patients is required for at least 24h [B].[5] Other types of treatment should be applied following specialist advice (β-blockers etc.).

- *Thrombolytic agents*—contraindicated and should not be used.[4]

Table 8.2 Post-operative AF—treatment

- *Principles*— follow same recommendations for AF in non-surgical patients [D].[4,6,7]
- *Haemodynamically unstable patient.*
  - *Features*—ventricular rate >150bpm, ongoing chest pain, or shock.[6]
  - *Start IV heparin* (heparin 5,000–10,000U IV) if no or subtherapeutic anticoagulation exists.
  - *Life-threatening cases*—use electrical cardioversion immediately [D].[6]
  - *Non-life-threatening unstable cases.*
    - *First-time AF (or unknown history)*—electrical cardioversion if readily available. Otherwise, use IV amiodarone (rhythm control) [D].[6]
    - *Known AF* (or known history of coronary symptoms, age >65, contraindications to anticoagulation or antiarrhythmias)—control ventricular rate (digoxin: loading dose 500μg/12h×2, followed by maintenance dose 0.125–0.25mg/24h) [D].[6]
      - Use β-blockers or rate-limiting calcium antagonists as alternative. Otherwise, use amiodarone.

- *Haemodynamically stable patient*
  - *Refer to a medical specialist.*
  - *Correct underlying abnormalities.*
  - *Anticoagulation*—start IV heparin as above for acute AF <48h (cardioversion for AF >48h is probably safe if no signs of cardiac thrombus exist). Consider warfarin in high-risk patients for recurrent AF, stroke (formal stroke risk assessment), or if AF persists >48h [D].[6]
  - *Persistent AF*—consider rhythm control or rate control.
    - Rhythm control for symptomatic, young, first-time patients.
    - Rate control for over 65, known coronary heart diseases, or contraindications to anticoagulation.[6]

- *Aetiology*—multifactorial. Commonly associated with sepsis, electrolyte disturbances (especially potassium and magnesium), hypoxia, hypovolaemia, and drug toxicity (mainly theophylline, adenosine, and digitalis). Other risk factors include hypertension (RR × 1.42),[3] recent or active MI (AF occurs in 6–10%),[9] rheumatic valvular disease, heart failure (AF occurs in 10–30%),[10] obesity (BMI >35kg/m²),[11] and in binge drinkers (AF occurs in 10–30%).[12]
- *Presentation*—many episodes are asymptomatic. Patients may complain of dizziness, weakness, palpitations, and dyspnoea. More serious presentations include angina, hypotension, and heart failure.
- *Diagnosis*—ECG should be performed in all patients,[6] and typically shows rapid and irregular atrial waves (350–600/min) with irregularly irregular ventricular response (90–170bpm). Look for evidence of left ventricular hypertrophy, bundle branch block, prior MI, and arrhythmias on earlier ECGs. Measure important intervals (P wave duration and morphology, RR, QRS, and QT). Other investigations include CXR, U&Es, ABGs, and echocardiogram.[6,7]
- *Prevention.*
  - Correct electrolyte abnormalities, anaemia, and hypoxia [D].[6] Keep potassium levels above 4mmol/L (common practice).[6] Correct magnesium levels as appropriate.[6]
  - Perioperative pain should be effectively controlled (see 📖 Chapter 19, pp.134–140).
  - Routine ECG and troponin check should always be considered in high-risk asymptomatic patients (see above).
  - Preoperative β-blockers and nitrates—never stop without alternatives [B].[4]
  - Prophylactic medications—recommended in cardiothoracic[6] and other high-risk operations (e.g. vascular surgery).[7] Consider using amiodarone [A],[6,7] β-blocker [A],[6] sotalol [A],[6] or a rate-limiting calcium antagonist [B].[6] Digoxin should not be used as prophylaxis [B].[6]
- *Treatment*—see Table 8.2 (see also 📖 OHCM p110).
  - *Thoracoscopic epicardial radiofrequency ablation for atrial fibrillation*—small series and short-term follow-up showed evidence of efficacy.[8] The procedure should only be performed within appropriate clinical governance setting and by well-trained physician. Patient selection should involve a multidisciplinary team.
    - Indications—when drug treatment is ineffective or not tolerated.
    - Efficacy—within limited patient numbers and follow-up period, 81–93% of patients were in sinus rhythm at 6–18mo.
    - Safety—few complications were reported, including atria-oesophageal fistula, pleural effusion, and pneumothorax.[8]

Further reading

1. Devereaux PJ, Goldman L, Yusuf S, Gilbert K, Leslie K, Guyatt GH (2005). Surveillance and prevention of major perioperative ischaemic cardiac events in patients undergoing non-cardiac surgery: a review. *CMAJ* 173, 779–88.
2. Bursi F, Babuin L, Barbieri A et al. (2005). Vascular surgery patients: perioperative and long-term risk according to the ACC/AHA guidelines, the additive role of post-operative troponin elevation. *Eur Heart J* 26, 2458–60.
3. Krahn AD, Manfreda J, Tate RB, Mathewson FA, Cuddy TE (1995). The natural history of atrial fibrillation: incidence, risk factors, and prognosis in the Manitoba Follow-up Study. *Am J Med* 98, 476–84.
4. Scottish Intercollegiate Guidelines Network (2004). Postoperative management in adults. Available from: http://www.sign.ac.uk/pdf/sign77.pdf.
5. Scottish Intercollegiate Guidelines Network (2007). Acute coronary syndromes. Available from: http://www.sign.ac.uk/pdf/sign93.pdf.
6. National Institute for Health and Clinical Excellence (2006). Atrial fibrillation. Available from: http://www.nice.org.uk/nicemedia/pdf/cg036fullguideline.pdf.
7. ACC/AHA/ESC (2006). Guidelines for the management of patients with atrial fibrillation—executive summary: a report of the American College of Cardiology/American Heart Association Task Force on Practice Guidelines. *J Am Coll Cardiol* 48, 854–906.
8. National Institute for Health and Clinical Excellence (2009). Thoracoscopic epicardial radiofrequency ablation for atrial fibrillation. Available from: http://www.nice.org.uk/nicemedia/pdf/IPG286Guidance.pdf.
9. Wong CK, White HD, Wilcox RG et al. (2000). New atrial fibrillation after acute myocardial infarction independently predicts death: the GUSTO-III experience. *Am Heart J* 140, 878–85.
10. Dries DL, Exner DV, Gersh BJ, Domanski MJ, Waclawiw MA, Stevenson LW (1998). Atrial fibrillation is associated with an increased risk for mortality and heart failure progression in patients with asymptomatic and symptomatic left ventricular systolic dysfunction: a retrospective analysis of the SOLVD trials. Studies of Left Ventricular Dysfunction. *J Am Coll Cardiol* 32, 696–703.
11. Wang TJ, Parise H, Levy D et al. (2004). Obesity and the risk of new-onset atrial fibrillation. *JAMA* 292, 2471–7.
12. Ettinger PO, Wu CF, De La Cruz C Jr, Weisse AB, Ahmed SS, Regan TJ (1978). Arrhythmias and the 'Holiday Heart'. Alcohol-associated cardiac rhythm disorders. *Am Heart J* 95, 555–62.

Respiratory complications

Key guidelines

- Scottish Intercollegiate Guidelines Network (2004). Postoperative management in adults.
- American College of Physicians (2006). Risk assessment for and strategies to reduce perioperative pulmonary complications for patients undergoing non-cardiothoracic surgery.
- Scottish Intercollegiate Guidelines Network (2008). British guideline on the management of asthma.
- Resuscitation Council (UK) (2008). Emergency treatment of anaphylactic reactions.

Post-operative atelectasis

- *Incidence*—very common.[1] Most likely cause of transient hypoxaemia post-operatively, which complicates the recovery of 30–50% of patients following abdominal surgery.[5,7] Endotracheal intubation and mechanical ventilation may be required in 8–10% of cases.
- *Pathophysiology*—atelectasis refers to collapse or loss of lung volume (clinically or radiologically) without evidence of respiratory infection.[1] This results from altered compliance of lung tissue, impaired regional ventilation, and retained airway secretions in the perioperative period.[4] Post-operative pain (especially in abdomino-thoracic surgery) contributes significantly to the reduction of functional residual capacity (FRC) and the development of atelectasis.
- *Presentation*—may remain asymptomatic, or progresses into respiratory infection or respiratory failure.
- *Diagnosis*—suspect in patients with abnormal respiratory rate (>25 or <10 breaths/min), tachycardia (>100bpm), or reduced conscious levels [CS].[1] Diagnosis is based on clinical examination, ABGs, sputum culture, and ECG. CXR should be reserved for patients with major lung collapse [CS].[1]
- *Prevention*—most important (see Ch. 6). Consider continuous positive airway pressure (CPAP) in selected cases.[1,2]
- *Treatment.*
  - Early mobilization and breathing exercises are sufficient for most cases.[1]
  - Extensive lobar or pulmonary collapse (unresponsive to respiratory therapy)—consider extraction of secretions using bronchoscopy (unproven efficiency).[1]
  - Respiratory infection—maintain oxygenation, clear blocked airways, expand collapsed alveoli, and clear infection.
  - Oxygen therapy—can be delivered using nasal catheters (variable performance and low flow), Venturi masks (high flow; oxygen concentrations up to 60%), and reservoir masks (up to 70% oxygen delivery). Patients with type 2 respiratory failure due to COPD require special attention as they have chronic CO_2 retention, and therefore, are dependent on hypoxic drive. Oxygen is required to return SpO_2 to its normal (or subnormal, but acceptable) level.[1]

Bronchospasm and asthma-like reaction[1,3]

- *Incidence*—common in the post-operative period.
- *Pathophysiology*—abnormal constriction of bronchial smooth muscles, triggered by aspiration of gastric contents, medications (tubocurarine, morphine, atracurium), suctioning, endotracheal intubation, and/or exacerbation of underlying COPD or asthma.
- *Presentation.*
  - Acute severe cases—patient unable to complete a sentence in one breath, wheezy, tachycardic (>110bpm), tachypnoeic (>25rpm), and have low peak expiratory flow (PEF) if spirometry in use (33–50% of predicted).
  - Life-threatening cases—patient exhausted, confused, in coma, silent chest, cyanotic, bradycardic, hypotensive, and hypoxic (SpO$_2$ <92%, PEF <33% of best or predicted).
- *Management*—see Table 8.3 (see also 📖 OHCM p794).

Anaphylactic reaction[1,3]

- *Definition*—severe, life-threatening, generalized or systemic hypersensitivity reaction that may cause death.[4,7] Anaphylaxis is a much broader syndrome than 'anaphylactic shock'.
- *Pathophysiology*—sudden, systemic degranulation of mast cells or basophils with release of mediators (histamine etc.) into the circulation.
  - Might be immunologic-mediated (IgE, IgG, immune complex) or non-immunologic-mediated (no immunoglobulin involved).
  - Organ dysfunction results from abnormal systemic vascular response (increases vascular permeability, coronary artery vasospasm, etc.), respiratory compromise (upper airway oedema, petechial haemorrhages, bronchospasm, and mucus plugging), mucocutaneous vascular changes (generalized hives, flushing, pruritus, swollen lips-tongue-uvula), and increased consumption of oxygen in peripheral tissues despite decreased perfusion, leading to rapid onset of anaerobic metabolism.
- *Presentation.*
  - *First impression*—suspect in any patient who becomes suddenly ill (usually within minutes) upon exposure to a trigger (allergen).[4]
  - *Signs and symptoms.*
    - Skin—up to 90% of cases. Present with generalized itching, flushing, urticaria, periorbital oedema, and conjunctival swelling.
    - Respiratory—up to 70%. Present with nasal congestion, voice changes, choking sensation, cough, wheezing, and short of breath.
    - Gastrointestinal—up to 40%. Present with abdominal cramps, nausea, vomiting, and diarrhoea.
    - Cardiovascular—up to 35%. Presents with dizzy feeling, tachycardia, hypotension, and peripheral collapse.
  - *Criteria of diagnosis*—the presence of the following three criteria makes the diagnosis of anaphylaxis most likely.[4]
    - Timing—sudden onset and rapid progression.
    - ABC compromise—life-threatening disorder in airways, breathing, and/or circulation.
    - Mucocutaneous—skin and/or mucosal changes.

- • Supportive (but not essential) to diagnosis is the recent exposure to allergen. Notice that skin changes alone cannot be considered a confirmation criteria if unaccompanied by the other two.
  - • *Laboratory diagnosis*—mast cell tryptase for recurrent idiopathic anaphylaxis. This is useful in follow-up, but should not delay initial assessment and management.
- • *Treatment*—follow ABCDE protocol. See Table 8.4 (see also 📖 OHCM p781).
  - • Follow-up—keep patient for 6h in a clinical area where facilities are available for treating life-threatening conditions.
  - • Early recurrence (biphasic reaction) occurs in 1–20% of cases. Patient might require 24h observation.
  - • Consider antihistamine and steroids for 3d, especially in the presence of urticaria.

Table 8.3 Management of bronchospasm

- • *Immediate management*.
  - • *Acute severe cases*.
    - • Oxygen 40–60%.
    - • *Salbutamol* 5mg (or terbutaline 10mg) via nebuliser.
    - • *Ipratropium* 0.5mg via nebuliser.
    - • Consider for very ill patients—IV *hydrocortisone* 100mg or oral *prednisolone* 40–50mg or both; *CXR* if consolidation is expected.
    - • Sedatives are contraindicated.
  - • *Life-threatening/persistently severe cases*.
    - • Involve ITU team.
    - • Increase nebulisers' frequency—salbutamol 5mg/15–30min or 10mg continuously hourly.
    - • Magnesium sulphate 1.2–2g IV over 20min.
    - • Consider (experienced staff)—IV β2 agonist, IV aminophylline, or mechanical ventilation.
- • *Follow-up management*.
  - • Keep the patient on:
    - • Oxygen 40–60%.
    - • *Salbutamol* and *ipratropium* nebulisers 4–6 hourly.
    - • *Prednisolone* 40–50mg daily or IV *hydrocortisone* 100mg 6 hourly.
  - • Monitor for 24h, then give advice. Full instructions to GP to follow.

Table 8.4 Management of anaphylaxis

- **Position the patient**—supine, comfortable with elevated legs. Patient may prefer to sit up (easier for breathing), might require recovery position (unconscious) or left side position (pregnancy).

- **Remove the trigger**—if possible. Stop suspected drug, remove the bee stinger, and do not attempt to induce vomit in food anaphylaxis.

- **ABCDE protocol**—apply as appropriate (see 📖 Chapter 15, pp.102–106).
  - **Oxygen**—high oxygen flow if necessary with Venturi system.
  - **Crystalloid fluid bolus**—500–1000mL IV. Repeat as needed.
  - **Monitor**—pulse oximetry, ECG, and blood pressure.

- **Specific immediate management**.
  - **Adrenaline**—give 300–500µg (0.3–0.5mL of 1:10000) IM. Repeat as required (every 3–5min). Consider IV for refractory cases (experienced staff).

- **Consider also (second line)**.
  - **Chlorpheniramine (H1 blocker)**—IM or slow IV, 5–10mg (age >6y), especially for itching.
  - **Hydrocortisone**—IM or slow IV, 100–200mg (age >6y).
  - **Bronchodilators**—for wheezing (asthma-like) symptoms.

Further reading

1. Qaseem A, Snow V, Fitterman N et al. (2006). Risk assessment for and strategies to reduce perioperative pulmonary complications for patients undergoing non-cardiothoracic surgery: a guideline from the American College of Physicians. Ann Intern Med 144, 575–80.
2. Scottish Intercollegiate Guidelines Network (2008). British guideline on the management of asthma. Available from: http://www.sign.ac.uk/pdf/sign101.pdf.
3. Resuscitation Council (UK) (2008). Emergency treatment of anaphylactic reactions. Available from: http://www.resus.org.uk/pages/reaction.pdf.
4. Platell C, Hall JC (1997). Atelectasis after abdominal surgery. J Am Coll Surg 185, 584–92.
5. Squadrone V, Coha M, Cerutti E et al. (2005). Continuous positive airway pressure for treatment of post-operative hypoxaemia: a randomized controlled trial. JAMA 293, 589–95.
6. Scottish Intercollegiate Guidelines Network (2004). Postoperative management in adults. Available from: http://www.sign.ac.uk/pdf/sign77.pdf.
7. Sampson HA, Munoz-Furlong A, Campbell RL, et al (2006). Second symposium on the definition and management of anaphylaxis: summary report–Second National Institute of Allergy and Infectious Disease/Food Allergy and Anaphylaxis Network Symposium. J Allergy Clin Immunol 117:391.

Renal complications

Key guidelines
- The Renal Association (2002). Treatment of adults and children with renal failure.
- BMJ Clinical Evidence (2008). Acute renal failure.
- BMJ Clinical Review (2006). Acute renal failure.

Acute renal failure (ARF)

- **Incidence**—accounts for 1% of all hospital admissions and complicates 5–7% of inpatient episodes.[1,6] Cases requiring dialysis have in-hospital mortality rate of 50% or more, especially when associated with sepsis in critically ill patients.[1,6]
- **Definition and classification**—ARF is the abrupt and sustained decline (over hours or days) in renal excretory function, with resultant accumulation of urea and other chemicals in the blood.[1,2,6] Based on the degree of change in serum creatinine concentration and severity of oliguria, RIFLE classification can reliably be used (Table 8.5).[2]
- **Pathogenesis**—most in-hospital cases (>70%) are due to pre-renal (decreased renal perfusion) or acute tubular necrosis (ATN).
  - *Pre-renal.*
    - *Fluid loss*—gastrointestinal (diarrhoea, vomiting, bleeding), renal (diuretics, osmotic diuresis), skin or respiratory (sweat, burns), third space (crush injury). Hypotension—severely decreased blood pressure can result from shock (myocardial or septic) or treatment of severe hypertension.
    - *Decreased perfusion*—severe hypotension and shock, congestive heart failure, nephrotic syndrome, and cirrhosis.
    - *Renal ischaemia*—bilateral renal artery stenosis and hepatorenal syndrome.
  - *ATN*—results from severe persistent pre-renal diseases or the presence of nephrotoxins (aminoglycosides, radiocontrast media, haemopigments, and others).
  - *Other causes*—post-renal urinary tract obstruction (10%), acute glomerulonephritis, vasculitis, atheroemboli, etc.
- **Clinical presentation**—asymptomatic, oliguria and dark urine, signs of renal failure (oedema, hypertension, weakness, fatigue, anorexia, mental changes), and/or signs of underlying causative disorder (shock, sepsis, etc).
- **Diagnosis.**
  - *Careful history and scrutiny of charts*—best method to find the most likely underlying factor, and the timing and pattern of progression.
  - *Standard blood tests*—U&Es, FBC, coagulation screen, and urine test. Consider testing for CRP, ABGs, immunologic tests, virology tests, and kidney-ureter-bladder (KUB) ultrasound scan.
  - *Estimated GFR*—this is only reliable in stable kidney disease and is not accurate enough in ARF. The change in values of estimated GFR is a useful marker for progression.

- *Urine index* (fractional excretion of sodium (FENa))—is the most accurate diagnostic test to differentiate between pre-renal (reversible) disease and ATN.[2,3]
  - Start by measuring the serum sodium (PNa), serum creatinine (PCr), urine sodium (UNa), and urine creatinine (UCr).
  - Use the following formula to calculate FENa.

$$FE\ Na\ (\%) = \frac{UNa \times PCr}{PNa \times UCr} \times 100$$

  - FENa <1 suggests a pre-renal condition, FENa >2 suggests ATN.
- *Management*—see also 📖 OHCM p293.
  - Seek specialist advice if necessary.
  - Treat precipitating factors.
  - Good hydration with added *N*-acetylcysteine has been shown in some, but not all, studies to reduce contrast nephropathy compared with hydration alone.[2]
  - Using low osmolality contrast medium is less nephrotoxic than the standard media.[2]
  - Using a single dose aminoglycosides is less nephrotoxic and appears to have similar benefits.[2]
  - Data does not support using other agents (mannitol, theophylline, and calcium channel blockers) in ARF.[2]
  - Fluid management.
    - IV sodium chloride (0.9%)—can reduce the incidence of ARF in high-risk patients when compared with unrestricted oral fluid regime.[2]
    - Loop diuretics plus fluids have adverse effect on renal function.[2]
  - Treat/protect from complications—infection, hyperkalaemia, pulmonary oedema, bleeding.
  - Consider dialysis in appropriate cases—refractory pulmonary oedema, severe metabolic acidosis (pH <7.2 or base excess <10), severe persistent hyperkalaemia (K$^+$ >7mmol/L), uraemic encephalopathy, or pericarditis.
    - There is no supportive evidence for prophylactic renal replacement therapy with haemofiltration in reducing the risk of contrast nephropathy.

Table 8.5 RIFLE classification of ARF

	GFR criteria*	Urine output criteria
Risk	• Increased serum creatinine ×1.5 • Decreased GFR >25%	<0.5mL/kg per h for 6h
Injury	• Increased serum creatinine ×2 • Decreased GFR >50%	<0.5mL/kg per h for 12h
Failure	• Increased serum creatinine ×3 • Decreased GFR >75% • Serum creatinine >4mg/dL	<0.5mL/kg per h for 24h, anuria for 12h
Loss	• Complete loss of kidney function for >4wk	
ESRD	• Complete loss of kidney function for >3mo	

* GFR = actual (not estimated) glomerular filtration rate

Further reading

1. The Renal Association (2002). Treatment of adults and children with renal failure. Available from: http://www.renal.org/Standards/RenalStandards_2002b.pdf.
2. Kellum J, Leblanc M, Venkataraman R (2008). Acute renal failure. *BMJ Clin Evid* 9, 2001.
3. Bellomo R, Ronco C, Kellum JA, Mehta RL, Palevsky P (2004). Acute renal failure—definition, outcome measures, animal models, fluid therapy and information technology needs: the Second International Consensus Conference of the Acute Dialysis Quality Initiative (ADQI) Group. *Crit Care* 8, 204–12.
4. Bagshaw SM, Langenberg C, Wan L, May CN, Bellomo R (2007). A systematic review of urinary findings in experimental septic acute renal failure. *Crit Care Med* 35, 1592–8.
5. Pepin MN, Bouchard J, Legault L, Ethier J (2007). Diagnostic performance of fractional excretion of urea and fractional excretion of sodium in the evaluations of patients with acute kidney injury with or without diuretic treatment. *Am J Kidney Dis* 50, 566–73.
6. Hilton R (2006). Acute renal failure. Clinical review. *BMJ* 333, 786–90.

Neurological complications

Key guidelines

- Royal College of Physicians (2006). Stroke programme.
- Scottish Intercollegiate Guidelines Network (2002). Management of patients with stroke.
- BMJ Clinical Evidence (2008). Stroke management.

Transient ischaemic attack (TIA) and stroke

- *Incidence*—infrequent in surgical practice, but remains the third most common cause of death in most developed countries.[3] About 0.3–3.5% of in-hospital general surgical patients develop a stroke, depending on the age and the presence of atherosclerotic risk factors. Most cases (85%) occur post-operatively, and few intraoperatively.[4]
- *Pathogenesis*—mostly due to occlusive ischaemic injury to the brain following thromboemboli rather than haemorrhage.[3] Possible sources of emboli are cardiac (AF) or carotid stenotic lesion (see ◻ Chapter 45, pp.341–348).
- *Clinical presentation*—rapid development of focal or generalized loss of cerebral function (lasting >24h in stroke) and/or leading to death.
- *Outcome*—about 10% die within 30d of onset. Nearly half of survivals experience some level of disability developing over 6mo period.[3]
  - *Clinical disabilities*—may include arm, hand or leg weakness, sensory loss, aphasia, dysarthria, visual field defect, and cognitive impairment.[2]
  - *Physical limitations*—walking, dressing, toileting, feeding, and bathing. Urinary and faecal incontinence are common.[2]
  - *Common complications*—depression, anxiety, general pain, epileptic seizures, pressure sores, venous thromboembolism, and chest and urinary tract infection.[2]
- *Diagnosis*—see also ◻ OHCM p.462.
  - Seek specialist advice [B].[1]
  - *CT scan*—the first investigation of choice [B].[1]
    - *Indications*—all patients.
    - *Timing*—as soon as possible. Maximum waiting should not exceed 24h of onset [B].[1] Urgently in patients with coagulation issues (anticoagulant treatment, bleeding tendency, possibility for thrombolysis), severe neurological defect (depressed level of consciousness, progressive or fluctuating symptoms, papilloedema or stiff neck, fever or severe headache on initial presentation.[1]
  - *MRI scan*—reserve for patients with uncertain cause or equivocal results on CT scan.
  - *Other assessments*—risk of aspiration (50mL water swallow screening test), moving and handling requirements, and risk of pressure ulcers [B, C].[1]
- *Treatment*—should be provided in specialized unit (Table 8.6) [A].[1]

Table 8.6 Treatment of stroke

General management*		
Vital functions	• Maintain arterial oxygenation, blood glucose, hydration, and temperature within normal.	[B]
Blood pressure	• Only modest lowering of BP is indicated in the acute phase.[1,3] Very high BP (mean BP >110 and diastolic BP >90) increases mortality (× 1.6). Rapid drop of BP may increase cerebral ischaemia.[3]	[B]
Mobilization	• As soon as possible.	[B]
Special arrangements[1]		
Antiplatelets	• Aspirin (300mg od)—for all patients, orally or rectally, following exclusion of haemorrhage (CT or MRI—delay treatment if there is a large cerebral infarct).[3]	[A]
	• Clopidogrel (75mg od)—acceptable alternative.	
	• Dipyridamole MR (200mg) bd ± low dose aspirin [B] for intolerant patients.	
Anticoagulation	• Start in every patient with AF (persistent or paroxysmal) if not contraindicated.	[A]
Statin	• Simvastatin 40mg. for every patient if not contraindicated.	[A]
Surgical interventions		
Carotid endarterectomy	• Carotid artery territory stroke in patients with no severe disability should be considered for carotid endarterectomy.[1]	[A]
	• Timing—as soon as the patient is fit for surgery. Usually in 2wk of TIA (see 📖 Chapter 45, pp.341–348 for details).	

* Other types of assessment, physiotherapy, interventions, and follow-up should be organized and provided by the specialist unit.

Further reading

1. Royal College of Physicians (2006). Stroke programme. Available from: http://www.rcplondon. ac.uk/clinical-standards/ceeu/Current-work/Pages/Stroke-programme.aspx.
2. Scottish Intercollegiate Guidelines Network (2002). Management of patients with stroke. Available from: http://www.sign.ac.uk/pdf/sign64.pdf.
3. Alawneh J, Clatworthy P, Morris R, Warburton E (2008). Stroke management. *BMJ Clin Evid* 9, 201.
4. Bell R, Merli G (1998). Perioperative assessment and management of the surgical patient with neurologic problems. In: Merli G, Weitz H, eds. *Medical management of the surgical patient*, pp. 283–311, WB Saunders, Philadelphia.

Diagnosis
- Criteria in Tables 9.2 and 9.3 are adopted with modification from the international, multidisciplinary Delphi group consensus statement recruited by EWMA.

Table 9.2 Diagnostic criteria for wound infection*

Diagnostic	Possible	Non-diagnostic
Acute wound		
• Pus/abscess • Cellulitis	• Delayed healing • Erythema ± induration • Exudate—haemopurulent, seropurulent, malodour • Wound breakdown/ enlargement • Pocketing	• Increase in local skin temperature • Oedema • Pain/tenderness
Diabetic foot (adding to the above)		
• Purulent exudate • Lymphangitis • Phlegmon	• Joint crepitus • Swelling with increase in exudates • Localized pain in a normally asensate foot • Probes to bone	• Spreading dry necrosis • Exposed bone or tendon • Friable granulation tissue easily bleeds

* See original guidelines for full list

Table 9.3 Diagnostic criteria for superficial surgical site infection (SSI)

- All suspected infections (localized pain or tenderness, localized swelling, redness, or heat) *involving only* the skin or subcutaneous tissue around the incision *within 30d* of procedure, with *at least one* of the following:
  - Purulent discharge from the superficial incision.
  - Pathogenic organisms isolated from an aseptically obtained culture of fluid or tissue from the superficial incision.
- The following are not reported as superficial SSI:
  - Stitch abscess (minimal inflammation and discharge confined to the points of suture penetration).
  - Infection of an episiotomy or neonate's circumcision site.
  - Infected burn wound.
  - Incisional SSI that extends into the facial and muscle layers (deep SSI).

- Swabs for culture and sensitivity—must be obtained from relevant infected sites (separately) using aseptic technique.[2]

Risk for osteomyelitis
- Suspect in the presence of exposed bone (or easily probed), open fracture, underlying internal fixation, gangrenous wound, persistent

sinus tract, and non-healing wound [B].[4] Plain X-ray, bone scan, and/or MRI scan should be considered to confirm and assess the extent of infection [B].[4]

- MRI scan is the procedure of choice to establish the diagnosis in clinically high suspicious cases [B].[4] Bone culture and biopsy should be obtained [B].[4]

Risk for endocarditis

- See 📖 Chapter 22, pp.161–166.

Treatment

- *Pain relief* and patient reassurance.
- *Surgical drainage and debridement*—for abscesses and necrotic infected tissues [B].[4] Severe life-threatening infections may require extensive debridement and possible amputation [B].[2] Severe osteomyelitis requires aggressive resection and coverage with well-perfused tissue (e.g. muscles) [B].
- *Systemic antibiotics*—in all established wound infections as per approved unit protocols [A].[2] Prudent use is important to reduce the risk of antibiotic induced diarrhoea.
  - Common microbial pathogens:[2]
    - Aerobic—β-haemolytic *Streptococci*, *Staphylococcus aureus* and MRSA, *Escherichia coli*, and *Klebsiella*.
    - Anaerobic—bacteroides, *Clostridium tetani*, and *Clostridium welchii* (gas gangrene).
  - Type and route of antibiotics—depends on expected pathogen, unit protocols, and severity of infection.[2,4] Commonly used regimes include cephalosporins, amoxicillin-clavulanic acid, macrolides, anti-staphylococcal penicillins, and fluoroquinolones [B].[4]
  - Topical antibiotics—only use with caution in selected cases and under regular review [B].[2,4] Possible indications include wounds with poor blood supply (systemic antibiotics may not reach thera-peutic levels), wounds with frequent contamination (e.g. faeces), unsuccessful long-term systemic antibiotics with bacterial resistance, antibiotic allergy, and planned delayed primary closure.[9]
- *Wound dressing*—select the most appropriate (see below) and apply daily.

Dressing selection

- *Ideal dressing*—should protect, cleanse, optimize, and promote the wound healing process (Table 9.4) [B].[1,2,3,4]
- *Dressing types*—differs in its source of origin and mechanism of action. They also have different capabilities to achieve one or more of the ideal dressing functions.
- *Selection of dressing*—depends on (Table 9.4):
  - Accurate assessment of wound—e.g. heavy or light exudative, odorous, sloughy, and/or infected.
  - Stage of healing process—e.g. wound requires assisted debridement of sloughs, high absorbing intact dressing for infected exudates, moist environment for granulation tissue, or promotion of the final healing and epithelialization stage.

Know your results

Compliance of bleeding risk assessment practice with current guidelines—audit areas

Does the assessment of bleeding risk follows appropriate guidelines?

- *Standards*—compliance with guidelines.
- *Indicators*—% of patients who are **not** tested, in compliance with the guideline; % of patients who **are** tested, in compliance with the guideline; % of patients who are **not** tested, against the recommendations of the guideline; % of patients who **are** tested, against the recommendations of the guideline; % of patients who are tested and for whom one or more reasons for testing are documented.
- Compare results with published recommendations.

Further reading

1. Chee YL, Crawford JC, Watson HG, Greaves M; British Committee for Standards in Haematology (2008). Guidelines on the assessment of bleeding risk prior to surgery or invasive procedures. *Br J Haematol* 140, 496–504.
2. Houry S, Georgeac C, Hay JM, Fingerhut A, Boudet MJ (1995). A prospective multicentre evaluation of preoperative haemostatic screening tests. The French Associations for Surgical Research. *Am J Surg* 170, 19–23.

Venous thromboembolism (VTE) prophylaxis

Venous thromboembolism (VTE) prophylaxis

Key guidelines

- National Institute for Health and Clinical Excellence (2007). Venous thromboembolism.
- Scottish Intercollegiate Guidelines Network (2005). Prophylaxis of venous thromboembolism.
- American College of Obstetricians and Gynaecologists (2000). Prevention of deep vein thrombosis and pulmonary embolism.
- Finnish Medical Society Duodecim (2006). Deep vein thrombosis.
- BNF 56. Anticoagulants and protamine (2008).
- Department of Health (2007). Report of the independent working group on the prevention of venous thromboembolism in hospitalized patients.

Basic facts

- Venous thromboembolism (VTE) (referring collectively to deep venous thrombosis (DVT) and pulmonary embolism (PE)) is the most common preventable cause of hospital death worldwide. VTE is responsible for about 25,000 and 200,000 deaths per year in the UK and US, respectively.[1,7]
- Massive PE, the sudden killer,[1] occurs in ~1% of all admissions (ranging from 0.5% of elective general to 7% of fractured hip replacement patients), and accounts for ~10% of all hospital deaths.[1,2,6]
- *Risk factors*—see Table 11.1. Virchow's triad (factors causing stasis in blood flow, venous endothelial injury, and/or hypercoagulable state of blood) is a good concise summary of major processes leading to VTE. It is important to ensure an ultimate 100% compliance with the requirement for risk assessment of every individual patient admitted to the hospital.[6]

Prophylaxis methods

- *General measures.*
  - *Early mobility and leg exercises*—effective in increasing venous return.[1] Bed rest has no proven benefits for any medical condition.[2]
  - *Adequate hydration*—dehydration strongly correlates with VTE and should be avoided.[1,2] Adequate hydration increases blood flow and reduces viscosity.[2]
- *Mechanical measures.*
  - *Graduated compression stockings (GCS)*—effective in increasing deep venous blood flow velocity by 75% when correct pressures are applied (British Standard Class II and European Standard Class I stockings).[1] How often stockings should be changed is uncertain and will depend on infection risk and local protocols. Not all patients are able to tolerate wearing stockings, e.g. gross oedema.

Table 11.1 Major risk factors for VTE[1,2,8,9]

Factor	Risk
Personal factors	
Age >60	×1.7 per each decade over 55
Obesity (BMI >30kg/m^2)	×3
Immobility (>3d bed rest, paralysis, plaster cast)	×10
Continuous traveller—trips >3h in the 4wk pre- or post-operatively	
Surgical factors	
Hospitalization (acute trauma, acute illness, surgery)	×10
Active cancer (or cancer treatment)	×7
CVP line *in situ*	
Severe infection	
Varicose veins with associated phlebitis	×1.5
Inflammatory bowel disease	
Medical factors	
Personal or family history of VTE	VTE recurrence rate ~5% per y
Recent myocardial infarction or stroke	
Others: paraproteinaemia, paroxysmal nocturnal haemoglobinuria, Behcet's disease, antiphospholipid syndrome, inherited thrombophilia, myeloproliferative diseases, nephrotic syndrome	
Reproductive factors	
Use of oral contraceptives, hormonal replacement therapy or tamoxifen	×3 (×6 for high-dose progesterone oils)
Pregnancy or puerperium	×10

Table 11.2 Current recommendations for VTE prophylaxis

Type of operation	No extra risk factors*	>1 extra risk factors
General surgery	Mechanical	Mechanical + LMWH/ fondaparinux**
Vascular	Mechanical	Mechanical + LMWH**

* See Table 11.1; ** If patient is not already on or requiring anticoagulation (therapeutic dose)

- *Intermittent pneumatic compression (IPC) devices*—periodically apply moderate pressure on the calf/thigh muscles. Effective in reducing DVT risk by ~65%.[1,2]
- Other mechanical methods—include mechanical foot pumps and electrical stimulation.
- **Pharmacological measures.**
  - *Low-dose heparin*—heparin is composed of heavy chains of polysaccharides that bind and accelerate the action of antithrombin and affects the other coagulation factors/enzymes (X, IX, XI, and XII).[1] Low-dose heparin reduces DVT risk by >50% (RR × 0.44), PE risk by 30% (RR × 0.70), and increases post-operative major bleeding risk by >46% (RR × 1.46).[1] Prolonged use increases the risk of thrombocytopaenia and regular platelets count check should be performed.
  - *Low molecular weight heparin (LMWH)*—short chains of heparin that bind less avidly to heparin binding proteins and allow for lower effective doses and more predictable levels.[1,2] LMWH reduces DVT risk by >50% (RR × 0.49), PE risk by >60% (RR × 0.36), and increases post-operative major bleeding risk by >75% (RR × 1.77) when given preoperatively as compared to giving immediately before or early after surgery.[1] The risk of thrombocytopaenia is less on using LMWH.
  - *Fondaparinux and idraparinux*—synthetic pentasaccharides that specifically and indirectly inhibit the activated factor Xa through its potentiation of antithrombin.[1] Fondaparinux reduces DVT risk by 48% (RR × 0.52), PE risk by >60% (RR × 0.70), and increases the risk of major bleeding post-operatively compared to LMWH (RR × 1.49).[1]
- **Other measures—vena caval filters** should be considered for surgical inpatients with recent (within 1mo) or existing VTE, and in whom anticoagulation is contraindicated.[1]

Current recommendations

- **General approach**—depends on the type of operation (Table 11.2, Fig. 11.1).
- **All medical patients**—should, as part of a mandatory risk assessment, be considered for thromboprophylaxis measures. LMWH is the preferred prophylactic method.[6] Aspirin is not recommended for thromboprophylaxis in medical patients.[6]
- **Special precautions.**[1,2]
  - *Before admission*—assess risk factors for each individual patient, advise on considering the cessation of combined oral contraceptive pills for 4wk before elective surgery, and provide patients with verbal and written information on VTE.
  - *On admission*—offer all patients thigh-length GCS (or knee-length GCS if thigh-length not available) if not contraindicated. Wearing stockings requires active help by trained staff members. Best practice is to keep GCS on until discharge.

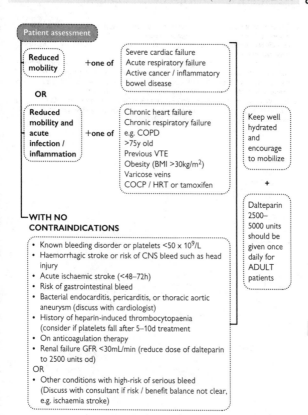

Fig. 11.1 A decision tool for VTE prophylaxis. Adapted with kind permission from Leicester Royal Infirmary guidelines

Further reading

1. National Institute for Health and Clinical Excellence (2007). Venous thromboembolism. Available from: http://www.nice.org.uk/nicemedia/pdf/VTEFullGuide.pdf.
2. Scottish Intercollegiate Guidelines Network (2002). Prophylaxis of venous thromboembolism. Available from: http://www.sign.ac.uk/pdf/sign62.pdf; (2005). Proposed review of SIGN guideline. Available from: http://www.sign.ac.uk/pdf/2005DVTreport.pdf.
3. The Seventh ACCP Conference on Antithrombotic and Thrombolytic Therapy (2007). Available from: http://www.guideline.gov/summary/summary.aspx?doc_id=11429. Accessed May 2009.
4. Finnish Medical Society Duodecim (2006). Deep vein thrombosis. Available from: http://www.guideline.gov/summary/summary.aspx?doc_id=9314.
5. BNF 56. Anticoagulants and protamine (2008).

6. Department of Health (2007). Report of the independent working group on the prevention of venous thromboembolism in hospitalized patients. Available from: http://www.dh.gov. uk/en/Publichealth/Healthprotection/Bloodsafety/VenousThromboembolismVTE/DH_073963 Accessed May 2009.

7. Horlander KT, Mannino DM, Leeper KV (2003). Pulmonary embolism mortality in the United States 1979–1998: an analysis using multiple-cause mortality data. *Arch Intern Med* 163: 1711–7.

8. Kikura M, Takada T, Sato S (2005). Preexisting morbidity as an independent risk factor for perioperative acute thromboembolism syndrome. *Arch Surg* 140, 1210–7.

9. Tsai AW, Cushman M, Rosamond WD, Heckert SR, Polak JF, Folsom AR (2002). Cardiovascular risk factors and venous thromboembolism incidence: the longitudinal investigation of thromboembolism aetiology. *Arch Intern Med* 162, 1182–9.

Prevention of infective endocarditis (IE)*

---

* The guidelines on this chapter have been sourced and summarized from different UK, Europe, and international government sources, professional organizations, and medical specialty societies. Leading guidelines have been listed in the Key guidelines box.

Prevention of infective endocarditis (IE)

Key guidelines
- National Institute for Health and Clinical Excellence (2008). Antimicrobial prophylaxis against infective endocarditis.
- The Royal College of Physicians (2004). Prophylaxis and treatment of infective endocarditis in adults: concise guidelines.
- European Society of Cardiology (2004). Infective endocarditis: guidelines on prevention, diagnosis, and treatment.
- American Heart Association (2007). Prevention of infective endocarditis.

Basic facts
- *Definition*—IE is an infection affecting one or more of the cardiovascular structures facing the bloodstream.[3] The term can be used to refer only to infection in the endocardium or, more broadly, to include infections affecting native or prosthetic valves, atrial or ventricular endocardium, patent ductus arteriosus, arteriovenous shunts, pacemakers, and surgically created conduits.[1,3]
- *Incidence*—about 2–6 annual cases per 100,000 population[4] Male-to-female ratios range from 3:2 to 9:1. More than 50% of current cases occur in patients over 60.[5]
- *Predisposing factors*—see Table 12.1.
- *Microbial pathogens*—viridans streptococci (50–70%), *Staphylococcus aureus* (25%), and enterococci (10%).[1]
- *Clinical presentation*—suspect in any patient with a well-recognized predisposing cardiac lesion who develops fever and heart murmur. Should also be suspected in patients with evidence of embolic events of unknown origin or patients with characteristic skin lesions (e.g. conjunctival or splinter haemorrhages).[4]
- *Diagnosis*—depends on a thorough history, clinical findings, laboratory studies (especially blood cultures), and echocardiogram. Diagnosis can be confirmed using different criteria (e.g. Duke criteria).
- *Treatment*—appropriate antibiotics. Surgery is occasionally required.

Prophylaxis
General concepts[1]
- Historically, IE, a serious condition that may result from bacteraemia, should be prevented in any exposure to invasive procedure, especially in high-risk patients.[1]
- *Current understandings.*
  - There is **no** consistent association between interventional procedures (dental or non-dental) and the development of IE.
  - The risk is greater during regular toothbrushing than in patients undergoing a single dental procedure.
  - Antibiotic prophylaxis has no solid proven effectiveness in protecting against IE.
  - Fatal anaphylaxis resulting from antibiotic usage may cause more deaths than the theoretical death caused by the possible risk of sustaining IE, and is not cost-effective.

Current recommendations[1]

- Antibiotics should **NOT** be offered to people undergoing dental or non-dental procedure to protect them from IE, even if they were from the high-risk group.[1]
- Prophylactic antibiotics (that covers IE) should only be considered in patients at risk of IE if the operative site is suspected to be infected,[1] and therefore, significant bacteraemia is to be induced **[C]**.[2] This applies mainly to microorganisms that have the potential to cause bacterial endocarditis.[4]
- This practice has not been adopted yet by some European organizations where prophylaxis is still considered for high-risk patients.[3]

Table 12.1 Predisposing factors to IE

- IV drug abusers.
- Acquired valvular heart diseases causing stenosis or regurgitation.*
- Prosthetic heart valve replacement.[6]
- History of previous IE* (recurrence occur in about 5%).[7]
- History of hypertrophic cardiomyopathy.*
- Haemodialysis patients (risk increases by 30–100 times).[8]
- Others—ventriculo-atrial shunts and patients undergoing liver, heart, and heart-lung transplantation.
- Structural congenital heart disease.* Patients with isolated atrial septal defect, fully repaired patent ductus arteriosus or ventricular septal defect, and those with endothelialized closure devices are **not** at high risk.

* = high risk

Know your results

Endocarditis prophylactic practice—audit areas

Compliance of prevention of IE policy/practice with NICE guidelines

- *Standards*—adherence to prophylaxis current recommendations.
- *Indicators*—% of patients with high-risk factors for endocarditis in a cohort of surgical patients, % of those patients receiving prophylactic antibiotics for the purpose of prevention of endocarditis, % of surgeons (juniors, seniors) who are aware of the new guidelines.

Further reading

1. National Institute for Health and Clinical Excellence (2008). Antimicrobial prophylaxis against infective endocarditis. Available from: http://www.nice.org.uk/guidance/index. jsp?action=byID&o=11938.
2. The Royal College of Physicians (2004). Prophylaxis and treatment of infective endocarditis in adults: concise guidelines. Available from: http://www.rcplondon.ac.uk/pubs/contents/ b99be9a0-eb8b-40e5-99fa-48e656e45e65.pdf.
3. European Society of Cardiology. Endocarditis. (EU) Available from: http://www.escardio.org/ guidelines-surveys/esc-guidelines//Pages/infective-endocarditis.aspx. Accessed May 2009

4. Wilson W, Taubert KA, Gewitz M et al. (2007). Prevention of infective endocarditis. *Circulation* 116, 1736–54.

5. Hill EE, Herijgers P, Claus P, Vanderschueren S, Herregods MC, Peetermans WE (2007). Infective endocarditis: changing epidemiology and predictors of 6-month mortality: a prospective cohort study. *Eur Heart J* 28, 196–203.

6. Tornos MP, Permanyer–Miralda G, Olona M, Gil M, Galve E, Almirante B, Soler–Soler J (1992). Long-term complications of native valve infective endocarditis in non-addicts. A 15-year follow-up study. *Ann Intern Med* 117, 567–72.

7. Ireland JH, McCarthy JT (2003). Infective endocarditis in patients with kidney failure: chronic dialysis and kidney transplant. *Curr Infect Dis Rep* 5, 293–9.

Principles of blood transfusion*

* The guidelines on this chapter have been sourced and summarized from different UK, Europe, and international government sources, professional organizations, and medical specialty societies. Leading guidelines have been listed in the Key guidelines box.

Principles of blood transfusion

Key guidelines

- Scottish Intercollegiate Guidelines Network (2005). Perioperative blood transfusion for elective surgery.
- The Association of Anaesthetists of Great Britain and Ireland (2005). Blood transfusion and the anaesthetist.
- Department of Health (2005). Indication code for transfusion—an audit tool.
- The British Committee for Standards in Haematology (2007). Current guidelines on blood transfusion.

Red cell blood transfusion

- *Benefits*—to increase the oxygen-carrying capacity of blood, with resultant more efficient delivery of oxygen to vital and non-vital organs.
- *Risks*—associated with blood transfusion, see Table 13.1.
- *Indications for transfusion*—always should weigh the expected benefits against possible risks. Clear valid justification for blood transfusion should always be available and documented in the patient's notes **[D]**.[1]
  - Acute blood loss.
    - Acute blood volume loss can usually be replaced using crystalloids or synthetic colloids.[1] Red cell transfusion to replace the oxygen-carrying capacity may be required only in later stages of shock.
    - Blood transfusion is beneficial for class III shock (30–40% blood loss, i.e. 1500–2000mL) as initial modality.[1] Less severe cases (classes I and II shock) do **NOT** require red cell transfusion for the only purpose of enhancing the blood oxygen-carrying capacity. Decision should be based on individual cases (e.g. patients over 65, those with pre-existing anaemia or reduced cardiorespiratory reserve may require red cell transfusion at an earlier stage).[1]
  - Low levels of haemoglobin.
    - Red cell transfusion is **NOT** required or justified if the level of current (or anticipated) Hb is >10g/dL **[D]**.[1] Transfusion is required if Hb level is <7g/dL **[D]**.[1]
    - Patients with poor tolerance to anaemia (e.g. age >65, cardiovascular problems) requires red cell transfusion when Hb drops below 9g/dL **[C]**.[1]
    - The number of units required depends on the clinical situation. Each unit of packed blood cells (300mL) in an adult would raise the Hb by ~1g/dL (within 15min of finishing the transfusion up to 12h) if no continued bleeding exists.[7]
    - Blood transfusion has no significant effect on cancer recurrence or perioperative infection rate **[B]**.[1]

Table 13.1 Risks of blood transfusion[1,5]

Transfusion transmitted infections (TTI)

- *Definition*—diagnosis made if no infection present prior to transfusion, the recipient has infection following the transfusion, and the blood component is contaminated or the donor of this component has evidence of the same infection.[5]

- *Viral*—HIV, HCV, HBV. Very low risk. Estimate risk for hepatitis C or HIV transmission: 1 in 1–2 million units transfused in UK and US.

- *Bacterial*—higher incidence. Estimated risk: 1 in 400,000 units of platelets transfused in UK and US.

- *Others*—prions (CJD—very rare), protozoa.

Transfusion reaction

- **Acute immune-mediated haemolysis—MEDICAL EMERGENCY.**
  - *Mechanism*—results from complement-mediated intravascular haemolysis, where the recipient's plasma has existing antibodies (anti-A, anti-B, or rarely anti-Rh) to the donor's red blood cells (RBCs), causing rapid RBC destruction.
  - *Risk*—may lead to disseminated intravascular coagulation (DIC), circulatory shock, and acute tubular necrosis with acute renal failure.
  - *Clinically*—agitation, anxiety, fever, flushing, abdominal, back and chest pain, abnormal bleeding from puncture sites, tachycardia, hypotension, tachypnoea.
  - *Treatment.*
    - *STEP 1*—stop infusion, check identity, start ABCDE management Plan (see ☐ Chapter 15, pp.101–106).
    - *STEP 2*—send bloods for FBC, U&Es, clotting, and culture. Send urine sample.
    - *STEP 3*—inform the haematologist.

- **Delayed haemolytic reaction.**
  - *Mechanism*—delayed antibody response after re-exposure to foreign red cell antigen. Occurs within 2–10d. Less severe.
  - *Clinically*—failing Hb, mild fever, slight increased bilirubin in serum.
  - *Treatment*—non-specific. Special care for future transfusions.

- **Febrile non-haemolytic reactions**—most common reaction.
  - *Mechanism*—cytokines (interleukin (IL)-1, IL-6, IL-8, tumour necrosis factor-alpha (TNFα)) generated and accumulated during blood components' storage process.[6]
  - *Clinically*—fever and chills within 1–6h of transfusion.
  - *Treatment*—stop infusion, exclude acute haemolysis, use paracetamol.

- **Anaphylactic reaction—LIFE-THREATENING CONDITION** (see Ch. 8).

- **Other reactions**—urticarial reaction, post-transfusion purpura, transfusion-related acute lung injury, immunomodulation.

Procedural errors[1]

- Human errors can occur in one or more of the minimum 40 steps of transfusing blood to patients. The estimated incidence is 71:24,000 transfusions. Transfusion best practice should always be followed [D].

- *Preoperative blood transfusion.*
  - Avoid transfusion if possible, especially if Hb is >10.[1] Possible causes for anaemia should be investigated and treated preoperatively if possible [C].[1]
- Erythropoietin—offers new and alternative route for improving Hb concentrations, and should be used when appropriate (e.g. patients with objections to allogeneic transfusions) [D].[1,6]
- Blood-sparing strategies (autologous transfusion)—should be made available for all patients undergoing major blood losing surgery [G].[1]
- Preoperative autologous blood transfusion should be offered only where patients are guaranteed an admission date for surgery [D].[1]

Fresh frozen plasma (FFP) transfusion

- *Preparation*—donors' whole blood using hard centrifugation or aphaeresis.[1,4] Subject to strict quality monitoring, e.g. FFP should be rapidly frozen to −30°C to maintain the activity of labile coagulation factors. Level of electrolytes, platelet, and leukocyte depletion are monitored. Handling of the frozen brittle plastic bags requires special care. Any discoloration or leak when subjecting the FFP pack to pressure should be investigated promptly.[1]
- *Benefits*—FFP contain the same spectrum of haemostatic factors found in healthy blood. Level of each factor differs with time and method of preparation.[1]
- *Risks*—hypersensitivity reaction (1–3%), leukocyte depletion, infection, and graft-versus-host defence.
- *Indications*—limited in surgical practice.
  - *Coagulation factor deficiencies and DIC.*
    - Multi-factor deficiencies in association with severe bleeding and/ or DIC require FFP (guided by coagulation tests).
      Not indicated where there is no evidence of bleeding.
  - *Reversal of warfarin effect*—see 📖 Chapter 14, pp.97–100.
    - Vitamin K deficiency in intensive care unit (ICU)—start with vitamin K supplements as a first-line choice.[1,4] FFP are not indicated to correct prolonged clotting time in ICU setting.
  - *Liver disease with prolonged PT time.*
    - FFP may be useful, but the response is unpredictable and repeated coagulation screening is essential to guide treatment.[1,4]
  - *Surgical bleeding and massive transfusion.*
    - FFP may be indicated based on the coagulation status. FFP is not indicated to replace volume depletion in massive bleeding.

Know your results

Blood transfusion practice—audit areas[1]

Compliance of blood transfusion policy/practice with published guidelines

- *Standards*—adherence to indications.
- *Indicators*—amount of blood transfused per operation (adjusted to surgeon's grade), % cross-matched to transfusion rate, level of Hb pre- and post-operatively and on discharge, training on safe transfusion practice.

Further reading

1. Scottish Intercollegiate Guidelines Network (2001). Perioperative blood transfusion for elective surgery. Available from: http://www.sign.ac.uk/pdf/sign54.pdf; updated in: Proposed review of SIGN guideline 2005. Available from: http://www.sign.ac.uk/pdf/2005bloodtransfusionreport.pdf.
2. The Association of Anaesthetists of Great Britain and Ireland (2005). Blood transfusion and the anaesthetist. Available from: http://www.aagbi.org/publications/guidelines/docs/bloodtransfusion06.pdf.
3. Department of Health (2005). Indication code for transfusion—an audit tool. Available from: http://www.dh.gov.uk/en/Publichealth/Healthprotection/Bloodsafety/Bloodsafetygeneralinformation/DH_4083545?IdcService=GET_FILE&dID=10835&Rendition=Web.
4. The British Committee for Standards in Haematology (2007). Current guidelines on blood transfusion. Available from: http://www.bcshguidelines.com/publishedHO.asp?tf=Blood%20Transfusion&status=.
5. Williamson LM, Lowe S, Love EM *et al.* (1999). Serious hazards of transfusion (SHOT) initiative; analysis of the first two annual report. *BMJ* 319, 16–9.
6. Enright H, Davis K, Gernsheimer T, McCullough JJ, Woodson R, Slichter SJ (2003). Factors influencing moderate to severe reactions to PLT transfusions: experience of the TRAP multicentre clinical trial. *Transfusion* 43, 1545–52.
7. Wiesen AR, Hospenthal DR, Byrd JC, Glass KL, Howard RS, Diehl LF (1994). Equilibration of haemoglobin concentration after transfusion in medical inpatients not actively bleeding. *Ann Intern Med* 121, 278–80.

Perioperative anticoagulation management*

* The guidelines on this chapter have been sourced and summarized from different UK, Europe, and international government sources, professional organizations, and medical specialty societies. Leading guidelines have been listed in the Key guidelines box.

Perioperative anticoagulation management

Key guidelines
- British Committee for Standards in Haematology (2008). Guidelines on the assessment of bleeding risk prior to surgery or invasive procedures.
- European College of Cardiology (2005). Antithrombotic therapy in patients with mechanical heart valves.

Background
- **General concept**—anticoagulant therapy is common among patients undergoing elective or emergency surgery. Perioperative effective management should balance the benefits of anticoagulation against the risk of causing significant bleeding.

Risk of thrombosis on stopping warfarin
- **Efficiency of warfarin.**
  - The risk of recurrent DVT during the first month of acute DVT is ~50% if no warfarin was taken, compared to 8–10% for patients taking warfarin (4–5% after 3mo period).[7,8]
  - *Warfarin* reduces the risk of embolism by more than two thirds (from 4% to 1% in patients with prosthetic heart valve, and from 0.5% to 0.2% in patients without). Arterial embolism event is fatal or severely disabling in about 60% of patients.[9,10]
- **Anticoagulation dynamics**—on stopping warfarin, most patients will drop the INR below 2.0 in about 4d.[4] Once warfarin is restarted, about 3d elapse before the INR reaches the level of 2.0. Patients can therefore be expected to have a sub-therapeutic INR for about 2d before surgery and 2d after. Partial protection against thromboembolism event is still expected during this period.

Risk of bleeding on using heparin
- **Heparin-related bleeding**—2d of IV heparin can increase the risk of major post-operative bleeding by ~3% compared to similar group with no heparin.[4] This bleeding is fatal in ~3% of episodes and causes permanent disability in ~1.5% of cases.[4]
- **Factors affecting perioperative bleeding**—include the type, extent, and duration of operation or procedure, the use of antiplatelets, and the presence of other comorbidities that have a potential effect on haemostasis (see 📖 Chapter 10, pp.75–80).

Recommendations
- **General approach**—patients with a target INR of 2.0 to 3.0 undergoing elective surgical procedure should stop oral anticoagulants for 5d before the procedure (4 clear days). The target INR should be around 2.0 on the day of surgery [B].[1] If immediate preoperative INR was <2.5, the surgeon can safely proceed to surgery.

- **In high-risk operations** (e.g. neurosurgery or vascular surgery)—where bleeding might have dramatic effect on outcome, a period of no anticoagulation is preferable [B].[1]
- **If INR is >2.5 on the day of surgery**—the risk of bleeding should be weighed against the urgency and required timing of the procedure by both the surgeon and anaesthetist.
  - If *rapid reversal* of warfarin anticoagulation is required, warfarin should be stopped and a small dose (e.g. 0.5–1.0mg) of IV vitamin K1 should be used [B].[1] The INR is expected to drop to 1.4 or less in over 50% of patients within a median duration of 27h.[6]
- *High-risk patients*—include all patients with thrombogenic prosthetic valve in the mitral position (see Table 14.1), recent episode of venous thromboembolism within the last 4wk, or patients with active malignancy. Those patients should be considered for alternative prophylactic measures (e.g. LMWH) when INR drops below 2 [C].[1,11]
- **Vena caval filter**—should be considered if an absolute contraindication to therapeutic anticoagulation (or a failure of anticoagulation) exists associated with acute proximal venous thrombosis.

Table 14.1 A sample of recommended management plan for anticoagulation warfarin bridging for prosthetic heart valves in the perioperative period**

- Stop warfarin 5d preop (4 clear days).
- Commence dalteparin on d3 at 100U/kg twice daily, providing normal renal function.
- Reduce the dose to 5,000U on the evening before surgery.
- Omit dalteparin on morning of operation.
- Restart dalteparin at 5,000U, 6h post-op provided haemostasis is secure.
- Increase dalteparin to 100U/kg twice daily the following morning, after reassessment and exclusion of post-op bleeding complications.
- Recommence warfarin at USUAL MAINTENANCE DOSE on day after surgery, (no loading doses).
- Continue dalteparin 100U/kg bd with WARFARIN until INR is within therapeutic range on two consecutive tests, taken at least 24h apart. Teach injection technique if domiciliary self-medication required.
- Prior to discharge, ensure follow-up arrangements for repeat INR.
- Attention to hydration and mobilization as for routine thromboprophylaxis.
- This anticoagulation plan should be kept with the drug chart at all times.

** Adapted with kind permission from Leicester Royal Infirmary guidelines

Further reading

1. Chee YL, Crawford JC, Watson HG, Greaves M; British Committee for Standards in Haematology (2008). Guidelines on the assessment of bleeding risk prior to surgery or invasive procedures. *Br J Haematol* 140, 496–504.
2. European College of Cardiology (2005). Antithrombotic therapy in patients with mechanical heart valves. Guideline summary. Available from: http://www.uptodate.com/online/content/image.do;jsessionid=6B4CFC6CED886CF75F27328FF7803492.0603?imageKey=card_pix/esc_rx_m.htm.

3. Dunn AS, Turpie AG (2003). Perioperative management of patients receiving oral anticoagulants. A systematic review. *Arch Intern Med* 163, 901–8.

4. Kearon C, Hirsh J (1997). Management of anticoagulation before and after elective surgery. *N Engl J Med* 336, 1506–11.

5. Torn M, Rosendaal FR (2003). Oral anticoagulation in surgical procedures: risks and recommendations. *Br J Haematol* 123, 676–82.

6. Shields RC, McBane RD, Kuiper JD, Li H, Heit JA (2001). Efficacy and safety of intravenous phytonadione (vitamin K1) in patients on long-term oral anticoagulant therapy. *Mayo Clin Proc* 76, 260–6.

7. Levine MN, Hirsh J, Gent M et al. (1995). Optimal duration of oral anticoagulant therapy: a randomized trial comparing four weeks with three months of warfarin in patients with proximal deep vein thrombosis. *Thromb Haemost* 74, 606–11.

8. Research Committee of the British Thoracic Society (1992). Optimum duration of anticoagulation for deep vein thrombosis and pulmonary embolism. *Lancet* 340, 873–6.

9. Cerebral Embolism Task Force (1986). Cardiogenic brain embolism. *Arch Neurol* 43, 71–84.

10. Lin HJ, Wolf PA, Kelly–Hayes M et al. (1996). Stroke severity in atrial fibrillation. The Framingham Study. *Stroke* 27, 1760–4.

11. O'Donnell MJ, Kearon C, Johnson J et al. (2007). Brief communication: preoperative anticoagulant activity after bridging low molecular weight heparin for temporary interruption of warfarin. *Ann Intern Med* 146, 184–7.

Principles of care of critically ill patients*

* The guidelines on this chapter have been sourced and summarized from different UK, Europe, and international government sources, professional organizations, and medical specialty societies. Leading guidelines have been listed in the Key guidelines box.

   The authors would like to thank the Welsh Institute for Minimal Access Therapy (WIMAT) Medicare centre in Cardiff, and Mr. Louis Fligelstone, Head of School & Associate Dean, the CCrISP course director at WIMAT. Their dedication, enthusiasm and vision have contributed significantly to the concepts detailed in this chapter.

Principles of care of critically ill patients

Key guidelines
- National Institute for Health and Clinical Excellence (2007). Acutely ill patients in hospital.
- Anderson I (2003). Care of the critically ill surgical patient (CCrISP) manual.
- American College of Surgeons (2004). Advanced trauma and life support (ATLS) program for doctors.
- Society of Critical Care Medicine. Learn ICU.
- The Intensive Care Society.
- European Society of Intensive Care Medicine. Guidelines.

'Key' definitions
- *Critical care*—concerned with the provision of life support or organ support systems in patients who are critically ill and who usually require intensive monitoring and/or intervention.[7]
- *Critically ill patients.*
  - Patients with no existing critical illness, but who are at higher risk to develop life-threatening condition (e.g. extreme age groups, significant comorbidities, high-risk operations),
  - Patients with existing but compensated critical illness (e.g. pre-shock patients with peripheral shutdown and tachycardia, but no end-organ failure, pre-respiratory failure patients with normal PaO_2 on high-flow oxygen),
  - Patients with existing critical illness (e.g. shock with end-organ failure, respiratory failure requiring ventilation).[2]
- *Level of care*—the level of monitoring and intervention required for the individual patient critical case (Table 15.1).[5]
- *Organ failure*—altered organ function (reversible or irreversible) requiring intensive intervention to achieve homeostasis (Table 15.2).

Recommended approach
- *Immediate management*—see Fig. 15.1.
  - Always follow the ABCDE approach in the initial assessment of any sick patient (A: **A**irways, B: **B**reathing, C: **C**irculation, D: **D**isability, E: **E**xposure).[2,3,4] (See also ▢ OHCM p767.)
  - Remember to assess and manage simultaneously (e.g. identify tension pneumothorax and treat immediately; identify the shock state and commence fluid management).
  - This stage ends once the patient is physiologically stable enough and not in immediate danger.[2] Airways should be secured, breathing and oxygenation should be effective (oxygen saturation >90–94%),[2,3] and circulation should be fully assessed and fluid management established.

Table 15.1 Levels of care for critically ill surgical patients

- **Level 0**—normal ward in acute hospital. Provides basic physiologic monitoring and a fairly low nurse-to-patient ratio.

- **Level 1**—acute ward with higher nurse-to-patient ratio and additional support from critical care (outreach) team, e.g. the Surgical Extended Care Unit (SECU).

- **Level 2**—more advanced physiologic monitoring and high nurse-to-patient ratio, with the ability to support a single failing organ system, e.g. the High Dependency Unit (HDU).

- **Level 3**—advanced physiologic monitoring and respiratory support with high nurse-to-patient ratio. Ability to support two failing organ systems or more, e.g. the Intensive Care Unit (ICU).

Table 15.2 Organ failure—diagnostic criteria

- **Cardiovascular**—inadequate organ perfusion with resultant hypoxia.[2,8] Clinical criteria include:
  - *Hypotension*—BP <90mmHg or fall of >30–40mmHg.
  - *Decreased renal perfusion*—oliguria <20mL/h.
  - *Decreased cerebral perfusion*—confusion or restlessness.
  - *Decreased limb perfusion*—dry mucous membranes, cold peripheries.

- **Respiratory**—failure of gas exchange resulting from inadequate function of one or more components of the respiratory system.[6] Clinical criteria include:
  - *Hypoxaemia*—PO_2 <8kPa[2] (or <60mmHg)[8] at sea level.
  - *Hypercarbia*—PCO_2 >7kPa[2] (or >45mmHg).[8]
  - PaO_2/FIO_2 <250 (or <200 in the presence of pneumonia).[10]
  - Or (more frequently) a combination of more than one criteria.

- **Renal**—a significant decline in glomerular filtration rate (GFR) with retention of nitrogenous waste products, and disturbance of body fluid volume, electrolyte and acid-base balance.[2,9] Clinical criteria include:
  - *Oliguria*—urine output <0.5mL/kg/h or <45mL every 2h despite adequate resuscitation.[10]
  - Raised creatinine >0.5mg/dL or 44.2µmol/L.[10]
  - Decreased GFR.

- **Coagulopathy**—INR >1.5 with the absence of anticoagulants or platelet count <100,000.[10]

- **Other parameters**—lactate ≥4mmol/L.

- *Full patient assessment*—follows the previous step and aims at gathering as much information as needed to establish a working diagnosis of the current problem and to formulate an effective management plan.[2]
  - *History and systematic examination*—should be thorough and focused. Holistic approach is required, including significant comorbidities, patient's current quality of life, and family members' opinion. Repeated examination and revisiting the history (e.g. ten minutes later) maximizes the chance of picking up on missed information and is a recommended practice.[2]
  - *Chart review*—be systematic in your approach (e.g. R: **R**espiratory, C: **C**irculation, S: **S**urgical).[2] Look specifically on the absolute values and trends. Check drug charts for both prescribed and delivered medications (e.g. missed antihypertensives in uncontrolled hypertension crises).
  - *Notes and results review*—including routine bloods, recent investigations, and documented reviews. Maximize your chance of getting the blood results on time by maintaining a forward organization of your team. Waiting at the end of the bed to get the results from computers is more effective practice than promising to review later.[2]
- *Decision and plan*—following the thorough review (and management of life-threatening conditions), the management strategy depends on the stability of the patient.
  - *Stable patient*—should be haemodynamically stable enough and progressing as expected. A full management plan should ensure clear instructions on the required monitoring schedule (and level of care necessary for the day, see Table 15.1), fluid balance, required and urgency of investigations, care of the surgical site (dressing, drains), medications, and other significant instructions for the day (e.g. physiotherapy, referrals, nutrition).
  - *Unstable patient*—include those with unstable vital signs, inappropriate progression, unexpected level of pain, and slow but established deterioration. Arrange appropriate (soon or immediate) investigations or procedure, request specialist opinion immediately, and decide on the level of care required.
- *Documentation*—essential final (or interval) step and should be done properly (see 📖 Chapter 2, pp.11–16).
- Further management of each organ failure is discussed further in 📖 Chapter 16, pp.107–114.

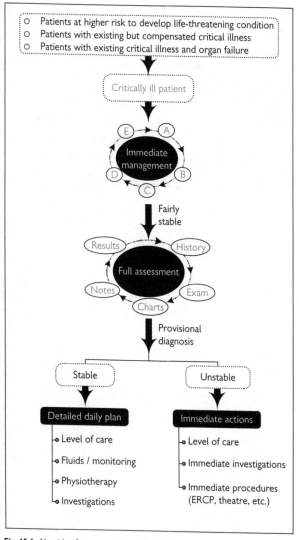

- O Patients at higher risk to develop life-threatening condition
- O Patients with existing but compensated critical illness
- O Patients with existing critical illness and organ failure

Critically ill patient

E → A
Immediate management
D ← C ← B

Fairly stable

Results — History
Full assessment
Notes — Charts — Exam

Provisional diagnosis

Stable

Unstable

Detailed daily plan

- Level of care
- Fluids / monitoring
- Physiotherapy
- Investigations

Immediate actions

- Level of care
- Immediate investigations
- Immediate procedures (ERCP, theatre, etc.)

Fig. 15.1 Algorithm for approaching critically ill surgical patients

Further reading

1. National Institute for Health and Clinical Excellence (2007). Acutely ill patients in hospital. Available from: http://www.nice.org.uk/Guidance/CG50.
2. Anderson I (2003). *Care of Critically Ill Surgical Patient*, 2nd edition. Hodder Arnold, London.
3. American College of Surgeons (2004). *Advanced trauma and life support program for doctors*, 7th ed. American College of Surgeons, Chicago.
4. Society of Critical Care Medicine. Learn ICU. Available from: http://www.learnicu.org/Pages/default.aspx.
5. The Intensive Care Society. Available from: http://www.ics.ac.uk/.
6. European Society of Intensive Care Medicine. Guidelines. Available from: http://www.esicm.org/Data/ModuleGestionDeContenu/PagesGenerees/06-publications/0D-guidelines-recommendations/92.asp.
7. Wikipedia. Intensive care medicine. Available from: http://en.wikipedia.org/wiki/Intensive_care_medicine.
8. Webb AJ, Shapiro MJ, Singer M, Suter PM (1999). *Oxford Textbook of Critical Care*, Oxford University Press, Oxford.
9. Fauci AS, Braunwald E, Kasper DL et al. (2008). *Harrison's Principles of Internal Medicine*, 17th ed, McGraw–Hill Professional, Maidenhead.
10. Dellinger RP, Levy MM, Carlet JM et al. (2008). Surviving Sepsis Campaign: international guidelines for management of severe sepsis and septic shock. *Crit Care Med* 36, 296–327.

Sepsis and septic shock*

---

* The guidelines on this chapter have been sourced and summarized from different UK, Europe, and international government sources, professional organizations, and medical specialty societies. Leading guidelines have been listed in the Key guidelines box.

Sepsis and septic shock

Key guidelines

- Dellinger RP, Levy MM, Carlet JM et al. (2008). Surviving Sepsis Campaign.
- Anderson ID (2003). Care of the critically ill surgical patient.

Basic facts

- **Definitions**—sepsis is a syndrome of systematic inflammatory process caused by infection. The spectrum ranges in severity from mild sepsis to refractory septic shock (Table 16.1).[1]
- **Incidence**—sepsis accounts for over 25% of potentially preventable in-hospital deaths.[1] Septic shock is associated with >40–50% mortality rate.[3]
- **Clinical features**—related to the severity of sepsis and organ dysfunction (Table 16.1; Table 15.2, p.103).

Recommended management plan[1,2]

- **Immediate resuscitation**—should start promptly (first 6h) once sepsis has been recognised [C].[1] Resuscitation should follow agreed protocols and aims at achieving identifiable targets (goal-directed) [C] (Fig. 16.1).[1] Sepsis-related mortality can be reduced significantly using this approach (reduction by >15%).[4]
- **Confirm the source, type, and site of infection**—using appropriate cultures (e.g. blood, sputum, wound, and urine—Table 16.2) and imaging (± aspiration of potential source of infection) [C].[1]
- **Infection source control.**
  - *Antimicrobial therapy*—should start promptly (Table 16.3) following appropriate cultures (within the first hour in septic shock [B]).[1,5] Each hour of delay in starting antibiotics in the first 6h can reduce survival rate by ~8%.[5]
  - *Source control*—should be achieved as soon as possible (e.g. operative management of peritonitis, endoscopic management of cholangitis) [C].[1] This is best done within the first 6h of identification in severe septic cases [D].[1] Minimal invasive procedures are always preferable when appropriate [D].[1]
- **Circulatory support.**
  - *Fluid therapy*—using colloids or crystalloids (no significant difference) [B]. Goal-targeted fluid therapy [C], fluid challenge technique [D], and reduction of fluid administration upon reaching the target [D] are recommended practices.[1]

Table 16.1 Definitions in sepsis[1,2]

- **Infection**—inflammatory response to microorganism invasion.

- **Systemic inflammatory response syndrome (SIRS)**—the presence of two or more of the following:
  - Temperature >38.3°C or <36.0°C; heart rate >90bpm (or >2SD of normal value for age); respiratory rate >20 breaths/min; positive fluid balance (>20mL/kg in 24h); change in mental state.
  - WBC count >12,000 cells/mL or <4,000 cells/mL or >10% immature (band) forms; CRP >2SD of normal values; hyperglycaemia (blood glucose >7.7mmol/L) in non-diabetic patients.

- **Sepsis**—SIRS in the presence of documented infection (e.g. positive culture for blood, urine, sputum, or normally sterile body fluid; clear focus of apparent infection).

- **Severe sepsis**—sepsis with signs of organ dysfunction of moderate severity (e.g. oliguria or change in mental status).

- **Septic shock**—severe sepsis with inadequate tissue perfusion refractory to fluid management (e.g. mean BP <60mmHg after 40–60mL/kg normal saline solution, the need for norepinephrine or epinephrine of >0.25µg/kg/min to maintain mean BP >60mmHg).

Table 16.2 Blood culture—good practice[1,2]

- **Timing**—before commencing antibiotics.

- **Number**—two or more.

- **Site.**
  - One percutaneously and one from each vascular access that has been inserted 48h or more.

- **Volume**—10mL or more.

Table 16.3 Antibiotic usage—good practice

- **Timing**—soon (within 1h of identifying severe sepsis).

- **Type**—start empirical antibiotics that have known broad enough activity against most likely pathogen/s (and against MRSA where this is prevalent) [B].[1] Avoiding antibiotic resistance by reducing the spectrum is not recommended initially. Combination therapy should be considered in individual cases. Narrow the antibiotic spectrum once specific pathogen is identified.

- **Review**—daily (more safe and cost-effective) [C].[1]

- **Duration**—7 to 10d, then stop (unless immunosuppressed or slow clinical response) [D].[1]

- *Vasopressors*—should be considered to maintain the mean arterial pressure (MAP) at 65mmHg or above when fluid therapy fails to achieve this goal [C].[1] MAP of ≥65mmHg is associated with adequate blood flow and acceptable tissue perfusion (Table 16.4).[6]
- *Inotropes*—dobutamine should be considered for patients with myocardial dysfunction [C].[1] Increasing oxygen delivery to supranormal levels has no beneficial effect and is not recommended [B].[1]
- *Blood products*—indicated when Hb drops below 7g/dL [B].[1] The target Hb should be 7–9g/dL [B] (see 📖 Chapter 13, pp.91–96).[1]
- **Respiratory support.**
  - Mechanical ventilation, when indicated, should aim at achieving adequate tidal volume of 6mL/kg [B] and plateau pressure of ≤30cmH$_2$O [C].[1]
- **Renal support.**
  - Renal replacement, when indicated, can be applied intermittently or continuously (no significant difference) for acute renal failure [B].[1] Continuous dialysis is recommended for accurate fluid management in unstable patients [D].[1]
- **Other interventions in septic patients.**
  - *Steroid therapy*—indicated only in cases of refractory hypotension to fluid and vasopressor management [C].[1] (Table 16.5)
  - *Recombinant human activated protein C (rhAPC)*—recommended for patients with severe sepsis and high risk of death (e.g. APACHE II score ≥25 or multi-organ failure) [B], but not for low risk of death (e.g. APACHE II score <20 or one organ failure) [A].[1] The average total mortality reduction is ~6%.[7]
  - *Sedation, analgesia, and neuromuscular blockade*—sedation using agreed protocols (intermittent bolus or continuous with daily interruption) is recommended for ventilated patients (significant decrease of ventilation duration and tracheostomy rates) [B].[1] Neuromuscular blockade causes more harm (prolonged neuromuscular blockade) than benefits and should be avoided if possible [B].[1]
  - *Glucose control*—using agreed protocols (sliding scale) to maintain serum glucose level at <150mg/dL is highly recommended (average mortality reduction of ~45% and absolute mortality reduction of 4–10%) [B].[1,8]
  - *Bicarbonate therapy*—not recommended for the sole purpose of improving the haemodynamic status in acidotic patients [B].[1]
  - *Prophylaxis*—is recommended against DVT [A] and stress ulcers (using H$_2$ blockers [A] or proton pump inhibitors [B]).[1]
- See also 📖 OHCM p778.

Table 16.4 Vasopressors—good practice[1]

- Insertion of arterial catheter is recommended for accurate titration of vasopressors [D].
- Noradrenaline and dopamine are recommended initially [C], with epinephrine used as alternative for refractory cases [C].
- Renal—protection dose of dopamine is not recommended routinely [A].

Table 16.5 Steroids—good practice[1]

- No role for ACTH stimulation test—no clear clinical significance [B].
- No role for dexamethasone if hydrocortisone exists [B].
- No role for steroids once vasopressors have been discontinued [D].
- No role of high doses (comparable to over 300mg hydrocortisone) as a treatment option for septic shock [A].
- No role for treating sepsis without the presence of septic shock [D].

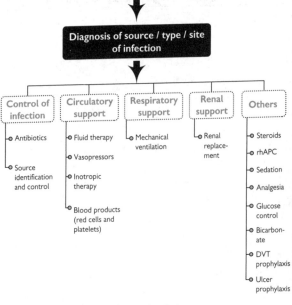

Severe sepsis / Septic shock
(hypotension, unresponsive to fluid, lactate ≥4mmol/L)

Immediate resuscitation (first 6h)

> *Monitor* – BP, P, UO, oxygenation, central venous pressure, and other physiologic parameters as appropriate.
> *Fluid therapy* – use crystalloids or colloids, with challenge boluses (1L crystalloid or 0.3–0.5L colloid over 30min or faster if required) and attention to cardiac filling pressure (reduce rate if no consistent response).[1]
> *Consider also* – oxygen therapy, packed red cell transfusion.
> *Goals* – mean arterial BP >65; urine output >0.5mL/kg/h; CVP 8-12; PvO₂ >70% (central venous).[1]

Diagnosis of source / type / site of infection

Control of infection	Circulatory support	Respiratory support	Renal support	Others
Antibiotics	Fluid therapy	Mechanical ventilation	Renal replacement	Steroids
Source identification and control	Vasopressors			rhAPC
	Inotropic therapy			Sedation
	Blood products (red cells and platelets)			Analgesia
				Glucose control
				Bicarbonate
				DVT prophylaxis
				Ulcer prophylaxis

Fig. 16.1 Recommended approach to septic patients

Further reading

1. Dellinger RP, Levy MM, Carlet JM et al. (2008). Surviving Sepsis Campaign: international guidelines for management of severe sepsis and septic shock. *Crit Care Med* 36, 296–327.
2. Anderson ID, ed. (2003). *Care of the critically ill surgical patient*, 2nd ed, Hodder Arnold, London.
3. Sasse KC, Nauenberg E, Long A, Anton B, Tucker HJ, Hu TW (1995). Long-term survival after intensive care unit admission with sepsis. *Crit Care Med* 23, 1040–7.
4. Rivers E, Nguyen B, Havstad S et al. (2001). Early goal-directed therapy in the treatment of severe sepsis and septic shock. *N Engl J Med* 345, 1368–77.
5. Kumar A, Roberts D, Wood KE et al. (2006). Duration of hypotension prior to initiation of effective antimicrobial therapy is the critical determinant of survival in human septic shock. *Crit Care Med* 34, 1589–96.
6. LeDoux D, Astiz ME, Carpati CM, Rackow EC (2000). Effects of perfusion pressure on tissue perfusion in septic shock. *Crit Care Med* 28, 2729–32.
7. Bernard GR, Vincent JL, Laterre PR et al. (2001). Efficacy and safety of recombinant human activated protein C for severe sepsis. *N Engl J Med* 344, 699–709.
8. van den Berghe G, Wouters P, Weekers F et al. (2001). Intensive insulin therapy in critically ill patients. *N Engl J Med* 345, 1359–67.

Antibiotic prophylaxis in surgery*

* The guidelines on this chapter have been sourced and summarized from different UK, Europe, and international government sources, professional organizations, and medical specialty societies. Leading guidelines have been listed in the Key guidelines box.

Antibiotic prophylaxis in surgery

Key guidelines

- Scottish Intercollegiate Guidelines Network (2008). Antibiotic prophylaxis in surgery.
- National Institute for Health and Clinical Excellence (2008). Surgical site infection: prevention and treatment of surgical site infection.
- British National Formulary 57 (2009). Summary of antibacterial prophylaxis.
- The National Surgical Infection Prevention Project (2005).

Background

- **Main objectives**—to reduce the incidence of surgical site infection (SSI), a common and potentially avoidable problem in surgical practice.[1] Emergency procedures with contaminated fields should be treated as established infection.[1]
- **Definitions**—SSIs refer to infections affecting surgical wounds, body cavities, bones, joints, and other tissues within the surgical field, including infection of prosthetic implants.[1,5] Prevalence of SSIs ranges from 2 to 20% depending on different factors (see below).
- **Impact of SSIs**—increased length of hospital stay (by ~7–10d), increased rate of admission to intensive care (by ~60%), increased hospital readmission rate (×5), and increased mortality rate (×2).[1,4] The costs of treating SSIs are substantial.
- **Efficiency**—properly used, prophylactic antibiotics can reduce the risk of SSIs by up to 6 times compared to controls.[6]

Risk factors for developing SSIs[1,4,7]

- **Operative field contamination**—operative procedures can be classified into four groups (Table 17.1) with incremental risk of SSI.
- **Comorbidities, patient's health, and ASA Grade**—ASA grade ≥2 has significant effect on SSI risk.
- **Surgical skills and technique**—e.g. operations taking longer than the 75th percentile for similar type of procedure have significantly higher SSI rate.
- **Risk index**—more reliable in estimating SSI risk than each factor alone (Table 17.2).[1,7]

Risk of prophylactic antibiotics[1]

- **Antibiotic resistance**—rates increase significantly with increased total antibiotic exposure.
- **Antibiotic-associated colitis** (C. difficile infection)—risk increases with even a single dose of prophylactic antibiotics (especially third generation cephalosporins), and becomes significantly more common when antibiotics are given for >24h (see 📖 Chapter 18, pp.123–132).
- **Increased cost of treatment.**
- **Adverse drug reactions**—e.g. allergy, toxicity.

Table 17.1 Types of surgical wounds

Type	Description
Clean	No breach to a potentially contaminated organ (respiratory, alimentary, or genitourinary tracts). No inflammatory process or sepsis are found or entered, and no break to aseptic techniques.
Clean contaminated	Entering the respiratory, alimentary, or genitourinary tracts without significant spillage.
Contaminated	Operating on acute inflammatory process but no pus, or the presence of gross contamination of the wound (e.g. gross spillage from a hollow viscus).
Dirty	Operative field has gross pus, or operating on old (>4h) compound/open injuries.

Table 17.2 Risk index for developing SSIs*

Type of surgery	No extra factors**	One extra factor**	Two extra factors**
Clean	1%	2.5%	5.5%
Clean contaminated	2%	4%	10%
Contaminated	3.5%	7%	14%

* Numbers represent probability of wound infection rounded to the nearest 0.5. ** Extra factors include: 1. ASA grade ≥2, 2. duration of operation more than the 75th percentile

Current antibiotic prophylaxis recommendations

- *Which procedure*—any clean operation involving the use of prosthesis or implant, clean contaminated, and contaminated operations.[2]
- *Antibiotics choice* (Table 17.3).
  - Consider using for prophylaxis the same antibiotics used for active treatment of infections in this site.
  - The choice must reflect the local information on common pathogens and their antimicrobial sensitivity.
  - Infections occurring post-operatively usually are caused by the same bacteria that prophylactic antibiotics were given to protect against. Consider using different type of antibiotics if first prophylaxis did not achieve its targets.[1]
- *Dose*—single dose should be the same as usual therapeutic dose [G].
- *Timing*—IV prophylactic antibiotics should be given <30min before the incision is made or on starting the anaesthesia [B].[1,2]
- *Duration of effect*—the half-life of selected antibiotic should be sufficient to cover the operating time. Prolonged surgery or when significant blood loss has occurred would indicate a second dose.[1,2,3]
- *Stopping the antibiotics*—post-operative doses of prophylaxis antibiotics (>24h) should not be given for any operation [A].[1,3,4] All doses should be administered immediately before or during the operation. Continuing antibiotics for prophylaxis reasons should be clearly justified (blood loss >1,500mL, haemodilution [B], or treatment of established infection).
- *Penicillin allergy history*—any anaphylactic reaction, urticaria, or rash occurring immediately after previous penicillin administration increases the likelihood that immediate hypersensitivity to penicillins exists. Beta-lactam antibiotic should be avoided in such cases [B].[1]
- *MRSA*—a glycopeptide (e.g. vancomycin or teicoplanin) should be considered for prophylaxis in the carriers of MRSA undergoing high-risk surgery. Intranasal mupirocin may be used in MRSA carriers pre- and/or post-operatively to minimize carriage and the risk of subsequent infection (see 📖 Chapter 18, pp.123–132).

See also 📖 OHCM p556.

Table 17.3 Types of surgical wounds

Operation	Common pathogens	R*	Type and dose[3]	Grade
Gastric/oesophageal surgery	Enteric gram −ve bacilli, gram +ve cocci	b	Single dose ** of: gentamicin (IV) or cefuroxime (IV)	A, D
Colorectal surgery	Enteric gram −ve bacilli, enterococci, anaerobes	a	Single dose of: gentamicin (IV) + metronidazole (IV or PR) or cefuroxime (IV) + metronidazole (IV) or co-amoxiclav (IV) alone	A
Appendicectomy	Enteric gram −ve bacilli, enterococci, anaerobes	b	Single dose of: gentamicin (IV) + metronidazole (IV or PR) or cefuroxime (IV) + metronidazole (IV or PR) or co-amoxiclav (IV) alone	A
Biliary surgery (open)	Enteric gram −ve bacilli, enterococci, *clostridia*	b	Single dose of: cefuroxime (IV) + metronidazole (IV or PR) or gentamicin (IV) + metronidazole (IV or PR)	A
Laparoscopic cholecystectomy		N***		A
ERCP	[Enteric gram −ve bacilli, enterococci, *clostridia*]	?	Single dose of: gentamicin (IV) or ciprofloxacin (IV or PO)	D
Vascular surgery	S. aureus, S. epidermidis, anaerobes in diabetes, gangrene, or undergoing amputation	b	Single dose of: Cefuroxime (IV) or ciprofloxacin (IV) Add metronidazole (IV) for suspected anaerobic infection	A

Table 17.3 Contd.

Operation	Common pathogens	R*	Type and dose[3]	Grade
Lower limb amputation/ major trauma		b	Benzylpenicillin 300–600mg qds for 5d or (for penicillin-allergic) metronidazole 400–500mg tds	A
Breast surgery		b	–	C
Inguinal/femoral hernia repair (open)		N	–	A
Inguinal/femoral hernia repair (laparoscopic)		N	–	B
Surgery using mesh (e.g. gastric band)		N***	–	B
Clean contaminated procedures		b	–	D

* R = level of recommendation: a = highly recommended (unequivocal benefits), b = recommended (highly likely to be beneficial), c = usually recommended but may be withdrawn as per local policy, N = not recommended (likely to cause harm more than benefit).
** Add extra dose for prolonged operations (>2–4h).[1,3] *** Consider for high-risk patients.

Beyond the guidelines and the future

Although some examples of appropriate agents have been shown in Table 17.3, many centres have extensively revised their antibiotic regimens in an attempt to reduce the incidence of *C. difficile*. In particular, the use of cephalosporins and quinolones for both treatment and prophylaxis has been markedly reduced.

Although some vascular and orthopaedic surgeons favour multiple dose/24h regimens, the trend is towards single dose prophylaxis for all surgical procedures. *Dr. Andrew Swann, Consultant Microbiologist*

Know your results

Antibiotic prophylaxis in surgery—audit areas
Compliance of antibiotic prophylaxis with current published guidelines (2008)
• *Standards*—type, timing, dose, frequency, and duration of antibiotic usage.
• *Data collection*—see SIGN 104.[1]
• *Indicators*—% of patients receiving prophylactic antibiotics who **should** receive antibiotics, % of patients receiving prophylactic antibiotics who should **not** receive antibiotics, % of patients **not** receiving prophylactic antibiotics who should receive antibiotics, % of patients **not** receiving prophylactic antibiotics who should **not** receive antibiotics.

Further reading

1. Scottish Intercollegiate Guidelines Network (2008). Antibiotic prophylaxis in surgery. A national clinical guideline. Available from: http://www.sign.ac.uk/pdf/sign104.pdf.
2. National Institute for Health and Clinical Excellence (2008). Surgical site infection: prevention and treatment of surgical site infection. Available from: http://guidance.nice.org.uk/CG74.
3. British National Formulary 57 (2009). Summary of antibacterial prophylaxis. Available from: http://www.bnf.org/bnf/bnf/current/104928.htm.
4. Bratzler DW, Houck PM; Surgical Infection Prevention Guideline Writers Workgroup (2005). Antimicrobial prophylaxis for surgery: an advisory statement from the National Surgical Infection Prevention Project. *Am J Surg* 189, 395–404.
5. The Society for Hospital Epidemiology of America; the Association for Practitioners in Infection Control; the Centres for Disease Control; the Surgical Infection Society (1992). Consensus paper on the surveillance of surgical wound infections. *Infect Control Hosp Epidemiol* 13, 599–605.
6. Classen DC, Evans RS, Pestotnik SL, Horn SD, Menlove RL, Burke JP (1992). The timing of prophylactic administration of antibiotics and the risk of surgical wound infection. *N Engl J Med* 326, 281–6.
7. Culver DH, Horan TC, Gaynes RP *et al.* (1991). Surgical wound infection rates by wound class, operative procedure, and patient risk index. National Nosocomial Infections Surveillance System. *Am J Med* 91(3B), 152S–157S.

Principles of infection control*

* The guidelines on this chapter have been sourced and summarized from different UK, Europe, and international government sources, professional organizations, and medical specialty societies. Leading guidelines have been listed in the Key guidelines box.

Principles of infection control

Principles of infection control

Key guidelines

- Department of Health (2008). The Health Act 2006: code of practice for the prevention and control of health care associated infections.
- Department of Health (2008). Clean, safe care: reducing infections and saving lives.
- epic2: national evidence-based guidelines for preventing health care-associated infections in NHS hospitals in England (2007).
- National Institute for Health and Clinical Excellence (2003). Infection control: prevention of health care-associated infection in primary and community care.
- World Health Organization (2004). Practical guidelines for infection control in health care facilities.
- Centres for Disease Control and Prevention (2007). Infection control guidelines.
- MRSA guidelines (Europe, UK)
- Department of Health/Public Health Laboratory Service Joint Working Group (1994). *Clostridium difficile* infection: prevention and management.
- Department of Health (2007). A simple guide to *Clostridium difficile*.
- Healthcare Commission (2005). Management, prevention and surveillance of *Clostridium difficile*.

Background

- *Definitions*—health care-associated infections (HCAIs—also known as nosocomial infections) are infections acquired in hospitals or as a result of health care interventions.[2] Infection control is a strategy that applies epidemiologic and scientific principles to achieve effective prevention or reduction in HCAIs.
- *Prevalence*—the overall prevalence of HCAIs in England has remained relatively constant at about 8% over the last 25y.[2] The particular challenge in management and cost from MRSA and *Clostridium (C.) difficile* infections has recently taken the infection control strategies to the top of the agenda.[2] Infection with, e.g. *C. difficile*, can cost the hospital an extra £4,000–10,000 per patient,[2] and cost the patients their lives!
- *Medico-legal issues*—prevention and control of infection is a legal obligation for the Department of Health, NHS Trusts, and their staff.[1] Under the Health Act of October 2006, if a patient, visitor, or health care worker can prove that they acquired an infection in hospital that resulted in harm, they may be able to claim damages (e.g. for loss of earnings).[1]
- *Common types of HCAIs*—include urinary tract infection (~40% of cases), surgical site infection (~10%), chest infection (~10%), and skin and mucous membrane infection (~10%).[3–6]
- *The five main routes of transmission*—include direct and indirect contact (dressing, contaminated gloves), droplets (coughing, sneezing), airborne (air conditioner, dust), common vehicle (food, water), and vector-borne (mosquitoes, flies).[3–6]

- *Transmission*—occurs via transiently contaminated hands of hospital staff, contaminated environmental surfaces, and the direct contact with colonized or infected individuals.[7]

Table 18.1 MRSA management

- *Decolonization.*
  - *Indications*—recommended for certain patient groups under the advice of infection control team. This may include patients with documented recurrent MRSA infections, patients undergoing operative procedure, and carrier staff during outbreak time.
  - *Techniques*—nasal (mupirocin 2% in a paraffin base to the inner surface of each anterior nares three times a day for 5d), throat (systemic antibiotics), skin (4% chlorhexidine body wash/shampoo, 7.5% povidone iodine or 2% triclosan), and clean clothing, bedding, and towels after completion.[7]

- *Strict infection control measures.*

- *Physical setting*—patient isolation is recommended depending on available facilities. Patient movement should be kept to the minimum. Patient equipment (stethoscopes, sphygmomanometers) should be single use or decontaminated before used for other patients. Topical and systemic prophylaxis (+/– prophylactic antibiotics) should be considered prior to performing any procedure (including placing patients at the end of theatre list). No special arrangements for prolonged eradication protocol on discharge from the unit are usually required.[7]

Table 18.2 C. difficile risk factors[9,21]

- *Antibiotics*—main risk factor.
  - *Most frequent*—broad-spectrum penicillins and cephalosporins, clindamycin, and fluoroquinolones. Receiving multiple antibiotics and long duration treatment increases the risk significantly.
  - *Occasional*—trimethoprim and sulphonamides.
  - *Rare*—metronidazole and vancomycin (usual treatment for C. difficile), aminoglycosides, and chloramphenicol.

- *Hospital admission factors*—hospitalization of elderly, ICU stay, long hospital stay.

- *Disease- and procedure-related factors*—severe underlying disease, gastrointestinal procedures, use of NGT, and receiving anti-ulcer drugs.

- *Development of outbreak*—depends on the ability of a high infectivity C. difficile strain to cause more than one new case in patients surrounded by individuals with high risk factors (hospitalized elderly treated with antibiotics in the same ward) where standards of infection control are low (high cross-contamination).

- *Screening*—should be performed on all high-risk patients admitted to general units and on all general patients admitted to high-risk units.[7] Regular screening (weekly or monthly) should be performed on all patients in high-risk units.[7]
  - *Screening sites*—anterior nares, groin and perineum, skin lesions and wounds, IV catheters sites, urine catheters, tracheostomy, and sputum from productive cough.[7]
  - *Staff screening*—not recommended routinely. Screening is indicated if new MRSA carriers are found in the unit, and if transmission in the unit continued despite active control measures.[7]
- *Management* (Table 18.1).
- *Prevention.*
  - *Strict infection control measures*—are essential.
  - *Surveillance*—must be performed regularly by infection control team.
  - *Strict antibiotic policy.*

Clostridium difficile-associated diarrhoea

- *Definition*—C. difficile is an anaerobic, Gram positive, spore-forming bacterium, capable of producing enterotoxins, and resulting in occasionally life-threatening antibiotic-associated colitis.[8–10,21]
- *Prevalence*—C. difficile colonizes <5% of normal population (up to 20–50% of hospitalized elderly patients), and is usually kept under control by normal bacterial flora.[21,22] About 20% of hospitalized patients become infected during their stay (cross infection)[9], up to a third of them develop diarrhoea due to C. difficile toxins.[22] Some types of C. difficile strains (type 027) can cause major outbreaks.
- *Risk factors* (Table 18.2).
- *Clinical presentation*—ranges from mild diarrhoea to severe pseudomembranous colitis, severe sepsis, and bowel perforation.
- *Diagnosis and treatment approach*—see Fig. 18.1.
- *Prevention*—six key measures can significantly reduce the burden of C. difficile within hospital setting: judicious antibiotic prescribing policy, early isolation of infected (or suspected) cases, enhanced environmental cleaning, strict hand hygiene, appropriate use of personal protective equipment, and staff education and training.[23]

Management of short-term urinary catheters[3]

- Only to be used if absolutely necessary, always with full asepsis, and with the smallest gauge and 10mL balloon. Remove catheter as soon as possible [D].
- A single-use sterile lubricant should be used and a sterile closed drainage system which should be at a lower level than the bladder, but not in contact with the floor [D].
- When possible, self-catheterization should be encouraged. Relatives and carers must be educated on best practice and routine personal hygiene encouraged [D].

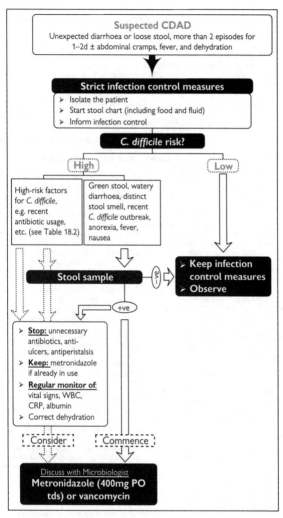

Fig. 18.1 Management algorithm for suspected *C. difficile*-associated diarrhoea (CDAD)

130 CHAPTER 18 **Principles of infection control**

Further reading

1. Department of Health (2008). The Health Act 2006: code of practice for the prevention and control of health care associated infections. Available from: http://www.dh.gov.uk/en/Publicationsandstatistics/Publications/PublicationsPolicyAndGuidance/DH_081927.

2. Department of Health (2008). Clean, safe care: reducing infections and saving lives. Available from: http://www.dh.gov.uk/en/Publicationsandstatistics/Publications/PublicationsPolicyAndGuidance/DH_081650.

3. Pratt RJ, Pellowe CM, Wilson JA *et al.* (2007). epic2: national evidence-based guidelines for preventing health care-associated infections in NHS hospitals in England. *J Hosp Infect* 65 Suppl1, S1–64.

4. National Institute for Health and Clinical Excellence (2003). Infection control: prevention of health care-associated infection in primary and community care. Available from: http://www.nice.org.uk/nicemedia/pdf/CG2fullguidelineinfectioncontrol.pdf.

5. World Health Organization (2004). Practical guidelines for infection control in health care facilities. Available from: http://www.searo.who.int/LinkFiles/Publications_PracticalguidelinSEAROpub-41.pdf.

6. Centres for Disease Control and Prevention (2007). Infection control guidelines. Available from: http://www.cdc.gov/ncidod/dhqp/guidelines.html.

7. The Groupement pour le Depistage, l'Etude et la Prevention des Infections Hospitalieres (1993). Guidelines for control and prevention of methicillin-resistant *Staphylococcus aureus* transmission in Belgian hospitals. Available from: http://www.escmid.org/fileadmin/src/media/PDFs/4ESCMID_Library/2Medical_Guidelines/other_guidelines/Staphylococcus_Aureus.pdf; Coia JE, Duckworth GJ, Edwards DI *et al.* (2006) Guidelines for the control and prevention of meticillin-resistance Staphylococcus aureus (MRSA) in health care facilities. *J Hosp Infect* 63 Suppl1, S1–44. Gemmell CG, Edwards DI, Fraise AP (2006) Guidelines for the prophylaxis and treatment of methicillin-resistant Staphylococcus aureus (MRSA) infection in the UK. *J Antimicrob Chemither* 57, 589–608. European: Link: http://www.escmid.org/fileadmin/src/media/PDFs/4ESCMID_Library/2Medical_Guidelines/other_guidelines/Staphylococcus_Aureus.pdf. Accessed May 2009.

8. Department of Health/Public Health Laboratory Service Joint Working Group. Clostridium Difficile Infection – Prevention and Management. 1994 (UK). Available from: http://www.hpa.org.uk/web/HPAwebFile/HPAweb_C/1194947325732 Accessed May 2009.

9. Department of Health (2007). A simple guide to *Clostridium difficile*. Available from: http://www.dh.gov.uk/en/Publicationsandstatistics/Publications/PublicationsPolicyAndGuidance/DH_4115883.

10. Healthcare Commission (2005). Management, prevention and surveillance of C. Difficile. (UK). Available from: http://www.hpa.org.uk/web/HPAwebFile/HPAweb_C/1194947368363. Accessed May 2009.

11. Haley RW, Culver DH, White JW *et al.* (1985). The efficacy of infection surveillance and control programs in preventing nosocomial infections in the US hospitals. *Am J Epidemiol* 121, 182–205.

12. Pittet D, Mourouga P, Perneger TV (1999). Compliance with handwashing in a teaching hospital. Infection Control Program. *Ann Intern Med* 130, 126–30.

13. Voss A, Widmer AF (1997). No time for handwashing!? Handwashing versus alcoholic rub: can we afford 100% compliance? *Infect Control Hosp Epidemiol* 18, 205–8.

14. Quraishi ZA, McGuckin M, Blais FX (1984). Duration of handwashing in intensive care units: a descriptive study. *Am J Infect Control* 12, 83–7.

15. Pittet D, Hugonnet S, Harbarth S *et al.* (2000). Effectiveness of a hospital-wide programme to improve compliance with hand hygiene. Infection Control Programme. *Lancet* 356, 1307–12.

16. Alrawi S, Houshan L, Satheesan R, Raju R, Cunningham J, Acinapura A (2001). Glove reinforcement: an alternative to double gloving. *Infect Control Hosp Epidemiol* 22, 526–7.

17. Voss A, Milatovic D, Wallrauch-Schwarz C, Rosdahl VT, Braveny I (1994). Methicillin-resistant *Staphylococcus aureus* in Europe. *Eur J Clin Microbiol Infect Dis* 13, 50–5.

18. Cosgrove SE, Sakoulas G, Perencevich EN, Schwaber MJ, Karchmer AW, Carmeli Y (2003). Comparison of mortality associated with methicillin-resistant and methicillin-susceptible *Staphylococcus aureus* bacteraemia: a meta-analysis. *Clin Infect Dis* 36, 53–9.

19. Cosgrove SE, Qi Y, Kaye KS, Harbarth S, Karchmer AW, Carmeli Y (2005). The impact of methicillin resistance in *Staphylococcus aureus* bacteraemia on patient outcomes: mortality, length of stay, and hospital charges. *Infect Control Hosp Epidemiol* 26, 166–74.

20. Schneider–Lindner V, Delaney JA, Dial S, Dascal A, Suissa S (2007). Antimicrobial drugs and community-acquired methicillin-resistant *Staphylococcus aureus*, United Kingdom. *Emerg Infect Dis* 13, 994–1000.

21. Starr J (2005). *Clostridium difficile* associated diarrhoea: diagnosis and treatment. *BMJ* 331, 498–501.

22. Riggs MM, Sethi AK, Zabarsky TF, Eckstein EC, Jump RL, Donskey CJ (2007). Asymptomatic carriers are a potential source for transmission of epidemic and non-epidemic *Clostridium difficile* strains among long-term care facility residents. *Clin Infect Dis* 45, 992–8.

23. Health Protection Agency. *Clostridium difficile* guidelines. Available from: http://www.hpa.org.uk/webw/HPAweb&Page&HPAwebAutoListName/Page/1179745281238?p=1179745281238.

24. Surrey Primary Care Trust (2008). Guidance for the management of *Clostridium difficile*. Available from: http://www.transition.surreypct.nhs.uk/policies-and-procedures/clinical-policies/infection-control-guidelines/Management_of_Clostridium_Difficile._August_08.pdf.

Principles of pain management*

* The guidelines on this chapter have been sourced and summarized from different UK, Europe, and international government sources, professional organizations, and medical specialty societies. Leading guidelines have been listed in the Key guidelines box.

Principles of pain management

Key guidelines

- European Society of Regional Anaesthesia and Pain Therapy. Post-operative pain management—good clinical practice
- Clinical Knowledge Summaries. Palliative cancer care—pain management.
- NHS Quality Improvement Scotland (2004). Best practice statement: post-operative pain management.
- American Society of Anaesthesiologists Task Force on Acute Pain Management (2004). Practice guidelines for acute pain management in the perioperative setting.
- European Federation of Neurological Societies (2006). Guidelines on pharmacological treatment of neuropathic pain.
- The Pain Society (2004). Recommendations for the appropriate use of opioids for persistent non-cancer pain.

Basic facts

- **Definition of pain**—unpleasant sensory and emotional experience associated with potential or actual tissue damage.[14] Pain is a subjective conscious experience; 'Pain is whatever the experiencing person says it is, and exists whenever he says it does.'[15]
- **Pain types and transmission**—see Tables 19.1 and 19.2.

RECOMMENDED APPROACH

Post-operative pain

- **General approach**—should be multimodal. Management of post-operative pain requires a thorough preoperative assessment (with pre-emptive measures), post-operative assessment of vital organs and pain pattern, appropriate use (and adjustment) of analgesia, management of side effects, and proper discharge plan.
- **Preoperatively.**
  - *Directed pain history*—is essential (Tables 19.3 and 19.4).[1,4,16]
  - *Pre-emptive measures*—should be instituted appropriately to achieve effective post-operative pain control.
    - *Options*—include written and verbal information regarding the post-operative pain management procedures and routes (e.g. IV, PO, PCA), methods of non-pharmacologic interventions available (*distraction* including music and videos, *relaxation* including abdominal breathing and jaw relaxation, *physical agents* including cold and heat massage, and *hypnosis* including focused attention states), and full explanation of patient concerns with appropriate patient education [B].[1,4,16]
    - *Efficiency*—although literature is insufficient to evaluate the exact impact of such measures,[4] individualized preoperative education can favourably alter the pain experience and is a recommended practice.[1,4,16]

Table 19.1 Types and transmission of pain

- *Nociceptive pain*—any pain associated with tissue damage. Pain correlates well with the extent and location of damage.
    - *Nociceptive somatic*—stimulus is transmitted by somatic nerves. Pain is often described as well-localized, sharp, aching, throbbing, and/or pressure-like.
    - *Nociceptive visceral*—stimulus is transmitted by visceral nerves. Pain is usually poorly localized, cramping, or gnawing if tissue damage was in a hollow viscus, and aching or sharp if the damage was in a capsule or mesentery tissue.

- *Non-nociceptive pain*—(also known as neuropathic pain) results from direct effect of a lesion on the somatosensory system, causing abnormal function (without tissue damage) in the central or peripheral nerves. Usually presents with burning, stabbing, or lancinating pain; initiated spontaneously or by thermal, chemical, or mechanical stimulants. Common conditions causing this pain include diabetes, stroke, post-incision chronic pain, vascular diseases, and amputation.[7]

- *Idiopathic pain*—this pain cannot usually be explained by any obvious organic abnormality.

Table 19.2 Pain transmission—therapeutic implications

- *Steps of pain perception.*
    - *Transduction*—of signals from damaged tissue.
    - *Transmission*—of electrical impulses through spinal cord, to brain stem and thalamocortical regions.
    - *Modulation*—of initial nociceptive stimulus (amplification).
    - *Perception*—of nociceptive impulse stimulus (emotional and physical experience).

- *Management therapy*— should aim at attacking all four stages of nociception: NSAIDs for reducing inflammatory process at the damaged tissue, local anaesthesia and neural blockage for blocking transmission of stimulus, opiates to activate the inhibition process at the modulation level, and proper education to reduce anxiety at the perception level.

Table 19.3 Preoperative pain assessment

- *Pain history*—history of chronic pain, successful or unsuccessful pain control methods in the past, and previous side effects of pain management.

- *PC*—expected post-operative pain in the planned procedure, type of procedure (e.g. elective or emergency, minor or major), current preoperative severity of pain (if any).

- *PMH*—associated significant medical problems (e.g arthritis), history of neurologic disorders, prior trauma, infection or respiratory difficulties, history of spinal surgery, history of alcohol abuse or addiction.

- *DH*—anticoagulants, use of opiates for chronic pain, monoamine oxidase inhibitors (MAOIs), allergies to opiates, local anaesthetics or NSAIDs.

- *Others*—infection on site of needle insertion, anatomical abnormalities.

- *Post-operatively.*
  - *Immediate action*—should follow the ABCDE approach (see 📖 Chapter 15, pp.101–106).[1,2,3,4,16]
  - *Assess the pain and recognize its pattern.*
    - *In general*—the sudden increase in pain intensity or unexpected high degree of pain may indicate that a new condition or complication has developed which may require further investigation.[2,3]
    - *Pain assessment*—should be thorough and holistic (Table 19.4). Charting pain pattern should be undertaken with the same regularity as charting observations of other vital signs (the fifth vital sign) [B].[16,17]
  - *Review, initiate, and modify the pain management plan.*
    - *Educate the patient/carers*—on the importance of pain as a signal, the effectiveness of management options, and reinforce the basic pain management principles [B].[1,4,16]
    - *Effective non-pharmacologic procedures*—should be rechecked and applied as appropriate (e.g. distraction with films, raising a cellulitic limb, physiotherapy).[16]
    - *Pharmaceutical interventions (painkillers)*—checked for type, dose, route, frequency, interval, combination, and side effects. ▶ALWAYS GO MULTIMODAL AND STEPWISE (Table 19.5).
  - *Treat side effects.*[3,16]
    - *Nausea and vomiting*—can be effectively treated (following exclusion of serious underlying abnormality) by changing the dose, route or type of analgesia, and adding appropriate antiemetics.
    - *Sedation and lethargy*—can be effectively treated (following exclusion of serious underlying abnormality) by reducing the dose of analgesic agent and using reversal agent if necessary.
    - *Other side effects*—include itching, numbness, hallucinations, dysphoria, and urinary retention.
  - *Re-evaluate management plan*—at regular intervals.

Cancer pain

- *General approach*—should be based on a risk/benefit balance and tailored to each individual case.[8] A multimodal and stepwise (WHO analgesic ladder)[20] approach is recommended [B].[8] The same principles of approaching pain should be followed, i.e. ABCDE approach, proper pain assessment, appropriate use (and adjustment) of analgesia, management of side effects, and proper long-term plan.[8,10]
- *Origin of cancer pain*—may be directly related to cancer (most common), cancer complications (bedsore, muscles spasms), therapeutic modalities (radiotherapy, surgical scar), or resulting from associated disorders (arthritis).[21]

Table 19.4 Pain assessment[2,3,16]

- **Location**—e.g. operative site, deep, chest, joints, calf, forefoot.
- **Intensity**—mild, moderate, severe (or by using visual scale).
- **Frequency**—e.g. persistent, an hour or so before having the next analgesic injection, during the night.
- **Nature**—e.g. sharp, cramps, dull.
- **Associated symptoms**—e.g. nausea and vomiting.
- **Impact of pain**—depression, suicide thoughts.
- **Aggravating and alleviating factors**—e.g. certain positions, physio, distraction.
- **Presence of support**—for daily activities.

Table 19.5 Perioperative pain control options[16,18,19]

	Mild*	Moderate**	Severe***
Non-opioids†	P + local infiltration + NSAIDs (if not CI)	+	+
Weak opioids††	±	+ Regional block ± PRN weak opioids	+
Strong opioids†††	±	±	+ Major peripheral nerve block/plexus block/epidural local anaesthesia ± IV PCA

P = paracetamol; CI = contraindicated; PRN = when necessary; PCA = patient-controlled analgesia; * = mild pain (inguinal hernia repair, varicose vein operations); ** = moderate pain (hysterectomy, hip replacement); *** = severe pain (aortic surgery, thoracotomy); † = paracetamol, NSAIDs, gabapentin; †† = codeine, tramadol; ††† = morphine, pethidine, oxycodone

Table 19.6 Other therapeutic modalities for cancer pain

- **Neuropathic pain**—see below.
- **High-dose dexamethasone**—consider for severe bone pain, spinal cord compression, soft tissue swelling, etc. [C].
- **Anticancer systemic therapy**—consider aromatase inhibitors for metastatic breast cancer [A] and androgen blockade for prostate cancer [C].
- **Radiotherapy**—for painful bone metastasis [C].
- **Bisphosphate**—for multiple myeloma patients [A].
- **Coeliac plexus block**—for upper GI infiltrating cancer [A].

- *Patient education*—essential step to ensure appropriate compliance [A].[8,10]
- *Pain assessment*—should be holistic (e.g. physical, functional, psychosocial) and performed by the patient him/herself [B].[8,21,22]
- *Pain management plan*—should start at a level appropriate to the severity (and type) of pain (see also Table 19.5).[8,21]
  - *Mild pain*—non-opioids ± adjuvants [A].
  - *Mild to moderate pain*—non-opioids + weak opioid ± adjuvants [B].
  - *Moderate to severe pain*—opioids as a first-line [B]. Oral route is always recommended if possible.
- *Appropriate use of morphine*—should ensure effective initiation and titration (5–10mg of morphine, 4-hourly, titrated to control the pain with minimum side effects), effective management of breakthrough pain (one sixth of normal regular dose of oral morphine), active management of side effects (constipation, nausea and vomiting, oversedation), proper management of toxicity effects, and switching to parenteral administration (subcutaneous diamorphine) when necessary.[8,21]
- *Other types of treatment*—should also be considered (Table 19.6).

Neuropathic pain
- *Definition and aetiology*—see Table 19.1. Accurate diagnosis relies on a proper history and physical examination, supported by the use of validated assessment tools.[7]
- *General approach*—should be multimodal using proper patient education, pharmacological, and non-pharmacological therapies.[5,7]
- *Non-pharmacological therapies*—include avoiding bed rest if at all possible. Maintaining functional and active life is important.[7]
- *Pharmacologic therapy*—options include:[5,7]
  - Tricyclic antidepressants, gabapentin, or pregabalin—recommended first-line treatment [A].
  - Duloxetine and venlafaxine—second choice (but preferable to tricyclic antidepressants for patients with cardiovascular risk factors).
  - Opioids and tramadol—are the second/third-line options [A].
  - Capsaicin, mexiletine, topiramate, memantine, mianserin, and topical clonidine are of weak or no evidence of effectiveness [A, B]. Valproate has mixed evidence.[5,7]
- *Spinal cord stimulation (SCS)*—14 SCS devices manufactured by three companies have received European approval to market.[23] Patient selection should involve a multidisciplinary team, expert in managing chronic pain.
  - *Indications*—severe chronic pain (measuring at least 50 on visual analogue scale of 0–100) for over 6mo, which remains resistant to conventional medical management (CMM). SCS is not indicated for ischaemic pain unless within a robust clinical trial.
  - *Efficacy*—trials have shown ~50% reduction in pain (in over 50% of people in 6mo time) compared to ~10% in CMM patients, and ~35% in SCS vs 7% in CMM group at 12mo.[23]
  - *Safety*—serious complications are rare.[23]

Further reading

1. European Society of Regional Anaesthesia and Pain Therapy. Post-operative pain management—good clinical practice. Available from: http://www.esraeurope.org/PostoperativePainManagement.pdf.

2. Clinical Knowledge Summaries. Palliative cancer care—pain management. Available from: http://www.cks.library.nhs.uk/palliative_cancer_care_pain.

3. NHS Quality Improvement Scotland (2004). Best practice statement: post-operative pain management. Available from: http://www.nhshealthquality.org/nhsqis/files/Post_Pain_COMPLETE.pdf.

4. American Society of Anaesthesiologists Task Force on Acute Pain Management (2004). Practice guidelines for acute pain management in the perioperative setting: an updated report by the American Society of Anaesthesiologists Task Force on Acute Pain Management. Anaesthesiology 100, 1573–81.

5. Attal N, Cruccu G, Haanpää M et al. (2006). EFNS guidelines on pharmacological treatment of neuropathic pain. Eur J Neurol 13, 1153–69.

6. The Pain Society (2004). Recommendations for the appropriate use of opioids for persistent non-cancer pain. Available from: http://www.britishpainsociety.org/opioids_doc_2004.pdf.

7. CREST (2008). Guidelines on the management of neuropathic pain. Available from: http://www.crestni.org.uk/crest_-management_of_neuropathic_pain_guidelines-2.pdf.

8. Scottish Intercollegiate Guidelines Network (2008). Control of pain in adults with cancer. Available from: http://www.sign.ac.uk/guidelines/fulltext/106/index.html.

9. NHS Quality Improvement Scotland (2006). Best practice statement—management of chronic pain in adults. Available from: http://www.nhshealthquality.org/nhsqis/files/BPSManage_chronic_pain%20_adults%20(Feb06).pdf.

10. NHS Quality Improvement Scotland (2004). Best practice statement—the management of pain in patients with cancer. Available from: http://www.nhshealthquality.org/nhsqis/files/20372%20NHSQIS%20Best%20Practice.pdf.

11. NHS Quality Improvement Scotland (2003). Clinical standards—anaesthesia: care before, during and after anaesthesia. Available from: http://www.nhshealthquality.org/nhsqis/files/20372%20NHSQIS%20Best%20Practice.pdf.

12. European Association of Urology (2007). Guidelines on pain management. Available from: http://www.uroweb.org/fileadmin/user_upload/Guidelines/21_Pain_Management_2007.pdf.

13. Wounds UK (2004). Best practice statement—minimizing trauma and pain in wound management. Available from: http://www.wounds-uk.com/downloads/trauma_pain_statement.pdf.

14. Serpell M (2005). Anatomy, physiology and pharmacology of pain. Anaesth Intensive Care Med 6, 7–10.

15. McCaffery M (1972). Nursing management of the patient with pain, Lippincott, Philadelphia.

16. VHA/DoD Clinical Practice Guidelines for the management of postoperative pain (2006). Available from: http://www.guideline.gov/summary/Summary.aspx?ss=15&doc.id=10198&nbr=5382.

17. McCaffery M, Pasero C (1992). Assessment: underlying complexities, misconceptions, and practical tools. In: Pain: clinical manual, 2nd ed, Mosby.

18. British National Formulary 57. Available at: http://www.bnf.org/bnf/.

19. Hyllested M, Jones S, Pedersen JL, Kehlet H (2002). Comparative effect of paracetamol, NSAIDs or their combination in post-operative pain management: a qualitative review. Br J Anaesth 88, 199–214.

20. World Health Organization. WHO's pain ladder. Available from: http://www.who.int/cancer/palliative/painladder/en/.

21. World Health Organization (1990). Cancer pain relief and palliative care. Available from: http://www.who.int/bookorders/anglais/detart1.jsp?sesslan=1&codlan=1&codcol=10&codcch=804; WHO (1996). Cancer pain relief, 2nd ed, WHO Geneva. Available from: http://books.google.co.uk/books?id=Fhall7PMHZcC&dq=WHO+Cancer+Pain+Relief&pg=PP1&ots=te8gl4CW6d&sig=MMdO9v5E106l955jeJS1UWE0e8k&hl=en&sa=X&oi=book_result&resnum=4&ct=result#PPR1,M1.

22. Cancer Research UK (2008). Treating cancer pain. Available from: http://www.cancerhelp.org.uk/help/default.asp?page=5884.

23. National Institute for Health and Clinical Excellence (2008). Spinal cord stimulation for chronic pain of neuropathic or ischaemic origin. Available from: http://www.nice.org.uk/nicemedia/pdf/TA159QuickRefGuide.pdf.

Principles of nutritional support*

* The guidelines on this chapter have been sourced and summarized from different UK, Europe, and international government sources, professional organizations, and medical specialty societies. Leading guidelines have been listed in the Key guidelines box.

Principles of nutritional support

Basic facts
- **Definition**—malnutrition is a state of poor nutrition resulting in measurable adverse effects on body composition, function, or clinical outcome.[1,7,8]
- **Incidence**—some degree of significant malnutrition can be found in ~10–60% of in-hospital patients, compared to ≤5% of the general population at home.[1]
- **Risk factors**—commonly found in hospitalized patients (Table 20.1).
- **Effect of malnutrition**—see Table 20.2.
- **Clinical assessment**—should be thorough and holistic (Table 20.3).
  - *Clinical history*—any existing or potential risk factors for malnutrition (Table 20.1).
  - *Physical examination*—includes clinical appearance, weight and height, and anthropometrics (e.g. mid-arm circumference, triceps skinfold thickness).[1]
  - *Laboratory evaluation*—patients requiring nutritional support should be checked for FBC, urea and creatinine, glucose, LFTs, albumin, prealbumin, and CRP. Trace elements (Mg, PO_4, Ca, zinc, copper, folate, and B12) are required for total parenteral nutrition (TPN) commencement.[1]

Screening for malnutrition
- **Patient selection**—nutritional screening should be offered to all patients upon their hospital admission, first outpatient appointment, and if a clinical concern arises at any time (e.g. unexpected post-operative long-standing ileus) **[C]**.[1,2] Screening should be repeated weekly for inpatients.[1]
- **Method of screening**—includes a proper thorough clinical and laboratory assessment by appropriately trained health care professional (Table 20.3) **[D]**.[1] The Malnutrition Universal Screening Tool (MUST) (BMI + degree of unintentional weight loss + effect of acute disease) has been developed by British Association for Parenteral and Enteral Nutrition (BAPEN) to ensure a reliable, thorough, and reproducible technique for screening.[8]

Table 20.1 Malnutrition—risk factors

- *Original disease*—effect varies depending on the severity and type of disease: elective operations (SF* × 1.1), sepsis (SF × 1.35), pancreatitis (SF × 1.3–1.8), acute renal failure (SF × 1.3), major surgery with compromised cardiopulmonary functions (SF × 1.55).[9]

- *Poor intake*—depression, nausea, weakness, poor quality of food, inadequate food intake (patient unable to eat for >7d or has insufficient food intake (<60% of energy expenditure) for >10d).[3]

- *Poor digestion/absorption*—operations on GI tract.

- *Excess loss*—fistulae, stomas, drains, etc.

*SF = stress factor reflecting the estimated increase in calorie needs[9]

Table 20.2 Effects of malnutrition

- *Impaired immune defence*—e.g. the risk of bloodstream infection in critically ill patients increases (relative hazard × 1.27) when calorie intake is less than 25% of recommended.[10]

- *Poor wound healing*—with decreased rate of fibroblastic proliferation and neovascularization.[11] This leads to slower rates of wound healing,[11] but rarely leads to complete wound disruption.[12]

- *Reduced muscle strength*—skeletal, respiratory, etc.

- *Vitamin*—deficiencies.

- *Fluid and electrolytes*—disturbances.

- *Impaired psychosocial functions.*

Table 20.3 Malnutrition—diagnostic criteria

- *At risk*—poor eating for the last (or coming) 5d or more, existence of one or more risk factors:[1]
  - *Clinical appearance*—bitemporal wasting, thin extremities, low mid-arm circumference, low triceps skinfold thickness, hair loss, xerosis, glossitis, bleeding or sore on the gums and oral mucosa.[9]
  - *Laboratory findings*—low albumin (<33g/L), low prealbumin (<150g/L), low transferrin (<1,500mg/L), absent cutaneous hypersensitivity, decreased total lymphocyte count (<1,500 cells/L).[9]

- *Confirmed*—BMI ≤18kg/m² (or ≤20kg/m² with associated weight loss of >5% over 3–6mo), weight loss of >10% over 3–6mo.

Nutritional support—requirements
- The usual nutritional support should include adequate calories (total energy 25–35kcal/kg/d), protein (0.8–1.5g protein/kg/d), fluid (30–35mL fluid/kg), and electrolytes, micronutrients, minerals, and fibre where appropriate [D].[1]

Nutritional support—oral
- *Patient selection*—should be offered to all patients at risk or in existing malnutrition, providing the patient's swallowing function is intact and efficient [D].[1,2,3] Patients with impaired swallowing function should be referred to the swallowing assessment service [D].[1]
- *Method of support*—provide normal diet and fluid, with adequate quality and quantity, appropriate feeding aids, and encouraging environment to eat.[1,2] Modification of diet and fluid should be considered in individual cases (e.g. multivitamins, modified oral nutrition, mineral supplements) [D].[1,2,3]
- *Efficiency*—nutrition supplements can decrease the infection rate (ARR×10%) and length of hospital stay (by 2d) when compared to no supplements.[13] However, the quality of available trials is low and insufficient to conclude solid recommendations.[1,13]

Nutritional support—enteral
- *Patient selection*—should be offered to all patients at risk or in existing malnutrition who have inappropriate (or unsafe) oral route, but intact GI tract [B].[1,2] All patients undergoing major abdominal procedures should be considered for preoperative enteral nutrition support (preferably with immune-modulating substrates such as arginine, omega-3 fatty acids, and nucleotides) for 5–7d (but not within 48h of surgery) [A].[1,2]
- *Method of support*—special diet and fluid can be delivered preferably via a tube to the stomach (NG feeding tube, gastrostomy) [A], or to the duodenum or jejunum if stomach tube is inappropriate [D].[1,2] Confirmation of tube position is necessary [D].[1] Feeding can be delivered in boluses (gastric tube) or continuously (gastric or enteral tubes) over 16–24h [B].[1,2]
- *Efficiency*—enteral nutrition (using a tube) can decrease the infection rate (ARR×11%), but has no significant effect on the length of hospital stay when compared to no artificial nutrition.[13] When compared to parenteral nutrition, patients on enteral nutrition have decreased infections rate (ARR×11%), decreased complication rate (ARR × 6% for major complications), and shorter length of hospital stay (by ~1.7d).[13]

Nutritional support—parenteral
- *Patient selection*—should be offered to all patients at risk or in existing malnutrition who have inappropriate (or unsafe) oral route and disrupted (inaccessible, non-functional, or leaking) GI tract [D].[1,2]
- *Method of support*—best delivered via a dedicated central catheter. This can be inserted via peripheral access (for short-term feeding ≤14d) [B], non-tunnelled subclavian line (feeding requirement ≤30d) [D], or via a tunnelled subclavian line (feeding requirement >30d) [D].[1]

Feeding is best delivered continuously (or cyclical if nutritional requirement exceeds 2wk) **[D]**.[1]

- *Efficiency*—when compared to enteral nutrition, patients on parenteral nutrition have increased infections rate, increased complication rate, and longer length of hospital stay.[13] Parenteral nutrition should therefore be used judiciously to maximize benefits and minimize risks.

Further reading

1. National Institute for Health and Clinical Excellence (2006). Nutrition support in adults: oral nutrition support, enteral tube feeding and parenteral nutrition. Available from: http://www.nice.org.uk/CG32.

2. Arends J, Bodoky G, Bozzetti F et al. (2006). ESPEN guidelines on enteral nutrition: non-surgical oncology. Clin Nutr 25, 245–59.

3. Council of Europe Resolution Food and Nutritional Care in Hospitals (2003). 10 key characteristics of good nutritional care in hospitals. Available from: http://www.bda.uk.com/resources/071012CoEHospitalNutrition.pdf.

4. CREST (2004). Guidelines for the management of enteral tube feeding in adults. Available from: http://www.crestni.org.uk/tube-feeding-guidelines.pdf.

5. British Association for Parenteral and Enteral Nutrition. Available from: http://www.bapen.org.uk/.

6. American Society for Parenteral and Enteral Nutrition (2004). Nutrition requirements: safe practices for parenteral nutrition. Available from: http://guidelines.gov/summary/summary.aspx?doc_id=12510&nbr=006440&string=nutrition.

7. Cerra FB, Benitez MR, Blackburn GL. Applied nutrition in ICU patients. A consensus statement of the American College of Chest Physicians. Chest 111, 769–78.

8. Elia M, ed. (2003). The 'MUST' report. Nutritional screening for adults: a multidisciplinary responsibility. Development and use of the 'Malnutrition Universal Screening Tool' ('MUST') for adults. A report by the Malnutrition Advisory Group of the British Association for Parenteral and Enteral Nutrition, BAPEN, Redditch, UK.

9. Margenthaler J, Herrmann V (2002). Nutrition. In: The Washington manual of surgery, 3rd ed, Lippincott Williams & Wilkins.

10. Rubinson L, Diette GB, Song X, Brower RG, Krishnan JA (2004). Low caloric intake is associated with nosocomial bloodstream infections in patients in the medical intensive care unit. Crit Care Med 32, 350–7.

11. Haydock DA, Hill GL (1986). Impaired wound healing in surgical patients with varying degrees of malnutrition. JPEN J Parenter Enteral Nutr 10, 550–4.

12. Albina JE (1994). Nutrition and wound healing. JPEN J Parenter Enteral Nutr 18, 367–76.

13. Koretz RL, Avenell A, Lipman TO, Braunschweig CL, Milne AC (2007). Does enteral nutrition affect clinical outcome? A systematic review of the randomized trials. Am J Gastroenterol 102, 412–29.

Part 3

Oesophagus

Gastro-oesophageal reflux disease (GORD)*

* The guidelines on this chapter have been sourced and summarized from different UK, Europe, and international government sources, professional organizations, and medical specialty societies. Leading guidelines have been listed in the Key guidelines box.

Gastro-oesophageal reflux disease (GORD)

Key guidelines
- National Institute for Health and Clinical Excellence (2004). Dyspepsia: managing dyspepsia in adults in primary care.
- Scottish Intercollegiate Guidelines Network (2003). Dyspepsia.
- American College of Gastroenterology (2005). Updated guidelines for the diagnosis and treatment of gastroesophageal reflux disease.

Basic facts
- *Definition*—GORD is the sensation of stomach contents returning past the oesophageal sphincter, prolonging acid and pepsin exposure in the lower oesophagus and affecting patient well being.[1] Gastro-oesophageal acid reflux is a normal physiologic process; GORD occurs when symptoms or complications result from the reflux episodes.[1,4]
- *Incidence*—about 7% of the population in Europe and US experience heartburn on a daily basis, over 25% of them have symptoms suggestive of GORD. Oesophagitis affects ~10–16% of GORD patients.[1,2,5,6,12]
- *Risk factors*—loss of the 'high pressure zone' at the gastro-oesophageal junction (GOJ) (the antireflux barrier) is a universal 'denominator' for almost all physiological or pathological episodes. Most patients (>60%) have mechanically defective lower oesophageal sphincter (LOS) function, most commonly caused by anatomical disruption of the GOJ, often associated with a hiatus hernia (Table 21.1).[10,11]
- *Clinical presentation*—symptoms have low prediction power in estimating disease severity, underlying pathology, or the presence of complications (including Barrett's oesophagus).[1,3] This applies to 'ALARM' symptoms as well.[2] (Tables 21.2 and 21.3).

Recommended initial approach
- *General concepts*—investigations should follow a stepwise approach and sound clinical judgment (Fig. 21.1). 'ALARM' symptoms (Table 21.3) require urgent referral for investigation with endoscopy (2wk rule) (Table 21.4) [B].[1,2,3,12]
- *Simple reflux-like disease*—requires no specific initial investigations [A].[1,2,3,12]
  - *Initial advice*—begin with a comprehensive review of medications, practical lifestyle advice (healthy eating, weight reduction, and smoking cessation) [B], and proper advice to avoid known precipitants that attribute to reflux symptoms (e.g. chocolate and caffeine) [C].[1,2,3,12]
  - *Over-the-counter antacids*—useful in reducing the number of days with reflux symptoms and the median symptom score when compared with placebo, but have no significant effect on healing rate.[3,6] Useful as patient-directed therapy for mild GORD [C].[3]

Table 21.1 Risk factors for GORD

- **Obesity**—significant risk factor (OR × 2.15) for GORD, erosive oesophagitis, and oesophageal adenocarcinoma, but association remains vague.[6,7]

- **Social and dietary habits**—insufficient evidence on the precise role of each factor.[7] Possible implication of smoking, alcohol, dietary fat, mints, onions, citrus fruits, tomato, chocolate, and caffeine. Lifestyle changes are recommended for prevention (see later).[1]

- **Medications**—calcium channel blockers and anticholinergics can relax the LOS and promote GORD.[8] Research data is limited for definite conclusions.[7]

- **Genetics**—suggested by twin studies.[9]

Table 21.2 GORD symptoms and signs

- **Heartburn**—retrosternal burning discomfort triggered or aggravated by bending over or lying flat, and radiating occasionally to the neck.

- **Regurgitation**—sudden and effortless return of gastric or oesophageal contents into the pharynx, giving a sour or bitter taste ('acid brash').

- **Dysphagia**—difficulty swallowing in long-standing GORD. Might result from severe chronic oesophageal inflammation, impaired peristalsis, or development of strictures.

- **GORD-associated chest pain**—may mimic heart attack, lasts minutes to hours, and resolves spontaneously or with antacids. Usually postprandial and may be aggravated by emotional stress.

- **Water brash or hypersalivation**—patient foams at the mouth, producing salivary secretions as much as 10mL of saliva per minute.

- **Globus sensation**—constant feeling of a lump on throat.

- **Odynophagia**—painful swallowing.

Table 21.3 'ALARM' symptoms and signs[1]

- GI bleeding.

- Difficulty swallowing.

- Unintentional weight loss.

- Abdominal swelling.

- Persistent vomiting.

Table 21.4 Endoscopy for GORD—indications[1,2,12]

- Patients of any age with **ALARM symptoms**.

- Patients >55 with new onset of unexplained dyspepsia or reflux symptoms that have not responded to acid suppression treatment [B].

- Persistent symptomatic GORD despite adequate investigations and treatment (including *Helicobacter pylori* 'test and treat') in primary care (e.g. frequent relapses, severe symptoms) [B].

- *Proton pump inhibitors (PPIs)*—consider at full dose for 1mo in persistent mild to moderate symptoms [A].[1] PPIs promote healing in ~75% of patients with oesophagitis (NNT = 2), reduce relapse at 6–12mo in ~35% of patients, and eliminate symptoms in ~50% of patients with endoscopically negative reflux disease.[1,2,6,12]
  - *Helicobacter (H.) pylori 'test and treat'*—consider as alternative initial step in investigating dyspepsia of unknown cause [A].[1,2,12] Patients with proven GORD do not require this testing initially.[1,2,12]
- **Recurrent mild symptoms**—encourage patients to step down the PPI to the lowest dose necessary to control the symptoms, and to use treatment on an 'on demand' basis following good control [B].[1,2,3,12]
- **Special precautions**—further actions may be required in patients with complicated oesophagitis, history of bleeding ulcer, and regular NSAIDs therapy.[12]

Recommended secondary investigations

- **Endoscopy**—very reliable in detecting and stratifying pathological changes (Table 21.4). Absence of endoscopic features of GORD does not exclude the diagnosis or indicate an easy-to-control case.[3] Inter-observer variability exists and may affect the reliability of the investigation.[3,13] Commonly used classification systems are the Savary–Miller and Los Angeles classifications (Table 21.5).
  - *Endoscopy-negative reflux disease*—refers to patients with established reflux symptoms and normal endoscopic findings. Up to 75% of those patients have histological evidence of oesophageal injury and respond significantly to acid suppression.[14]
  - *Reflux oesophagitis*—is confirmed by finding inflammatory features in the oesophagus by endoscopy or biopsy.[1]
- **Double contrast barium meal studies**—are of limited use in current modern practice. May be helpful for investigating complicated GORD cases (sensitivity reaches over 80%). Should be tailored to individual patient needs.[3,13] Has relatively low sensitivity (~25%) and specificity (50%) compared to endoscopy in mild forms of GORD. Biopsies can not be taken for suspicious lesions.[1,3]
- **Ambulatory oesophageal pH studies**—consider in all patients with persistent symptoms who have no evidence of mucosal damage and have failed to respond to acid suppression management [C].[3,15] The test is reproducible, sensitive, and specific (96%) to confirm or exclude the presence of GORD.[3,15]
  - *Prospects*—two recent advances have potential significant impact on GORD approach: [3,15]
    1) *Combined impendence and acid testing*—allow for accurate measurement of acidity and volume of reflux.
    2) *Tubeless telemetric acid monitoring*—decreases patient's discomfort and allows for a longer monitoring period.

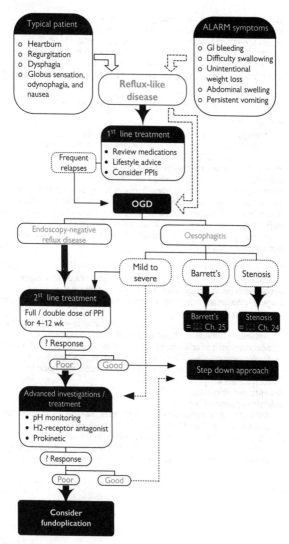

Fig. 21.1 GORD recommended approach

- *Oesophageal manometric testing*—has minimal role in making or confirming the suspected diagnosis of GORD [C].[3,16] Used mainly to assess the structural integrity of the LOS, to investigate and diagnose any motility disorder, to assess the accurate location of the upper border of the LOS for correct positioning of the pH electrode in ambulatory pH monitoring, and proper planning of antireflux surgery.[13]

RECOMMENDED TREATMENT OF RESISTANT CASES

Medical treatment

- *PPI therapy*—offer further PPI at full dose for 4–8wk [A].[1] Consider PPIs at a double dose for further 4wk in resistant or recurrent cases [C*].[1]
- *H2–receptor antagonist (H2RA) and prokinetics*—consider H2RA for patients with inadequate response to PPIs [B].[1] Prokinetics (metoclopramide or domperidone) may improve bloating and early satiety. Cisapride is no longer licensed to use in the UK,[1] but can be prescribed by a consultant on a named patient basis where appropriate.
- *Refractory cases*—check compliance, tolerability of treatment, and confounding factors. Consider advanced investigations (pH monitoring) and surgery if appropriate.

Antireflux surgery

- *Indications*—antireflux surgery cannot be recommended for every patient with recurrent symptoms. Current evidence suggests that surgery is no better than medical treatment in achieving remission from symptoms in the long term [A].[1,3,6,17]
  - Surgery is a good maintenance option for patients with significantly impaired quality of life (failed or partial responders) despite adequate dose of acid suppression for a reasonable period of time.[1]
  - Surgery may also be offered to those who require high dose of maintenance PPIs to control symptoms or those who failed to tolerate the drugs (e.g. diarrhoea).[1]
- *Benefits and risks*—see Table 21.6.
- *Selection of surgical technique.*
  - *Types of surgical techniques*—different types available. Fundoplication procedure introduced by Nissen in 1956 or its variants is the most commonly used antireflux operation in the world. Nissen fundoplication is performed by mobilizing the lower oesophagus and wrapping the fundus of stomach around the mobilized area.

Table 21.5 Savary–Miller classification of reflux disease[25]

Grade I	One or more non-confluent reddish spots (± exudate).
Grade II	Distal oesophagus non-circumferential erosive and exudative lesions that may be confluent.
Grade III	Circumferential distal oesophagus erosions covered with haemorrhagic and pseudomembranous exudates.
Grade IV	Chronic complications—including deep ulcers, stenosis, or scarring with Barrett's metaplasia.

Table 21.6 Antireflux surgery—benefits and risks

- *Main benefits.*
  - *Symptom relief*—significant improvement in oesophagitis and heartburn symptoms (about 85–90% of patients at 3y[1,18] and ~80% at 5y).[6] Studies are heterogeneous with odds ratios for improvement (compared to medical treatment) raging from 1.2 to 200, and NNT ranging from 1.2 to 58.[17]
  - *High patient satisfaction*—up to 95% for Nissen fundoplication when performed by experienced surgeons.[19]
- *Main risks.*
  - *Recurrence of symptoms*—about 62% of patients will require further acid-suppressant medications at 10y to control symptoms.[12]
  - *Operative morbidity*—including significant increase in early satiety, inability to belch, and inability to vomit.[17]
  - *Operative mortality*—small (0.1–0.5%) but significant.[1]

- Fundoplication can be total or partial, in anterior or posterior positions, and can be performed using open or laparoscopic techniques. Other surgical techniques include posterior and anterior partial fundoplication, Hill's procedure, Collis' procedure, and Angelchik prosthesis.
- *Choice of surgical technique*—the choice depends on the efficiency and complication rate of each technique as well as the individual patient case.[1,6,21]
  - Laparoscopic Nissen fundoplication (the gold standard procedure) has fewer overall complications and shorter recovery compared to open approach. There is no significant difference in recurrence rate of GORD or relief of heartburn [A].[1,6,21]
  - Nissen fundoplication and posterior partial fundoplication have no significant difference in post-operative dysphagia or recurrent GORD rate [B].[1,6,21]
  - Partial and anterior fundoplication have less post-operative wind-related complications compared to total fundoplication. Dysphagia is less common in anterior partial fundoplication [B].[1,6,21]
  - There is no difference in the outcome whether vagus nerves were included or excluded, and whether short gastric arteries were divided or left intact.

Newer interventional techniques
See Table 21.7.

Table 21.7 Newer antireflux techniques

- *Endoluminal gastroplication.*[22]
  - *Technique*—outpatient procedure. Using a standard endoscope and endoscopic sewing device, a plication (or pleat) is created at the LOS.
  - *Safety*—no major safety concerns according to current available evidence.
  - *Efficiency*—unknown. Procedure is at the early stages of development.
  - *Terms of use*—special arrangements should be undertaken for clinical governance, patient consent, audit, and review of all outcome results by a dedicated team.

- *Endoscopic injection of bulking agents.*[23]
  - *Technique*—patient sedated. Using a standard endoscope and fluoroscopic control, a needle catheter (filled with a bio-compatible polymer and solvent) is introduced into the GOJ. The polymer is injected (or implanted) into the GOJ (often four injections), along the muscle layer or deep submucosal layer of the cardia.
  - *Safety*—no major safety concerns, but side effects have been reported (chest pain in 50–90% of patients, dysphagia, fever, nausea). Current evidences are insufficient to support the use of this procedure without special arrangements in the unit.
  - *Efficiency*—unknown as the procedure is at the early stages of development.

- *Endoscopic radiofrequency ablation.*[24]
  - Guidelines are under construction.

- *Endoscopic augmentation of the LOS using hydrogel implants.*
  - Performed under sedation by using a special delivery system to apply suction on the GOJ mucosa and implant a hydrogel prosthesis. The prosthesis absorbs water and takes its full shape within 24h.[26] Current evidence raises concerns on the safety of this procedure, and its use is therefore NOT recommended outside a strict clinical governance setting by well-trained endoscopists.[26]

Beyond the guidelines and the future

GORD is a very common problem, in many instances related to lifestyle, and particularly, the rise in obesity which raises the intra-abdominal pressure leading to reflux of the gastric contents and acid into the oesophagus. This may also be related to the rise in detection of Barrett's oesophagus and oesophageal adenocarcinoma. Barrett's oesophagus is probably a protective mechanism, and may reduce the symptoms of GORD and delay the diagnosis of cancer.

First-line treatment should be attention to lifestyle, including weight and smoking.

For infrequent episodes of reflux, antacid treatment provides effective symptomatic relief.

H2–receptor antagonists reduce the acidity of the gastric secretions and are effective treatments, but the most effective medical treatment of GORD is the PPI class of drugs. These provide effective acid suppression throughout the day, and especially at night when the added effect of gravity exacerbates GORD symptoms. As such, PPI therapy should be first-line for symptomatic reflux disease. The neutralized gastric secretion does not cause the heartburn pain of GORD.

Prokinetic drugs help to reduce the exposure of the oesophagus to gastric secretion. Metoclopramide is probably the most effective, but has a wider side effect profile than the acid suppression treatments. Similarly, cisapride was an effective medication, but was withdrawn because of cardiac arrhythmias.

It seems unlikely that more effective acid suppression drugs will be developed. Drugs, which selectively work on a dysfunctional LOS, may be developed in future years.

Laparoscopic fundoplication with relatively minor variations in technique is the gold standard surgical treatment of GORD refractory to medical treatment or in younger patients where lifelong medical treatment is not desired.

Therapeutic endoscopic treatments are intuitively attractive in avoiding the risks of major surgery. Endoscopic treatments consist of three basic principles, namely suturing the mucosa at the GOJ to create a valve which prevents reflux, radiofrequency ablation at the GOJ to create scarring and achieve the same aim, and the injection of polymers at the GOJ. All the techniques remain experimental, and generally are less effective than conventional surgery with a greater risk of recurrent disease. Innovation continues to contribute to this field; however, these techniques have not become mainstream treatment. Hybrid techniques utilizing NOTES (**N**atural **O**rifice **T**ransluminal **E**ndoscopic **S**urgery), surgery conventionally performed through incisions being performed through natural orifices (mouth, anus, vagina), may stimulate advances in effective antireflux surgery. *Mr David Corless*

Further reading

1. National Institute for Health and Clinical Excellence (2004). Dyspepsia: managing dyspepsia in adults in primary care. Available from: http://guidance.nice.org.uk/CG17.
2. Scottish Intercollegiate Guidelines Network (2003). Dyspepsia: a national clinical guideline. Available from: http://www.sign.ac.uk/pdf/sign68.pdf.

3. DeVault KR, Castell DO; American College of Gastroenterology (2005). Updated guidelines for the diagnosis and treatment of gastroesophageal reflux disease. *Am J Gastroenterol* 100, 190–200.
4. Richter JE (1996). Typical and atypical presentations of gastroesophageal reflux disease. The role of oesophageal testing in diagnosis and management. *Gastroenterol Clin North Am* 25, 75–102.
5. Dent J, El-Serag HB, Wallander MA, Johansson S (2005). Epidemiology of gastro-oesophageal reflux disease: a systematic review. *Gut* 54, 710–7.
6. Moayyedi P, Delaney B, Forman D (2005). Gastro-oesophageal reflux disease. *Clin Evid* 14, 567–81.
7. Corley DA, Kubo A (2006). Body mass index and gastroesophageal reflux disease: a systematic review and meta-analysis. *Am J Gastroenterol* 101, 2619–28.
8. Lagergren J, Bergström R, Adami HO, Nyren O (2000). Association between medications that relax the lower oesophageal sphincter and risk for oesophageal adenocarcinoma. *Ann Intern Med* 133, 165–75.
9. Romero Y, Cameron AJ, Locke GR 3rd et al. (1997). Familial aggregation of gastroesophageal reflux in patients with Barrett's oesophagus and oesophageal adenocarcinoma. *Gastroenterology* 113, 1449–56.
10. Ott DJ, Gelfand DW, Chen YM, Wu WC, Munitz HA (1985). Predictive relationship of hiatal hernia to reflux oesophagitis. *Gastrointest Radiol* 10, 317–20.
11. Wright RA, Hurwitz AL (1979). Relationship of hiatal hernia to endoscopically proved reflux oesophagitis. *Dig Dis Sci* 24, 311–3.
12. PRODIGY Guidance - Dyspepsia – proven gastro-oesophageal reflux disease & dyspepsia - uninvestigated by endoscopy. 2008 URL: http://www.nelm.nhs.uk/en/NeLM-Area/Evidence/Guidelines/CKS-Topic-Review-Dyspepsia—proven-gastro-oesophageal-reflux-disease-GORD. Accessed May 2009
13. Reginald V, Lord N, Demeester TR. Reflux disease and hiatus hernia In: *Oxford Textbook of Surgery*. Chapter 22.2.1. 2nd edition, Oxford University Press, Oxford.
14. Reginald V, Lord N, Demeester TR (2001). Reflux disease and hiatus hernia. In: *Oxford Textbook of Surgery*, 2nd ed, Oxford University Press, Oxford.
15. Dent J (2007). Microscopic oesophageal mucosal injury in non-erosive reflux disease. *Clin Gastroenterol Hepatol* 5, 4–16.
16. Nichols JH, Taylor D, Varnholt H, Williams L (2006). pH testing. In: *Laboratory medicine practice guidelines: evidence-based practice for point-of-care testing*, pp. 120–5, National Academy of Clinical Biochemistry (NACB), Washington DC.
17. Pandolfino JE, Kahrilas PJ; American Gastroenterological Association (2005). American Gastroenterological Association medical position statement: clinical use of oesophageal manometry. *Gastroenterology* 128, 207–8.
18. Allgood PC, Bachmann M (2000) Medical or surgical treatment for chronic gastro-oesophageal reflux? A systematic review of published evidence of effectiveness. *Eur J Surg* 166, 713–21.
19. Dassinger MS, Torquati A, Houston HL, Holzman MD, Sharp KW, Richards WO (2004). Laparoscopic fundoplication: 5-year follow-up. *Am Surg* 70, 691–4.
20. Hagedorn C, Lönroth H, Rydberg L, Ruth M, Lundell L (2002). Long-term efficacy of total (Nissen–Rossetti) and posterior partial (Toupet) fundoplication: results of a randomized clinical trial. *J Gastrointest Surg* 6, 540–5.
21. Watson D, Jamieson G (2006). Treatment of gastro-oesophageal reflux disease. In: *Oesophagogastric surgery: a companion to specialist surgical practice*, 3rd ed. Elsevier Saunders Ltd Publications, London.
22. National Institute for Health and Clinical Excellence (2005). Endoluminal gastroplication for gastro-oesophageal reflux disease. Available from: http://www.nice.org.uk/guidance/index.jsp?action=byID&o=11161.
23. National Institute for Health and Clinical Excellence (2004). Endoscopic injection of bulking agents for gastro-oesophageal reflux disease. Available from: http://www.nice.org.uk/guidance/index.jsp?action=byID&o=11132.
24. National Institute for Health and Clinical Excellence (2009). Endoscopic radiofrequency ablation for gastro-oesophageal reflux disease. Available from: http://www.nice.org.uk/guidance/index.jsp?action=byID&o=11234.
25. Monnier P, Savary M (1984). Contribution of endoscopy to gastroesophageal reflux disease. *Scand J Gastroenterol* 19 (Suppl. 106), 26.
26. National Institute for Health and Clinical Excellence (2007). Endoscopic augmentation of the lower oesophageal sphincter using hydrogel implants for the treatment of gastro-oesophageal reflux disease. Available from: http://www.nice.org.uk/Guidance/IPG222.

Ingestion of foreign bodies*

* The guidelines on this chapter have been sourced and summarized from different UK, Europe, and international government sources, professional organizations, and medical specialty societies. Leading guidelines have been listed in the Key guidelines box.

Ingestion of foreign bodies

Key guideline

- American Society for Gastrointestinal Endoscopy (2002). Guideline for the management of ingested foreign bodies.

Basic facts

- **Incidence**—relatively common event; about 4% of children in the US swallow a coin during their childhood.[1,2]
- **Risk factors**—common sources are coins in children and meat bolus in adults (Table 22.1).[1]
- **Clinical presentation**—varies between different age groups (Table 22.2).

Recommended investigations (Fig. 22.1)

- **Biplane radiographs**—can identify most true foreign objects, steak bones, and free mediastinal or peritoneal air.[1] Lateral view helps in confirming the location in oesophagus and revealing the presence of more than one coin.[1] Some objects like fish or chicken bones, wood, plastic, most glass, and thin metal objects may not be readily seen.[1]
- **CT scan**—indicated if symptoms are not specific and foreign body is still suspected. Handheld metal detectors and cautious endoscopy can also be used.[1]
- **Contrast examination**—should not be performed routinely due to the risk of aspiration and coating of the foreign body which may compromises subsequent endoscopy.[1]

Recommended management (Fig. 22.1)

- **Natural history**—most will pass through the bowel with faeces (those that reach the stomach have ~80–90% chance of passing through).[3] Some may become lodged and cause damage to the GI tract.
- **Factors affecting treatment options**—age, severity of clinical condition, anatomic location, size and shape of ingested material, and technical skills of the endoscopist.[1]
- **Asymptomatic patient with negative radiographs**—no specific treatment required. The foreign body may have passed out of the oesophagus.[1]
- **Asymptomatic patient with proven foreign body**—use rigid or flexible oesophagoscopy to retrieve the foreign body from the oesophagus within a maximum of 24h.[1] Both types of instruments are safe and effective. Check extraction instruments before proceeding with endoscopy.[1] Under no circumstances should a foreign body be allowed to stay in the oesophagus for more than 24h.[1,5]

Table 22.1 Risk factors for ingestion of foreign bodies

- *Age*—more common in patients between 6mo and 5y.

- *Underlying conditions*—more common in the presence of oesophageal carcinoma, strictures, diverticulum, post-gastrectomy, hiatus hernia and achalasia.[3]

- *Special groups*—more common among mental illness patients, prisoners, and persons involved in smuggling of illicit drugs.

- *Common sources*—coins in children and meat bolus in adults. Fish or chicken bones, wood, plastic, glass, and other objects are familiar as well.[1]

Table 22.2 Clinical presentation

- Clinical presentation.
  - *Fully sensible adults and older children*—may give clear history and point to the location of maximum discomfort.
  - *Younger children and mentally impaired adults*—may not recognize the incident and present lately with non-specific symptoms and signs.[1]
  - *Most common symptoms*—acute dysphagia, inability to swallow, hypersalivation, retrosternal fullness, regurgitation of undigested food, and odynophagia.
    - *Oropharyngeal foreign bodies*—sensation of trapped, well-localized object (usually bones and toothpicks) in the throat. May be associated with mild to severe discomfort, inability to swallow, and occasional compromise of airways.
    - *Oesophageal foreign bodies*—sudden onset of severe dysphagia following the event in fully conscious patients.

- Physical examination.
  - May reveal swelling, erythema, tenderness, or crepitus in the neck if oropharyngeal or proximal oesophageal perforation occurred. Abdomen should be carefully examined for evidence of peritonitis or small bowel obstruction.[1]

- *Failed retrieval*—objects may be advanced into the stomach for easier grasping. If unable to retrieve from stomach, treat conservatively as outpatient.[1,5,6] Advise patient on regular diet and observation of stool. If patient remains asymptomatic, weekly radiographs are recommended to follow the progression of small blunt objects.[1,5]
- *Lodged objects*—objects failed to leave stomach within 3–4wk should be removed endoscopically. Objects remaining in the same location (after passing the stomach) for more than 1wk should be removed surgically.[1]
- *Sharp objects*—include chicken and fish bones, straightened paperclips, toothpicks, needles, bread bag clips, and dental bridgework.[1,7,8] Many are not visible on X-ray and should be carefully investigated by laryngoscopy or OGD.[1,7,8]
  - Sharp objects must be retrieved or carefully followed up by daily radiographs. The risk of developing complications is >35%.[1]
  - Objects failing to progress in three consecutive days requires surgical intervention.[1]
- *Disc battery ingestion*—high risk of causing liquefaction necrosis and perforation of oesophagus, with possible death. Disc batteries should be retrieved immediately using a basket or a net.[1,9,10]

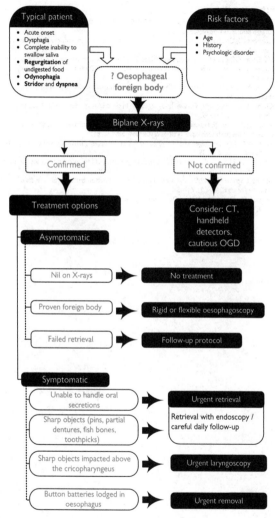

Fig. 22.1 Algorithm for approaching ingestion of foreign body

Further reading

1. Eisen GM, Baron TH, Dominitz JA et al. (2002). Guideline for the management of ingested foreign bodies. *Gastrointest Endosc* 55, 802–6.
2. Conners GP, Chamberlain JM, Weiner PR (1995). Paediatric coin ingestion: a home-based survey. *Am J Emerg Med* 13, 638–40.
3. Li ZS, Sun ZX, Zou DW, Xu GM, Wu RP, Liao Z (2006). Endoscopic management of foreign bodies in the upper GI tract: experience with 1,088 cases in China. *Gastrointest Endosc* 64, 485–92.
4. PatientPlus. Swallowed foreign bodies. Available from: http://www.patient.co.uk/showdoc/40024855/.
5. Cheng W, Tam PK (1999). Foreign body ingestion in children: experience with 1,265 cases. *J Pediatr Surg* 34, 1472–6.
6. Vicari JJ, Johansson JF, Frakes JT (2001). Outcomes of acute oesophageal food impaction: success of the push technique. *Gastrointest Endosc* 53, 178–81.
7. Webb WA (1995). Management of foreign bodies of the upper gastrointestinal tract: update. *Gastrointest Endosc* 41, 39–51.
8. Vizcarrondo FJ, Brady PG, Nord HJ (1983). Foreign bodies of the upper gastrointestinal tract. *Gastrointest Endosc* 29, 208–10.
9. Litovitz T, Schmitz BF (1992). Ingestion of cylindrical and button batteries: an analysis of 2,382 cases. *Pediatrics* 89(4 Pt 2), 747–57.
10. Gordon AC, Gough MH (1993). Oesophageal perforation after button battery ingestion. *Ann R Coll Surg Engl* 75, 362–4.

Achalasia*

---

* The guidelines on this chapter have been sourced and summarized from different UK, Europe, and international government sources, professional organizations, and medical specialty societies. Leading guidelines have been listed in the Key guidelines box.

Achalasia

Key guidelines

- The Society for Surgery of the Alimentary Tract (2006). Patient care guidelines: oesophageal achalasia.
- National Institute for Health and Clinical Excellence (2004). Dyspepsia.

Basic facts

- *Definition*—primary oesophageal motility disorder, characterized by failure of the lower oesophageal sphincter (LOS) to relax in response to swallowing and by the absence of peristalsis in the oesophageal body.[1,3]
- *Incidence*—about 0.5 cases/100,000 population per year.[3]
- *Pathogenesis*—poorly understood. Possibly results from the dysfunction of inhibitory neurons containing nitric oxide and vasoactive intestinal polypeptide in the distal oesophagus. Unknown aetiology.
- *Clinical presentation*—slow progressive dysphagia (almost all patients) and regurgitation (60%). This occurs more often in supine position, with higher risk of aspiration of undigested food. Other findings include weight loss (60%), chest pain (40%) usually at the time of meal, nocturnal regurgitation, and pneumonia.[1,3]

Recommended investigations (Fig. 23.1)

- *Routine blood tests*—iron deficiency anaemia may be detected.[4]
- *Plain chest radiograph*—may show widening of the mediastinum and posterior mediastinal air–fluid level. Signs of chronic aspiration may show on lung fields.[3]
- *Upper GI endoscopy and/or barium swallow*—are the initial investigations of choice, and should be performed urgently for patients with dysphagia (one of the 'ALARM' symptoms) [B].[5,6]
  - *Endoscopy*—can detect complications and reliably rule out cancer.[1,3] Retention oesophagitis may be found. Passage of the scope through the LOS often produces a characteristic 'pop' sensation.
  - *Barium swallow*—over 85% of cases have the characteristic dilated oesophagus with narrowing at the gastro-oesophageal junction (bird's beak deformity).[3]
  - *Disease severity*—can be determined by the oesophageal diameter (<4cm, 4–6cm, >6cm), amount of retained food, and degree of peristalsis.[3]
- *Oesophageal manometry*—confirms the diagnosis.[3]
  - *Classic findings*—absence of oesophageal peristalsis, and hypertensive or normotensive LOS that fails to relax completely in response to swallowing.[1]
- *Differential diagnosis*—Chagas' disease and pseudoachalasia accompanying carcinoma.

Recommended treatment (Fig. 23.1)

- *Main goals*—palliative. Mainly to eliminate the outflow resistance at the gastro-oesophageal junction.[1,3]
- *Minimally invasive surgery*—initial treatment of choice where experience exists.[1]
  - *Technique*—laparoscopic Heller myotomy and partial fundoplication. A generous myotomy of the lower oesophagus should be performed and extended well onto the gastric wall.
- *Medical treatment*—use only in patients unable to undergo standard treatment. Options include calcium channel blockers and nitrates (50% initial success).[3]
- *Pneumatic dilatation*—above 75% success rate. Advantages include relatively low cost and avoidance of general anaesthesia.[3] Possible complications include gastro-oesophageal reflux (25–35% of patients) and perforation (up to 5% of patients).[1]
- *Intrasphincteric injection of botulinum toxin.*
  - *Advantages*—about 60% success rate initially in relieving symptoms, but recurs within a year in the majority of patients.
  - *Disadvantages*—may cause inflammatory reaction at the gastro-oesophageal junction and obliterates anatomic planes. Less effective in recurrent cases.
- *Surveillance endoscopy*—should be offered to all patients due to increased risk for developing both squamous and adenocarcinoma of oesophagus.[1]

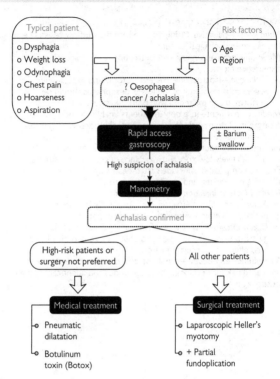

Fig. 23.1 Algorithm for achalasia approach

Further reading

1. The Society for Surgery of the Alimentary Tract (2006). SSAT patient care guidelines: oesophageal achalasia. Available from: http://www.ssat.com/cgi-bin/achalasia.cgi.
2. Morris PJ, Wood WC (2000). *Oxford Textbook of Surgery*, 2nd ed, Oxford University Press, Oxford.
3. Clinical Knowledge Summaries. Gastrointestinal (upper) cancer—suspected. Available from: http://cks.library.nhs.uk/gi_upper_cancer_suspected#-179345.
4. Kumar V, Abbas AK, Fausto N (2004). *Pathologic basis of disease*, 7th ed, Saunders, London.

Oesophageal cancer*

* The guidelines on this chapter have been sourced and summarized from different UK, Europe, and international government sources, professional organizations, and medical specialty societies. Leading guidelines have been listed in the Key guidelines box.

Oesophageal cancer

Key guidelines

- Association of Upper Gastrointestinal Surgeons of Great Britain and Ireland, British Society of Gastroenterology, British Association of Surgical Oncology (2002). Guidelines for the management of oesophageal and gastric cancer.
- National Institute for Health and Clinical Excellence (2004). Dyspepsia: managing dyspepsia in adults in primary care.
- Scottish Intercollegiate Guidelines Network (2006). Management of oesophageal and gastric cancer: a national clinical guidance.

Basic facts

- **Incidence**—ninth most common cancer in the UK. Most cases occur in elderly and very few below the age of 40. Most common types are squamous cell carcinoma (SCC) and adenocarcinoma (ACA). The male to female ratio is 3:2 for SCC and 5–10:1 for ACA.[4]
- **Risk factors**—for SCC include geographic location (more common in China and South Africa), people of African-American origin, excessive smoking (OR × 4 to 17), excessive alcohol consumption (OR × 2 to 10), and other factors (caustic oesophageal injury, etc.). Risk factors for ACA include long-standing reflux oesophagitis (RR × 2) and Barrett's oesophagus (OR × 44). Diet deficient in vegetables, fruit, dairy products, and diet with low contents of vitamin A, C, and riboflavin may have a role in the development of SCC.[1,2]
- **Clinical presentation**—transient 'sticking' of apples, meat, or bread may precede frank dysphagia (once lumen diameter is <13mm). Odynophagia, reflux oesophagitis, deep chest pain, cough, hoarseness, aspiration pneumonia, lymphadenopathy, unexplained anaemia (in chronic GI bleeding), anorexia, and hepatomegaly.

Recommended investigations (Fig. 24.1)

- **Upper GI endoscopy**—the first investigation of choice to confirm diagnosis and obtain sufficient tissue biopsies (Table 24.1) [B].[1,2,3]
  - *Referral guidelines*—patients with dysphagia or any other 'ALARM' symptoms (see 📖 Chapter 21, pp.149–160) should be investigated urgently using upper GI endoscopy [B].[1,2]
  - *Barium studies*—can be considered as the primary investigation if endoscopy is inappropriate [C].[1]
- **Pathologic confirmation**—multiple biopsies and brushings should always be obtained from suspicious lesions [B].[1,3,6]
  - *Biopsy detection rate*—ranges from 93% for one biopsy to 98% for seven biopsies.[7]
  - *Cytology*—complement histology and can increase accuracy to 100%.[7]

Recommended initial staging (Fig. 24.1)

- **Clinical assessment**—only those patients with an ASA score of 3 or less should be considered for surgery [B*].[1]

Table 24.1 Endoscopy for oesophageal cancer

- **Preparation**—withhold antacids and anti-secretory treatment if possible until after endoscopy to avoid any misdiagnosis.
- **Findings.**
  - **Early oesophageal cancer**—may appear as a superficial plaque or ulceration.
  - **Advanced cancer**—may appear as an ulcerated mass, diffuse ulceration, stricture, or circumferential lesion.

Table 24.2 TNM staging

T—primary tumour	
TX	Unable to assess the primary tumour
T0	No tumour evident
Tis	Carcinoma in situ
T1	Invasion reaching the lamina propria or submucosa
T2	Invasion reaching the muscularis propria
T3	Invasion reaching the adventitia
T4	Invasion reaching the adjacent structures
N—regional lymph nodes	
NX	Unable to assess the regional lymph nodes
N0	No evidence of regional lymph node involvement
N1	Evident regional lymph node metastasis
M—distant metastasis	
MX	Unable to assess the presence of distant metastasis
M0	No evidence of distant metastasis
M1	Distant metastasis

- *Basic investigations*—baseline haematological and biochemical profile, ABGs, pulmonary function tests (PFTs), CXR, and ECG [B].[1,2]
- *Spiral thoracic and abdominal contrast CT scan.*
  - *Indications*—first staging investigation of choice to evaluate the presence of metastatic disease [B].[1]
  - *Technique*—thin (5mm) slices and gastric distension with 600–800mL of water are recommended.
  - *Accuracy*—>85% accurate in detecting mediastinal or liver involvement.
  - *TNM staging*—see Table 24.3.
- *Nutritional assessment.*
  - *Effect on surgery*—risk increases in patients with BMI <18.5, BMI <90% of predicted value, recent weight loss of >20%, and low serum albumin (see Ch. 20).[1] Obesity increases the risk as well.
  - *Optimization*—essential part of the perioperative care. Nutritional support (enteral or parenteral) should be considered on all patients in the pre- and post-operative period [B].[1,2]
- *MDT discussion*—essential requirement prior to commencing any definitive staging or treatment [C].[1] Decisions are taken in the context of predicted prognosis and expected effect of any investigation or treatment intervention on quality of life.[1]
- *Breaking bad news*—should be done in a professional and effective way to ensure adequate compliance. The role of a cancer care nurse is essential.[1]
  - *Recommended points to discuss*—confirmation of diagnosis, available treatment options, expected perioperative experience, contact details, and sources for further information (including patient support groups). Discussion should be documented and communicated to other members of the team (e.g. GP, oncologists, and cancer care nurses).
- *Advanced staging*—only required if the patient is a good candidate for surgical resection.[1]

Recommended advanced staging (Fig. 24.1)

- *Patient selection*—all patients without evidence of metastatic disease on CT scan who are eligible for curative surgery should undergo endoscopic ultrasonography if available [B].[1,3]
- *Endoscopic ultrasonography (EUS).*
  - Superior to CT scan for local staging and more accurate in predicting resectability.[1,3] EUS can identify the five-layered structure of oesophageal wall (T staging), provide accurate and reliable N staging (features like well-defined margins of nodes over 1cm in diameter, rounded, and hypoechoic nodes are likely to correlate well with malignant infiltration[1,3]). It can demonstrate the presence of small volumes of ascites (M staging).[1]

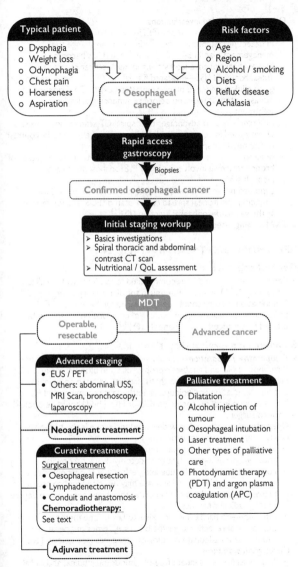

Fig 24.1 Algorithm for approaching the oesophageal cancer patient
(QoL = Quality of Life)

- *Other recommended investigations.*
  - *Positron emission tomography (PET)*—is superior to CT scan or EUS in detecting distant metastasis.[9] PET scan can change the management plan in 5–20% of cases,[9,10] and has become an essential part of advanced staging in many cancer centres.
  - *Transabdominal USS*—indicated if treatment options are limited and good clinical evidence of liver metastasis exists. Confirmation of disease extent is required before commencing palliative treatment [C].[1,3]
  - *MRI scan*—has no advantages over spiral CT scan in most cases. Usually used in certain individual cases such as allergy to IV contrast or the need for specific extra details [C].[1,3]
  - *Bronchoscopy*—recommended if CT scan and EUS raise suspicion of bronchotracheal involvement [D].[1,3] Bronchoscopy may be inconclusive.
  - *Laparoscopy*—recommended in the perioperative period for suspicious peritoneal spread on CT scan or EUS, and for cancers at the gastro-oesophageal junction [D].[1,3]
- *TNM staging*—see Table 24.2.

RECOMMENDED TREATMENT (Fig. 24.1)

General approach

- Radical surgery should be recommended for patients with localized tumours (T1, T2), who are fit enough to tolerate major surgery [D].[1,3] Combination therapy should be considered for T2 tumours. Other therapeutic modalities in the context of controlled trials should be offered to advanced cancer patients [D].[1,3]

Standards for surgical resection

- *Preoperative preparation*—should include psychological preparation, thromboembolic and antibiotic prophylaxis, and blood cross-matching.[1] Full communication with anaesthetist familiar with the complexity of one lung ventilation and epidural anaesthesia is recommended [C].[1,3] Depending on local protocols, an ICU or HDU bed should be booked prior to surgery.
- *Operative approach*—most widely used technique is the two-phase Lewis–Tanner (laparoscopic or open).
  - *Summary of technique*—the tumour is resected through lapa-rotomy/laparoscopy ± right thoracotomy/thoracoscopy, followed by construction of a gastric tube and performing of oesophagogastric anastomosis. A third cervical phase may be added in the case of proximally situated tumours in order to achieve appropriate degree of longitudinal clearance.[1,3]
  - *Efficiency*—no hard evidence exists to favour one method of oesophageal resection over the others. All types of operations should ensure adequate oncological standards (see below) [B].[1]
- *Oncological standards.*
  - *Main objectives*—adequate free-of-tumour longitudinal and radial resection margins, with appropriate lymphadenectomy [B].[1]
  - *Proximal extent of resection*—should ideally be 10cm above the macroscopic tumour and 5cm distal to it [D*].[1,3]

Table 24.3 TNM staging on CT scan

- *T staging.*
  - *T1 to T3*—unreliable in differentiating T1 from T2 cancers or in accurate estimation of microscopic invasion in T3.[1]
  - *T4*—can be identified by finding:
    - Intimate contact between tumour and contiguous organs
    - Focal loss of intervening fat plane
    - Clear CT scan evidence of direct organ invasion.[1]

- *N staging.*
  - *Accuracy*—node involvement can be identified in 38–70% of cases.[1]
  - *Criteria*—node size is the main criterion used for identification and still of low accuracy (48% sensitivity and 93% specificity if size >8mm was considered abnormal in coeliac axis).[1]

- *M staging.*
  - *Accuracy*—metastatic disease can be detected in 75–80% of 'truly positive' cases using newer techniques. Can only detect 50% of lesions with size <1cm.[1]

Table 24.4 Pathologic report minimum dataset

- Type of tumour.

- Depth of invasion.

- Resection margins involvement.

- Vascular invasion.

- Presence of Barrett's metaplasia.

- Number of nodes resected and number containing metastatic tumour.

- *Outcome measures*—anastomotic leakage rate <5%, Curative (R0) resection rates >30%, and overall in-hospital mortality <10% [B].[1,3]
- *Pathology report*—should follow the pathologic report minimum dataset (Table 24.4) [B].[1,3]

Recommendation for chemoradiotherapy

- Chemoradiation is the treatment of choice for localized SCC in the proximal oesophagus [B].[1]
  - *Adjuvant* chemotherapy*—has no clear beneficial role in oesophageal cancer [B].[1]
  - *Neoadjuvant chemotherapy* (cisplatin + 5-fluorouracil (5-FU))—improves the short-term survival when compared to surgery alone [B].[1]
  - *Preoperative radiotherapy*—has no evidence for a beneficial role in oesophageal cancer [B].[1]
  - *Preoperative chemoradiation*—improves the long-term survival [B].[1]

---

* Neoadjuvant therapy refers to chemo and/or radio therapy given to patients prior to surgery. Adjuvant therapy refers to treatment given postoperatively.

Recommendation for palliative treatment

- **General approach**—appropriate palliative treatment plan should be formulated at the MDT meeting for patients with inoperable cancers. A direct involvement of the palliative care team is recommended.
- **Options.**
  - **Dilatation**—indicated only for patients with predicted extremely short lifespan (4wk or less) who find difficulties in swallowing saliva. Consider also as a very short-term measure to relieve dysphagia while awaiting a more definitive treatment.[1,3]
  - **Alcohol injection of tumour**—considered in certain situations like eccentric or soft exophytic tumours that are difficult or risky to intubate, tumours lying too close to the cricopharyngeus (unsuitable for intubation), and tumour overgrowth at the ends of oesophageal prosthesis.[1,3]
  - **Oesophageal intubation**—the treatment of choice for palliation of firm stenosing tumours lying more than 2cm from the cricopharyngeus:[1,3]
    - Expandable metal stents preferable to plastic tubes—lower complication rate and shorter length of hospital stay.
    - Malignant tracheo-oesophageal fistulas or oesophageal perforation—use covered expandable metal stents or cuffed plastic tubes as the treatment of choice.
  - **Laser treatment**—indicated for exophytic tumours (or tumour overgrowth following intubation) to relieve dysphagia.[1,3]
  - **Other types of palliative care**—adjunctive external beam radiotherapy or brachytherapy and chemoradiation in patients with locally advanced metastatic cancer with good performance status.[2]
  - **Photodynamic therapy (PDT) and argon plasma coagulation (APC)**—are experimental.[1,3]

Know your results

Effectiveness of gastric cancer diagnosis and treatment—audit areas[8]

The National oesophagogastric cancer audit—setting good example.
- **Standards**—to measure the quality of care received by patients with oesophagogastric cancer in the UK, and to assess whether care is consistent with recommended practice.
- **Indicators**—the timescale of the process of care, determinants of treatment and outcomes, the factors that influence decisions about curative and palliative treatment, short-term outcomes of surgical treatment, and the survival at 1y, quality of life, and patient satisfaction with care.[8]

Further reading

1. Allum WH, Griffin SM, Watson A, Colin–Jones D; Association of Upper Gastrointestinal Surgeons of Great Britain and Ireland, British Society of Gastroenterology, British Association of Surgical Oncology (2002). Guidelines for the management of oesophageal and gastric cancer. *Gut* 50 Suppl. 5, v1–23.
2. National Institute for Health and Clinical Excellence (2004). Dyspepsia: managing dyspepsia in adults in primary care. Available from: http://guidance.nice.org.uk/CG17.

3. Scottish Intercollegiate Guidelines Network (2006). Management of oesophageal and gastric cancer: a national clinical guidance. Available from: http://www.sign.ac.uk/pdf/sign87.pdf.
4. Cancer Research UK. Available from: http://www.cancerresearchuk.org/.
5. Engel LS, Chow WH, Vaughan TL et al. (2003). Population attributable risks of oesophageal and gastric cancers. *J Natl Cancer Inst* 95, 1404–13.
6. Jacobson BC, Hirota W, Baron TH (2003). The role of endoscopy in the assessment and treatment of oesophageal cancer. *Gastrontest Endosc* 57, 817–22.
7. Graham DY, Schwartz JT, Cain GD, Gyorkey F (1982). Prospective evaluation of biopsy number in the diagnosis of oesophageal and gastric carcinoma. *Gastroenterology* 82, 228–31.
8. The Royal College of Surgeons of England (2008). National audit of oesophagogastric cancer report. Available from: http://www.rcseng.ac.uk/publications/docs/national-audit-of-oesophago-gastric-cancer-report-2008/.
9. Meyers BF, Downey RJ, Decker PA et al. (2007). The utility of positron emission tomography in staging of potentially operable carcinoma of the thoracic oesophagus: results of the American College of Surgeons Oncology Group Z0060 trial. *J Thorac Cardiovasc Surg* 133, 738–45.
10. Wallace MB, Nietert PJ, Earle C et al. (2002). An analysis of multiple staging management strategies for carcinoma of the oesophagus: computed tomography, endoscopic ultrasound, positron emission tomography, and thoracoscopy/laparoscopy. *Ann Thorac Surg* 74, 1026–32.

Barrett's oesophagus*

* The guidelines on this chapter have been sourced and summarized from different UK, Europe, and international government sources, professional organizations, and medical specialty societies. Leading guidelines have been listed in the Key guidelines box.

Barrett's oesophagus (columnar-lined oesophagus)

Key guidelines
- British Society of Gastroenterology (2005). Guidelines for the diagnosis and management of Barrett's columnar-lined oesophagus.
- National Institute for Health and Clinical Excellence (2007). Circumferential epithelial radiofrequency ablation for Barrett's oesophagus.
- National Institute for Health and Clinical Excellence (2004). Photodynamic therapy for high-grade dysplasia in Barrett's oesophagus.

Basic facts
- **Definition**—a condition that complicates chronic gastro-oesophageal reflux disease (GORD), in which any portion of the normal squamous lining of oesophagus is replaced by 'any' length of a histologically confirmed metaplastic columnar epithelium of intestinal type, visible macroscopically above the gastro-oesophageal junction (GOJ).[1] Barrett's oesophagus has recently been referred to as 'columnar-lined oesophagus (CLO)'. Short segment Barrett's refers to CLO with intestinal metaplasia that is less than 3cm in length.
- **Incidence**—in a catchment population of 250,000, the annual incidence is around 30 new cases per year.[1,6] Mean age at the time of diagnosis is 55. Male to female ratio is 2:1.[7] CLO is found in ~12% of patients undergoing endoscopy for GORD and 36% of patients with confirmed oesophagitis.[1,6,7]
- **Clinical presentation**—similar to chronic GORD. Heartburn, dysphagia, and bleeding are seen in ~50, 75, and 25% of CLO patients, respectively.[4] CLO is found more frequently in patients with severe and recurrent symptoms.[1] The metaplastic intestinal columnar metaplasia of Barrett's oesophagus causes no symptoms.[5]
- **Malignancy potential**—summarized in Table 25.1.

Recommended investigations

Upper GI endoscopy
- **Anatomical landmarks**—see Table 25.2.
- **Current diagnostic criteria.**
  - If the Z-line is located proximal to the GOJ line, a columnar-lined segment of oesophagus is diagnosed.
  - If biopsy specimens from this segment shows native oesophageal structures juxtapositioned to metaplastic glandular mucosa (whether intestinalized or not), Barrett's oesophagus (CLO) is diagnosed [C].
  - Histologic 'corroboration' (non-typical special histology) also represents high diagnostic possibility for CLO [C].[1]
  - In long segment CLO, the distance between Z-line and GOJ is ≥3cm; in short segment CLO, the distance is <3cm.
- **Accuracy and reliability**—see Table 25.3.

Table 25.1 Malignancy potentials of CLO[1,4,5]

- *Development*—GORD usually precedes CLO for up to 10y. About 30% of CLO patients develop ulcerations and strictures. Up to 5% of them develop dysplasia.
  - *Low-grade dysplasia*—progresses in 10–50% of patients into high-grade dysplasia within 2–5y.
  - *High-grade dysplasia*—will have a focus of invasive adenocarcinoma in 40–50% of cases at the time of diagnosis.
- *Risk factors for malignancy*—male patients, age >45, CLO segment >8cm, long duration of reflux symptoms, onset of GORD at early age, persistent GORD, presence of mucosal damage (ulceration and stricture), and possibly family history.
- *Overall malignancy risk*—30–fold above general population. The incidence of adenocarcinoma is 1–1.5% per y.

Table 25.2 Upper GI endoscopy—anatomic landmarks

- *GOJ*—imaginary line where the proximal limits of gastric folds are seen on retroflexing the endoscope and deflating the lumen.
- *Squamo-columnar junction (Z-line)*—the line where columnar epithelium (reddish, velvet-like area) joins the squamous epithelium (pale, glossy appearance area).
- *Lower oesophageal sphincter (LOS)*—difficult to reliably identify by endoscope and is not used for diagnosis purposes.

Table 25.3 Upper GI endoscopy—accuracy and reliability

- *Accuracy*—overall sensitivity and specificity of endoscopy with biopsy is ~80%.[1,5] Positive predictive value (correct correlation between detected CLO cases on endoscopy and definition) is ~35%. Negative predictive value (correct exclusion of CLO in negative endoscopy) is >95%.[1]
- *Reliability*—determined by the length of involved mucosa. Highly accurate and reliable if traditional Barrett's oesophagus definition with long segment CLO (>3cm) is used. Unreliable enough if short segment CLO is added to the definition.[1]

Recommended biopsy protocols
- No optimal protocol has been established. Most widely recommended protocol is to take quadrantic biopsies at 2cm intervals in the columnar segment together with biopsies of any visible lesion [C].[1]

Chromoscopy
- Does not give consistent sufficiently accurate results to justify its routine use in the diagnostic workout of CLO [C].[1]

Recommended treatment
General principles
- Management involves three main components: management of GORD, endoscopic screening for GORD patients, and treatment of proven CLO with and without dysplasia.

Management of GORD
- See 📖 Chapter 21, pp.149–161.

Endoscopic screening to detect CLO
- Not currently recommended for patients with chronic heartburn [C].[1] Diagnostic approach should follow the same principles as GORD.[1]

Recommended management of non-dysplastic CLO
- **Reflux symptoms control**—should follow the same GORD treatment principles (many have few or no symptoms). The absence of symptoms is not a reliable indicator for effective treatment [B].[1,4]
- **Proton pump inhibitors (PPIs)**—may require up to four times the standard daily dose to control symptoms and promote healing. Doses up to the maximal manufacturers' recommendations should be considered.[1]
- **Poorly controlled CLO** (poor symptom control and/or poor healing)—requires further assessment using pH monitoring [C].[1]
- **Surgical fundoplication**—indications should follow the same GORD approach. Surgical management is often more required in CLO patients (high-dose PPI therapy, higher incidence of hiatus hernia and LOS failure, reflux of duodenal contents). Fundoplication is currently NOT recommended on the sole basis of finding CLO in GORD patients [B].[1]
- **Endoscopic ablation**—effective in achieving squamous re-epithelialization, but remains experimental [C].[1]

Management of dysplastic CLO
- **Indefinite dysplasia**—a misleading diagnosis. Diagnosed if histologic changes suggest dysplasia, but definite diagnosis cannot be made due to inflammatory reaction. Treat aggressively with PPI and re-investigate early with new biopsies. If no definite dysplasia was detected in 6-month's follow-up, treat as 'CLO with no dysplasia' [C].[1]
- **Low-grade dysplasia**.
  - Treat aggressively with intensive acid suppression for 2–4mo, then re-biopsy [C].[1]
  - *Persistent low-grade dysplasia*—surveillance follow-up on 6-monthly bases. If regressed in two consequent occasions, increase surveillance to 2–3 yearly [C].[1]
- **High-grade dysplasia**—if persistent after intensive acid suppression.[1]
  - Confirm diagnosis by two expert pathologists.
  - Recommend oesophagectomy for fit patients [C].
  - Consider endoscopic ablation or mucosal resection for unfit patients [C].

Circumferential epithelial radiofrequency (RF) ablation[2]
- RF beam is used to obliterate a thin layer of oesophageal epithelium (containing CLO) for a few cm in length using endoscopy.
- The 12mo follow-up studies showed an overall efficiency of up to 69% with low transient morbidity.
- The procedure should only be used within the context of research due to insufficient evidence on safety and efficacy in the long term.[2]

Photodynamic therapy for high-grade dysplasia[3]

- A photosensitizing agent is administered, then activated using light beam to selected areas (containing CLO) to generate highly reactive oxygen molecules, leading to necrosis of the area.
- Follow-up studies showed an overall efficiency of 77–98% in downgrading the dysplasia, and 42–98% in eliminating the CLO. Strictures occurred in about a third of patients and photosensitivity (skin reaction) occurred in a third of them.
- The procedure has enough evidence to support its use in the clinical practice.[3] This should be done within a proper clinical governance framework as per NICE guidance.[3]

Further reading

1. British Society of Gastroenterology (2005). Guidelines for the diagnosis and management of Barrett's columnar-lined oesophagus. Available from: http://www.bsg.org.uk/pdf_word_docs/ Barretts_Oes.pdf.
2. National Institute for Health and Clinical Excellence (2007). Circumferential epithelial radiofrequency ablation for Barrett's oesophagus. Available from: http://www.nice.org.uk/ nicemedia/pdf/IPG244Guidance.pdf.
3. National Institute for Health and Clinical Excellence (2004). Photodynamic therapy for high-grade dysplasia in Barrett's oesophagus. Available from: http://guidance.nice.org.uk/IPG82.
4. Smith M, Soper N, Meyers B. Oesophagus. In: *The Washington manual of surgery*, 3rd ed, Lippincott Williams & Wilkins, Philadelphia.
5. UpToDate for patients (2008). Epidemiology, clinical manifestations and diagnosis of Barrett's oesophagus. Available from: http://www.uptodate.com/patients/content/topic.do? topicKey=~jGyGpYRK1NYDx.
6. Cameron AJ, Zinsmeister AR, Ballard DJ, Carney JA (1990). Prevalence of columnar-lined (Barrett's) oesophagus. Comparison of population-based clinical and autopsy findings. *Gastroenterology* 99, 918–22.
7. Cook MB, Wild CP, Forman D (2005). A systematic review and meta-analysis of the sex ratio for Barrett's oesophagus, erosive reflux disease, and non-erosive reflux disease. *Am J Epidemiol* 162, 1050–61.

Management of oesophageal variceal haemorrhage*

* The guidelines on this chapter have been sourced and summarized from different UK, Europe, and international government sources, professional organizations, and medical specialty societies. Leading guidelines have been listed in the Key guidelines box.

Management of oesophageal variceal haemorrhage

- Jalan R, Hayes PC (2000) UK guidelines on the management of variceal haemorrhage in cirrhotic patients.
- American Association for the Study of Liver Diseases, American College of Gastroenterology (2007) Prevention and management of gastro-oesophageal varices and variceal haemorrhage in cirrhosis.

Basic facts

- **Incidence**—affects ~25–40% of patients with cirrhosis, accounting for ~35% of all cirrhosis-related deaths. Varix bleeding is the source of upper GI bleeding in 50–90% of cases in cirrhosis patients.[1,4]
- **Pathogenesis**—varices develop as a decompression mechanism of hypertensive portal vein to return the blood to systemic circulation. They become apparent when the pressure gradient between portal and hepatic veins rises over 12mmHg. The average pressure gradient in bleeding varices is 20mmHg.[3]
- **Consensus definitions**—see Table 26.1.
- **Predicting 'at risk' patients.**
  - *Severity of liver dysfunction*—as estimated by Child classification. Bleeding occurs more frequently in severe cases.
  - *Patient history*—risk increases in active alcoholics, patients with previous history of variceal bleeding, and patients with ascites.
  - *Variceal pressure*—can be measured non-invasively during endoscopy. Bleeding risk increases from 0% at pressure <13mmHg to over 50% at pressure >15mmHg.
  - *Variceal size*—correlates well with the risk of bleeding. Varices can be small (straight), enlarged (tortuous varices occupying less than one third of the lumen), and large (coil-shaped, occupying more than one third of the lumen).
  - *Variceal location*—isolated gastric varices in fundus bleed more commonly than both gastro-oesophageal varices and isolated gastric varices in other sites.
  - *Appearance of varices*—risk increases with the presence of red wale marks (longitudinal red streaks on the varices), cherry red spots (discrete red cherry colour spots overlying the varices), haematocystic spots (raised discrete red spots overlying the varices), and diffuse erythema (diffuse red colour of the varices).

Recommended prophylaxis against first bleeding

- **Screening OGD**—recommended for all patients when diagnosis of cirrhosis is made [C].[1,2]
- **Cirrhotic patients with no varices**—repeat OGD in 3y interval [A]. Non-selective β-blockers are not recommended [B].[1,2]

Table 26.1 Consensus definitions in variceal bleeding

- *Time zero*—the time of first admission to a medical care centre.

- *Acute bleeding episode*—occurs when the bleeding events take place in the interval of 48h from time zero. Any bleeding during this time should be considered to reflect a failure of therapy rather than a re-bleeding event.

- *Clinically significant bleeding*—bleeding that requires a transfusion of ≥2 units of blood within 24h of time zero concurrently with a systolic BP of <100mmHg, a postural systolic change of >20mmHg, and/or a pulse rate of >100bpm at time zero.

- *Failure of therapy*—occurs in two time frames.
  - *0–6h*—transfusion requirement of >4 units and persistent systolic BP <70mmHg, inability to increase BP by 20mmHg, and/or persistent pulse rate >100bpm.
  - *Over 6h from time zero*—one or more events of haematemesis with increased pulse rate by 20bpm, drop in systolic BP of >20mmHg and the need for a transfusion of ≥2 units of blood to keep Hb at around 9g/dL.

- *Early re-bleeding*—occurs when the bleeding event occurs after 48h from the initial haemostasis counted from time zero, but less than 6wk.

- *Cirrhotic patients with small varices*—repeat OGD every 1–2y, depending on the presence or absence of signs of liver decompensation, the severity of cirrhosis, and the current use of β-blockers [A]. Non-selective β-blockers should be used for the prevention of first variceal haemorrhage in patients at very high risk [C]. Medium-risk patents can be considered for β-blockers, but long-term benefits remain unclear [B].
- *Cirrhotic patients with medium or large varices*—β-blockers should be instituted [A]. Endoscopic variceal ligation (EVL) is an acceptable alternative to β-blockers in high-risk patients, but remains inferior to β-blockers in low-risk patients [A].
- *Other treatment modalities*—nitrates (either alone or in combination with β-blockers), shunt therapy, or sclerotherapy have no proven role in the primary prophylaxis of variceal bleeding [A].

Recommended treatment for active bleeding (Fig. 26.1)[1,2]

- *Active resuscitation* [B].
  - Protect airways in severe, uncontrolled bleeding or severe encephalopathy.
  - Large bore peripheral IV lines or central line.
  - Cross-match 6 units of blood and replace blood loss with packed cells. Monitor carefully to avoid overtransfusion which may increase the risk of rebound portal hypertension and induced re-bleeding. Maintain the haemoglobin levels at about 8g/dL.
  - Replace clotting factors as needed.
  - Replace platelets if the count drops below 50,000/mm³ within the first 48h.
  - Monitor serum ionized calcium concentration in massive bleeding and replace as appropriate.

- *Prophylactic antibiotics.*
  - Short-term (maximum 1wk) antibiotic prophylaxis should be used in any patient with cirrhosis and GI bleeding. Oral or IV fluoroquinolone (ciprofloxacin) is recommended [A].
- *Control of bleeding.*
  - *OGD*—perform as soon as the patient is stable [A].
  - *EVL*—first treatment of choice [A]. Proper ligation is effective in over 90% of cases in controlling bleeding.
  - *Endoscopic variceal sclerotherapy*—should be used if EVL is technically difficult or unavailable [A]. Sclerotherapy is effective in 80% of cases in controlling bleeding.
  - *Somatostatin* (or its analogues octreotide)—use as soon as variceal haemorrhage is clinically suspected and there is no access to endoscopy (UK practice) [A].
- **Stent insertion for bleeding oesophageal varices**—has inadequate supporting evidence to recommend its use outside a strict clinical governance setting.

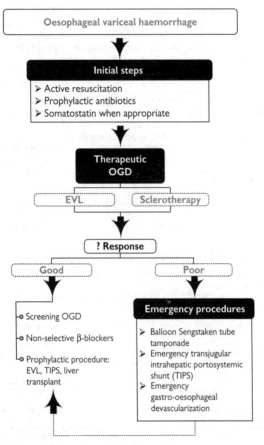

Fig 26.1 Approach to oesophageal variceal haemorrhage

- **Failure to control bleeding.**
  - *Balloon Sengstaken tube tamponade*—use temporarily (maximum 24h) in patients with uncontrollable bleeding until further definitive therapy (transjugular intrahepatic portosystemic shunt (TIPS) or endoscopic therapy) is instituted [B].
  - *TIPS*—consider in patients with difficult-to-control haemorrhage despite combined pharmacological and endoscopic therapy [B].

Recommended prevention of re-bleeding (Fig. 26.1)[1,2]

- **In general**—prophylaxis should be applied to all patients after surviving the episode of active bleeding [A].
- **Combination treatment: EVL (or sclerotherapy) + β-blocker.**
  - *EVL*—first method of choice [A]. Apply a single band on each varix at weekly intervals until all varices are eradicated [B]. Monitor with regular OGD at 3mo after obliteration, then every 6–12mo thereafter [A].
  - *Endoscopic variceal sclerotherapy*—should be used if EVL is technically difficult or unavailable [B]. Use the same interval protocols as above to treat each varix.
  - *β-blocker*—can be used alone in mild cases. Measure variceal pressure during treatment to ensure a safe level below 12mmHg [A].
- **TIPS**—more effective than endoscopic procedures, but does not increase survival. Consider in individual cases where expertise is available [A].
- **Liver transplant**—should be considered for eligible patients [C].

Further reading

1. Jalan R, Hayes PC (2000). UK guidelines on the management of variceal haemorrhage in cirrhotic patients. Available from: http://www.bsg.org.uk/pdf_word_docs/vari_hae.pdf.
2. American Association for the Study of Liver Diseases, American College of Gastroenterology (2007). Prevention and management of gastro-oesophageal varices and variceal haemorrhage in cirrhosis. Available from: http://www.guidelines.gov/summary/summary.aspx?doc_id=11370&nbr=005907&string=bleeding+AND+varices.
3. D'Amico G, Garcia-Pagán JC, Luca A, Bosch J (2006). Hepatic vein pressure gradient reduction and prevention of variceal bleeding in cirrhosis: a systematic review. *Gastroenterology* 131, 1611–24.
4. Odelowo OO, Smoot DT, Kim K (2002). Upper gastrointestinal bleeding in patients with liver disease. *J Natl Med Assoc* 94, 712–5.
5. National Institute for Health and Clinical Excellence (2008) Stent insertion for bleeding oesophageal varices. Available from: http://www.nice.org.uk/nicemedia/pdf/IPG265Guidance.pdf.

Part 4

Stomach and duodenum

Peptic ulcer disease*

* The guidelines on this chapter have been sourced and summarized from different UK, Europe, and international government sources, professional organizations, and medical specialty societies. Leading guidelines have been listed in the Key guidelines box.

Peptic ulcer disease

Key guidelines
- National Institute for Health and Clinical Excellence (2004) Dyspepsia: managing dyspepsia in adults in primary care.
- Scottish Intercollegiate Guidelines Network (2003) Dyspepsia: a national clinical guideline.
- University of Michigan Health System (2005) Peptic ulcer disease.

Basic facts
- *Definition*—abnormal gastrointestinal mucosal defect, caused by abnormal exposure to peptic juice, that extends through the muscularis mucosa layer, submucosa, or beyond.[1,5]
- *Incidence*—about 10% of the population in Europe and US suffer from an ulcer at some time in their life.[6] Peptic ulcers are found in 10–15% of patients investigated by endoscopy for dyspepsia.[1]
- *Risk factors*—three major risk factors attribute to 95% of cases: Helicobacter (H.) pylori infection, NSAIDs, and smoking (Table 27.1).[7]
- *Clinical presentation*—may remain asymptomatic, presents with typical or atypical symptoms, or present initially with complications (perforation, bleeding, or obstruction in ~20% of cases).[19] Symptoms have poor sensitivity, specificity, and predictive value for the presence of either duodenal ulcer (DU) or gastric ulcer (GU). Only 50% of patients with DU would have the classic ulcer-like dyspepsia, and only 15–25% of patients with ulcer-like dyspepsia would have an underlying peptic ulcer disease (gastroduodenitis is found in ~40% of such cases).[18]
  - *DU*—the typical 'hunger' pain occurs 90min to 3h after a meal, frequently relieved by antacids or food, and awakes patient from sleep between midnight and 3 am (most discriminating symptom that occurs in about two thirds of DU patients).[18]
  - *GU*—the pain typically precipitated by food, associated with nausea and weight loss (more commonly than DU). GU and DU patients can present with ill-defined burning or gnawing epigastric discomfort or ache.[18]

Recommended investigations (Fig. 27.1)
- *Initial approach*—should follow the general approach for dyspepsia (see Ch. 21). Confirmation of peptic ulcer by endoscopy or barium studies is neither necessary nor practical for every patient with dyspepsia in the absence of ALARM symptoms **[A]**.[1,2] Non-invasive H. pylori test is recommended as a first-line investigation in such patients.
- *Blood tests*—FBC, LFTs, and serum calcium are usually requested in patients with suspected peptic ulcer to exclude other diseases (e.g. liver disorders), and to identify patients with ALARM symptoms who require urgent endoscopy or other diagnostic testing.

Table 27.1 Risk factors for peptic ulcer

- *H. pylori infection*—presents in virtually all patients with DU and in ~70% of GU.[5] Eradication of H. pylori is associated with higher healing rate (92% vs 61% when H. pylori persists after treatment) and lower recurrence rate (21% vs 84% in a 12mo).[8–10]

- *NSAIDs*—within 90min of taking 300–600mg of aspirin, nearly everyone develops acute injury consisting of intramucosal petechiae and erosions.[11] GU and DU are found on endoscopy in 14–25% of NSAID users.[12] The overall RR is 2.74 for serious gastrointestinal event.[12]

- *Smoking*—when associated with H. pylori infection (RR × 2.2).[14]

- *Familial predisposition*—first-degree relatives of patients with peptic ulcer have ~3-fold increase in prevalence of ulcer.[15]

- *Blood group O*—indirect genetic link.[15,16]

- *High stress levels*—RR×3.2 in some, but not all studies.[14,17]

- *Corticosteroid use*

- *Others*—no clear evidence exists for exact diet or alcohol relation.

Table 27.2 H. pylori test—laboratory options

- *Carbon-13 urea breath test.*
  - *Preparation*—special arrangement for supervision required. Advise patients to keep fasting for a minimum of 6h before the test (if not diabetic where a special kit—diabact® UBT—should be used). Just before the test, patients should ingest citric acid or orange juice to slow gastric emptying.
  - *Performing the test*—two or three breath samples are tested before ingestion of the carbon-13 tablet. Patient should then blow through a straw into a series of glass screw-topped tubes. Another breath test should be repeated 30 minutes after carbon-13 ingestion.
  - *Breath samples*—should be sent for analysis by mass spectrometry. Results are available in ~24h.
  - *Accuracy*—very high (95% sensitivity and specificity).[1]

- *Stool antigen test*—cheaper test and no separate appointment required. Very high accuracy (95% sensitivity and specificity).

- *Laboratory-based ELISA serology test.*
  - *Indications*—acceptable alternative if validated appropriately.
  - *Accuracy*—sensitivity and specificity varies between different populations. Pay special precautions in interpreting results.

- *Campylobacter-like organism (CLO) test.*
  - *Indications*—patients undergoing endoscopy.
  - *Technique*—take biopsies and use the rapid urease test pot.
  - *Accuracy*—sensitivity and specificity are 85–90% and 98–100%, respectively.[1]

- *H. pylori test*—can be performed using different techniques depending on the setting and stage of the treatment.[1]
  - *Pre-treatment test* (before performing endoscopy)—best option is the carbon-13 urea breath test or stool antigen test (Table 27.2).
  - *Post-eradication testing*—best performed using a carbon-13 urea breath test only.[1]
  - *Special precautions*—reduce false negative results by stopping PPIs and antibiotics two and four weeks, respectively, before performing the *H. pylori* testing.
  - *Patients undergoing endoscopy*—use CLO test (Table 27.2).
- *Endoscopy*—the 'gold standard' investigation.
  - *Peptic ulcer appearance*—typically appears as mucosal defect with sharply demarcated edges and exposed underlying submucosa. Ulcer base is often clean and smooth, but can demonstrate eschar or adherent exudates in acute or bleeding cases. DU is more common in first part of duodenum.[18]
  - *Other benefits*—can take biopsies for suspicious lesions and test for *H. pylori*.
  - *Accuracy*—correctly diagnose the peptic ulcers (positive and negative predictive values) in >95% of cases.[20]
  - *Risks*—morbidity and mortality rates are low (1 in 200 and 1 in 2,000, respectively, in the UK).[1]
- *Barium studies*—still used in some cases (e.g. patient refusing endoscopy) as first-line test for confirming peptic ulcer disease where appropriate.[1]
  - *Accuracy*—depends on the skills, techniques, and interests of the radiologist, and the ability of patient to cooperate.[21] Single contrast studies can detect ~50% of DUs.[21] Double contrast studies can detect 80–90% of DUs. GU detection rate varies considerably depending on the technique used.[1,21]

Recommended treatment (Fig. 27.1)

- *General approach*—should be multimodal, including lifestyle adjustment, eradication of *H. pylori* infection, managing the NSAID, anti-secretory therapy, and/or surgery when indicated.[1]
- *Lifestyle adjustment*—advice for healthy eating, weight reduction, and smoking cessation.[1]
  - *Healthy eating*—benefits the general health as well and should be encouraged. Advise against any identifiable precipitating factor (e.g. alcohol, caffeine, chocolate, fatty or spicy foods).
  - *Smoking*—in the pre-*H. pylori* era, smokers were more likely to develop ulcers and have recurrence. Smokers post-eradication of *H. pylori* have similar rate of ulcer relapse (~3.6% for smokers vs 2% for non-smokers).[23]
  - *Reflux symptoms*—advise on eating smaller meals, avoiding meals before going to sleep, and raising the bed head.

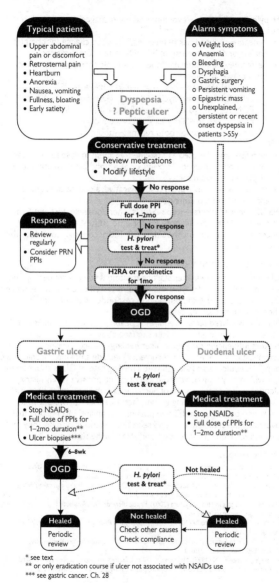

Typical patient
- Upper abdominal pain or discomfort
- Retrosternal pain
- Heartburn
- Anorexia
- Nausea, vomiting
- Fullness, bloating
- Early satiety

Alarm symptoms
- Weight loss
- Anaemia
- Bleeding
- Dysphagia
- Gastric surgery
- Persistent vomiting
- Epigastric mass
- Unexplained, persistent or recent onset dyspepsia in patients >55y

Dyspepsia ? Peptic ulcer

Conservative treatment
- Review medications
- Modify lifestyle

No response

Full dose PPI for 1–2mo

No response

H. pylori test & treat*

No response

H2RA or prokinetics for 1mo

Response
- Review regularly
- Consider PRN PPIs

No response

OGD

Gastric ulcer

Duodenal ulcer

H. pylori test & treat*

Medical treatment
- Stop NSAIDs
- Full dose of PPIs for 1–2mo duration**
- Ulcer biopsies***

Medical treatment
- Stop NSAIDs
- Full dose of PPIs for 1–2mo duration**

6–8wk

OGD

Not healed

H. pylori test & treat*

Healed
Periodic review

Not healed
Check other causes
Check compliance

Healed
Periodic review

* see text
** or only eradication course if ulcer not associated with NSAIDs use
*** see gastric cancer. Ch. 28

Fig. 27.1 Approach to patients with suspected/proven peptic ulcer

- *H. pylori eradication*—revolutionized the management and reduced the need for surgical intervention.[1]
  - *Benefits*—reduced risk of bleeding, increased chance for complete healing, and reduced risk of NSAID-related complications.
  - *Recommended treatment*—one-week triple therapy regimen with a PPI and two antibiotics.
    - Optimal regimes—PAC regimen (double dose PPI + amoxicillin 1g + clarithromycin 500mg, all given twice a day) or the PCM regimen (double dose PPI + clarithromycin 250mg + metronidazole 400mg, all given twice a day).[1]
    - Eradication rate for both regimes—about 82%.[1]
- *PPI.*
  - *Benefits*—may be used as first-line treatment in dyspepsia, as part of eradication therapy for *H. pylori*, or as a stand-alone treatment for *H. pylori*-negative ulcers.
  - *Indications*—if the *H. pylori* test is negative, a course of full dose PPI for 1–2mo is recommended.
- *NSAID-induced ulcers*—stop NSAIDs where possible, test and treat *H. pylori*, and start on full dose PPI for 2mo. Re-test for *H. pylori* is necessary and treatment should be tailored accordingly to reduce the recurrence rate.[1]

Recommended follow-up

- *GU*—re-scope 6–8wk after starting treatment to confirm healing and exclude malignancy. *H. pylori* should be re-tested to confirm clearance.[1]
- *DU*—re-test for *H. pylori* only in non-respondents to eradication therapy or for relapsing cases.[1]
- *NSAID-associated ulcer*—requires repeating endoscopy and *H. pylori* re-testing according to the ulcer site (see above).
- *Factors influencing the peptic ulcer healing*— (ulcer healing, complications, tendency for recurrence) include smoking, chronic usage of NSAIDs, ulcer size (the estimated healing rate of GU is about 3mm per wk), very young or very old age of onset, positive family history, alcohol abuse, consumption of human milk (which contains potentially protective factors, including growth factors, surface active phospholipids, and prostaglandin E2, and possibly has an anti-ulcer action that overrides the stimulation of acid secretion), stenosis or deformity of the duodenal bulb or ulcer bed, and stressful life situations.[7,10,14,17,22]

Further reading

1. National Institute for Health and Clinical Excellence (2004). Dyspepsia: managing dyspepsia in adults in primary care. Available from: http://guidance.nice.org.uk/CG17.
2. Scottish Intercollegiate Guidelines Network (2003). Dyspepsia: a national clinical guideline. Available from: http://www.sign.ac.uk/pdf/sign68.pdf.
3. University of Michigan Health System (2005). Peptic ulcer disease. Available from: http://www.guideline.gov/summary/summary.aspx?doc_id=7406.
4. Kumar V, Abbas AK, Fausto N (2004). *Robbins and Cotran Pathologic basis of disease*, 7th ed. Saunders, London.
5. Johnson A (2001). Peptic ulcer. stomach and duodenum. In: *Oxford Textbook of Surgery*, 2nd ed. Oxford University Press, Oxford.
6. Kurata JH, Nogawa AN (1997). Meta-analysis of risk factors for peptic ulcer, non-steroidal anti-inflammatory drugs, Helicobacter pylori, and smoking. *J Clin Gastroenterol* 24, 2–17.

7. Marshall BJ, Goodwin CS, Warren JR (1988). Prospective double-blind trial of duodenal ulcer relapse after eradication of Campylobacter pylori. *Lancet* 2, 1437–42.

8. Hopkins RJ, Girardi LS, Turney EA (1996). Relationship between Helicobacter pylori eradication and reduced duodenal and gastric ulcer recurrence: a review. *Gastroenterology* 110, 1244–52.

9. Laine L, Hopkins RJ, Girardi LS (1998). Has the impact of Helicobacter pylori therapy on ulcer recurrence in the United States been overstated? A meta-analysis of rigorously designed trials. *Am J Gastroenterol* 93, 1409–15.

10. Seager JM, Hawkey CJ (2001). ABC of the upper gastrointestinal tract: indigestion and non-steroidal anti-inflammatory drugs. *BMJ* 323, 1236–9.

11. Russell RI (2001). Non-steroidal anti-inflammatory drugs and gastrointestinal damage—problems and solutions. *Postgrad Med J* 77, 82–8.

12. Richy F, Bruyere O, Ethgen O (2004). Time-dependent risk of gastrointestinal complications induced by non-steroidal anti-inflammatory drug use: a consensus statement using a meta-analytic approach. *Ann Rheum Dis* 63, 759–66.

13. Räihä I, Kemppainen H, Kaprio J, Koskenvuo M, Sourander L (1998). Lifestyle, stress, and genes in peptic ulcer disease: a nationwide twin cohort study. *Arch Intern Med* 158, 698–704.

14. Hein HO, Suadicani P, Gyntelberg F (1997). Genetic markers for peptic ulcer. A study of 3,387 men aged 54 to 74 years: the Copenhagen Male Study. *Scand J Gastroenterol* 32, 16–21.

15. Sidebotham RL, Baron JH, Schrager J, Spencer J, Clamp JR, Hough L (1995). Influence of blood group and secretor status on carbohydrate structures in human gastric mucins: implications for peptic ulcer. *Clin Sci (Lond)* 89, 405–15.

16. Peters MN, Richardson CT (1983). Stressful life events, acid hypersecretion, and ulcer disease. *Gastroenterology* 84, 114–9.

17. Del Valle J (2005). Peptic ulcer disease and related disorders. In: *Harrison's Principles of Internal Medicine*, pp. 1747–62, 16th ed, McGraw-Hill Companies, Inc Publishing Group.

18. Pounder R (1989). Silent peptic ulceration: deadly silence or golden silence? *Gastroenterology* 96 (2 Pt 2 Suppl), 626–31.

19. Cotton PB, Shorvon PJ (1984). Analysis of endoscopy and radiography in the diagnosis, follow-up and treatment of peptic ulcer disease. *Clin Gastroenterol* 13, 383–403.

20. Levine MS (1995). Role of the double contrast upper gastrointestinal series in the 1990s. *Gastroenterol Clin North Am* 24, 289–308.

21. Eastwood GL (1997). Is smoking still important in the pathogenesis of peptic ulcer disease? *J Clin Gastroenterol* 25 (Suppl 1), S1–7.

22. Chan FK, Sung JJ, Lee YT et al. (1997). Does smoking predispose to peptic ulcer relapse after eradication of Helicobacter pylori? *Am J Gastroenterol* 92, 442–5.

Gastric cancer*

* The guidelines on this chapter have been sourced and summarized from different UK, Europe, and international government sources, professional organizations, and medical specialty societies. Leading guidelines have been listed in the **Key guidelines** box.

Gastric cancer

Basic facts

- *Incidence*—seventh most common cancer in the UK and second most common cause of cancer mortality worldwide.[4] Incidence rises steadily after the age of forty. Over 80% of cases are diagnosed after the age of 65.[1] The male to female ratio is 1.7:1.[4]
- *Risk factors*—usually related to external exposure (dietary habits, smoking), medical conditions (atrophic gastritis), and genetic factors (Table 28.1).
- *Clinical presentation*—over 85% of gastric cancers present initially with locally advanced or metastatic stage and poor resectability.[15,16] *Early gastric cancer* presents with dyspepsia in ~70% of cases and/or ALARM symptoms in ~10% of cases.[1,16] Dyspepsia in the general population is caused by cancer in only 1.6–4% of cases.[14] *Advanced cancers* present with palpable lymph nodes, ascites, jaundice, and/or palpable abdominal or pelvic mass (Table 28.2).[1,15,17–22]

Recommended investigations

- *General approach*—should follow dyspepsia pathway (see 📖 Chapter 21, pp.149–160) as appropriate.
- *Upper GI endoscopy*—first investigation of choice to confirm diagnosis and obtain sufficient tissue biopsies [B].[1]
  - *Endoscopic findings*—early gastric cancers appear as shallow ulcer, polypoid, flat, or plaque-like lesions. Advanced cancers appear typically as an ulcerated mass or a large ulcer with irregular beaded-like borders. The ulcer base is usually necrotic and shaggy.[23]
- *Pathologic confirmation*—multiple biopsies and brushings should always be obtained from suspicious lesions [B].[1,3,6]
  - *Biopsy detection rate*—ranges from 70% for one biopsy to 98% for seven biopsies.[24] Using a combination of strip and bite biopsy techniques for suspicious diffuse types of gastric cancer is recommended.[25]

Table 28.1 Risk factors for gastric cancer

- **Dietary factors**—very important role. More common in persons consuming diet rich in complex carbohydrates (egg, fava beans), smoked, salted or pickled foods, cooking oil, and dried fish.[1,6,7]

- **Smoking and alcohol**—possible link but magnitude of effect is unclear.[1]

- **Medical conditions.**
  - **Chronic atrophic gastritis**—with intestinal metaplasia. Precursor for gastric cancer. ~10% of patients develop gastric cancer.[1]
  - **H. pylori infection**—estimated relative risk (RR) × 2–6.[1,8]
  - **Pernicious anaemia**—RR 2–3.[9]
  - **Benign gastric ulcer**—incidence ratio over 9y is 1.8.[10]
  - **Subtotal gastric resection**—RR 1.5–3.[11]
  - **Gastric polyps**—over 2cm in size.[12]
  - **Barrett's oesophagus**—precursor for proximal gastric cancers (gastric cardia and distal oesophageal cancer). Estimated risk is 0.2–2% per y.[13]

- **Familial predisposition**—small (2–4 fold) increased risk in patients with first-degree relative with gastric cancer.[1]

- **Primary prevention**—may be achieved by encouraging increased fruit and vegetables consumption (up to 5 servings/day) and H. pylori detection and eradication.[1]

Table 28.2 Signs of advanced gastric cancer

- **Direct extension**—palpable abdominal mass (poor prognostic sign, but not in itself an indication of inoperable disease).[17]

- **Lymph node spread**—periumbilical nodule (Sister Mary Joseph's node), left supraclavicular adenopathy (Virchow's node).

- **Peritoneal spread**—enlarged ovary (Krukenberg's tumour), mass in the pelvic on rectal periotoneum examination (Blumer's shelf), ascites.

- **Liver metastasis**—palpable liver mass, elevated serum alkaline phosphatase, jaundice.

- **Paraneoplastic manifestations**—diffuse seborrhoeic keratoses (sign of Leser–Trelat), microangiopathic haemolytic anemia , membranous nephropathy, hypercoagulable states (Trousseau's syndrome).

Recommended initial staging

- **Clinical assessment**—only those patients with an ASA score of 3 or less should be considered for surgery [B*].[1]
- **Basic investigations**—baseline haematological and biochemical profile, ABGs on air, PFTs, CXR, and ECG [B]. Check results and optimize as appropriate.[1,3]
- **Spiral thoracic and abdominal contrast CT scan.**
  - *Indications*—first staging investigation to evaluate the presence of metastatic disease [B].[1]
  - *Technique*—thin (5mm) slices and gastric distension with 600–800mL of water are recommended.

- *Accuracy*—below 80% accuracy in identifying advanced disease in gastric cancer.
- *TNM staging*—see Table 28.3.
- **Nutritional assessment**
  - *Effect on surgery*—risk increases in patients with BMI <18.5, BMI <90% of predicted value, recent weight loss of >20%, and low serum albumin.[1] Obesity increases the risk as well.
  - *Optimization*—essential part of the perioperative care. Nutritional support (enteral or parenteral) should be considered on all patients in the pre- and post-operative period [B].[1,6]
- **MDT discussion**—essential requirement prior to commencing any definitive staging or treatment [C].[1] Decisions are taken in the context of predicted prognosis and expected effect of any investigation or treatment intervention on quality of life.[1]
- **Breaking bad news**—essential step to ensure adequate compliance. Should be done in a professional and effective way. The role of cancer care nurse is essential.[1]
  - *Recommended points to discuss*—confirmation of diagnosis, available treatment options, expected perioperative period experience, contact details, and sources for further information (including patient support groups). Discussion should be documented and communicated to other members of the team (GP, oncologists, breast care nurses, etc.).
- **Advanced staging**—only required if the patient is a good candidate for surgical resection.[1]

Table 28.3 TNM staging on CT scan

- **T staging.**
  - *T1 to T3*—unreliable in differentiating T1 from T2 cancers or in accurate estimation of microscopic invasion in T3, namely the differentiation between transmural extension and perigastric lymphadenopathy.[1]
  - *T4*—can be identified by finding:
    - Intimate contact between tumour and contiguous organs
    - Focal loss of intervening fat plane
    - Clear CT scan evidence of direct organ invasion.[1]

- **N staging.**
  - *Accuracy*—node involvement can be identified in 50–60% of cases.[1]
  - *Criteria*—node size is the main criterion used for identification and still of low accuracy (48% sensitivity and 93% specificity if size >8mm was considered abnormal in the coeliac axis).[1] The number of involved lymph nodes is more important than the distance from the primary tumour in the current TNM classification system.[1]

- **M staging.**
  - *Accuracy*—metastatic disease can be detected in 75–80% of cases using newer techniques. Can only detect 50% of lesions with size <1.5cm.[1]

Table 28.4 TNM staging on EUS

- *T staging*—can identify the different layer structure of stomach wall. Unable to delineate the omental reflections around the stomach clearly, and difficult or impossible to know if the carcinoma has penetrated the muscularis propria into the greater or lesser omenta (T2), but not breached the visceral peritoneum beyond (T3).[1,7] Accuracy does not exceed 77% for staging the depth of invasion.

- *N staging*—accurate and reliable. Features like well-defined margins of nodes over 1cm in diameter, rounded, and hypoechoic nodes are likely to correlate well with malignant infiltration.[1] Accuracy is ~69% for nodal stage.[27]

- *M staging*—small volumes of ascites can be demonstrated (possible diffuse peritoneal spread).[1]

Recommended advanced staging

- *Patient selection*—all patients without evidence of metastatic disease on CT scan, who are eligible for curative surgery, should undergo endoscopic ultrasonography (EUS), if available [B].[1,3]
- *EUS*—superior to CT scan for local staging of gastric cancer and more accurate in predicting resectability (Table 28.4).[1]
- *Laparoscopy*—recommended for all gastric cancer patients following CT and EUS prior to consideration of radical resection.
  - *Accuracy*—the only reliable method to detect peritoneal dissemination in apparently localized disease.[2] Can diagnose peritoneal metastases in ~25% of patients with clear CT scan.[28]
- *Other recommended investigations.*
  - Positron Emission Tomography (PET)—is superior to CT scan or EUS in detecting distant metastasis.
  - *Transabdominal USS*—indicated if treatment options are limited and good clinical evidence of liver metastasis exists. Confirmation of disease extent is required before commencing palliative treatment [C].[1,3]
  - *MRI scan*—has no advantages over spiral CT scan in most cases. Usually used in certain individual cases such as the allergy to IV contrast or the need for specific extra details [C].[1,3]
  - *Tumour markers*—have no practical use.
- *TNM staging*—Table 28.4

Recommended treatment

General approach

- Surgical resection with curative intent should be offered to all patients who are medically fit for surgery and who have a potentially resectable cancer [D].[1,3] Complete surgical resection with resection of adjacent lymph nodes represents the best opportunity for long-term survival. Only a small proportion of patients will be deemed suitable for potential complete curative treatment, and less than a third will be able to have a curative resection.[1]

Standards for surgical resection

- *Preoperative preparation*—should include psychological preparation, thromboembolic and antibiotic prophylaxis, and blood cross-matching.[1]
- *Resection extent*—see Table 28.5.
- *Outlines of recommended surgical approach*—see Table 28.6.

- *Oncological standards.*
  - *Main objectives*—to achieve a balance between macroscopic clearance and reduced morbidity. Well described by the Japanese classification for gastric cancer.[1,31]

Table 28.5 Stomach cancer resection—definitions

- *R0 (curative resection)*—surgery with no macroscopic or microscopic residual cancer at the resection margins. Less than a third of patients can have curative resection.[1,30]
- *R1*—surgery with positive margins due to microscopic residual cancer.
- *R2*—surgery with positive margins and gross (macroscopic) residual cancer.

Table 28.6 Stomach cancer resection—selection

- *Early or well-circumscribed cancers*—subtotal gastrectomy is recommended if the site of cancer allows a margin of >2cm proximally away from the cardia.
- *Infiltrative cancers*—require 5cm clearance. Total gastrectomy is recommended if clearance is deemed impossible and the tumour is diffuse (with submucosal infiltration).
- *Junctional tumours*—consider proximal oesophageal margin of 5cm. Lower cancers require total gastrectomy and abdominal lymphadenectomy.

Table 28.7 Lymph node dissection—definitions

- *D1 resection (limited lymphadenectomy)*—excision of primary cancer, omenta, and first tiers of lymph nodes (N1) which drain the affected area of the stomach.
- *D2 resection (systemic lymphadenectomy)*—excision of primary cancer, omentum, and first two tiers of lymph nodes (N1 and N2).
- *Extended lymphadenectomy*—excision of lymph nodes beyond the second tier (e.g. hepatoduodenal ligament lymph nodes).

Table 28.8 Lymph node dissection—selection

- **Extent of lymph node dissection**—remains controversial. In summary:
  - Multicentre trials have shown no clear-cut significant survival benefits for D2 over D1 resection for curable gastric cancer.
  - The International Gastric Cancer Association consensus recommends D2 resection for all respectable gastric cancers, although mortality seems to be higher.
  - Many US centres recommend removal of >15 lymph nodes to achieve adequate dissection.[30]
  - Surgeon experience, age and fitness of patient, stage of cancer, and workload of cancer centre should all be taken into consideration.[1,5,30]

- *Margins of resection*—about or over 5cm from the gross tumour is currently recommended by most cancer centres.[1,30,31] Transmural tumours (T4) may benefit from resection of adjacent organs if the patient is fit enough to tolerate radical surgery. No macroscopic residual disease should be allowed.
- *Lymph node resection*
  - Definitions—see Table 28.7.
  - Extent of lymph node dissection—see Table 28.8.
- *Reconstruction*—usually achieved with a Roux–en–Y or Billroth II gastrojejunostomy.
- **Outcome measures.**
  - *Curative resection (R0)*—achieved when all evidence of cancer is removed.
  - *Absolute curative resection*—achieved if at least one tier of nodes beyond those affected is removed.
- **Endoscopic mucosal resection (EMS)**—should be considered in early gastric cancer (T1, mucosal, and submucosal) if appropriate experience exists.[1,30] Indicated in well or moderately differentiated histology types, tumour of less than 30mm in size, and in the absence of ulceration or any other invasive features.[30]
- **Laparoscopic gastrectomy for cancer**—current evidence supports the use of this procedure by adequately trained laparoscopic surgeons for the management of operable gastric cancer patients.[34] The procedure should only be performed within appropriate clinical governance setting. Patient selection should involve appropriate multidisciplinary team (MDT).
  - *Indications*—most gastric cancers amenable to open surgical treatment.
  - *Efficacy*—when performed by a well-trained surgeon in an appropriate centre, laparoscopic surgery has similar efficiency to open surgery in terms of resection margins, cancer-free survival rate, and 30d mortality rate.[34] Laparoscopic surgery was found in a meta-analysis of 1,611 cases to be inferior to open surgery in terms of lymph node retrieval (mean difference 4.4 nodes, p<0.001).[34]
  - *Safety*—laparoscopic surgery has a lower complication rate (OR = 0.54) compared to open surgery.

Recommendation for chemoradiotherapy
- *Adjuvant chemotherapy*—increases survival (just marginal, OR = 0.80) when compared with surgery alone.[1,4,30] Insufficient evidence to recommend for all patients. Age, comorbidities, and expected beneficial effects should be considered in individual cases.
- *Neo-adjuvant chemotherapy*—improves 5y survival rate (36% in 'perioperative chemotherapy' groups vs 23% in 'surgery alone' group), but still inconclusive, and should only be considered in selected cases.
- *Chemoradiotherapy*—under investigation.

Recommendation for palliative treatment
- *General approach*—appropriate palliative treatment plan should be formulated at the MDT meeting for patients with inoperable cancers. Direct involvement of the palliative care team is recommended.
- *Options.*
  - *Endoscopic methods*—include oesophageal dilatation, alcohol injection therapy, oesophageal intubation, radiotherapy, and laser therapy.
  - *Limited surgical resection*—indicated in locally advanced incurable cancers complicated with bleeding, obstruction, or perforation.
  - *Chemotherapy*—offers a significant survival and quality of life benefits when compared with best supportive care alone.[1,30]

Recommended follow-up
- *Schedule*—no one optimal schedule. One accepted protocol is follow-up every 4–6mo initially for 3y, then annually thereafter.[30]
- *The visit*—take a detailed history and physical examination. Request FBC, multichannel serum chemistry analysis (SMA-12) tests, and endoscopy if clinically indicated. Supplement with vitamin B12 as appropriate for patients with proximal or total gastrectomy.[30]

Know your results

Effectiveness of gastric cancer diagnosis and treatment—audit areas[33]

The National Oesophagogastric Cancer audit—setting good example
- *Standards*—to measure the quality of care received by patients with oesophagogastric cancer in the UK, and to assess whether care is consistent with recommended practice.
- *Indicators*—the timescale of the process of care, determinants of treatment and outcomes, the factors that influence decisions about curative and palliative treatment, short-term outcomes of surgical treatment, survival at 1y, quality of life, and patient satisfaction with care.[33]

Further reading

1. Allum WH, Griffin SM, Watson A, Colin–Jones D; Association of Upper Gastrointestinal Surgeons of Great Britain and Ireland, British Society of Gastroenterology, British Association of Surgical Oncology (2002). Guidelines for the management of oesophageal and gastric cancer. *Gut* 50 (Suppl 5), v1–23.

2. National Institute for Health and Clinical Excellence (2004). Dyspepsia: managing dyspepsia in adults in primary care. Available from: http://guidance.nice.org.uk/CG17.

3. Scottish Intercollegiate Guidelines Network (2003). Dyspepsia: a national clinical guideline. Available from: http://www.sign.ac.uk/pdf/sign68.pdf.

4. Cancer Research UK. Available from: http://www.cancerresearchuk.org/.

5. BMJ Clinical Evidence. Gastric cancer, 2006. URL: http://clinicalevidence.bmj.com/ceweb/conditions/dsd/0404/0404.jsp. Accessed May 2009

6. Ngoan LT, Mizoue T, Fujino Y, Tokui N, Yoshimura T (2002). Dietary factors and stomach cancer mortality. Br J Cancer 87, 37–42.

7. Joossens JV, Hill MJ, Elliott P et al. (1996). Dietary salt, nitrate and stomach cancer mortality in 24 countries. European Cancer Prevention (ECP) and the INTERSALT Cooperative Research Group. Int J Epidemiol 25, 494–504.

8. Forman D, Newell DG, Fullerton F (1991). Association between infection with Helicobacter pylori and risk of gastric cancer: evidence from a prospective investigation. BMJ 302, 1302–5.

9. Hsing AW, Hansson LE, McLaughlin JK et al. (1993). Pernicious anaemia and subsequent cancer. A population-based cohort study. Cancer 71, 745–50.

10. Hansson LE, Nyren O, Hsing AW et al. (1996). The risk of stomach cancer in patients with gastric or duodenal ulcer disease. N Engl J Med 335, 242–9.

11. Tersmette AC, Offerhaus GJ, Tersmette KW et al. (1990). Meta-analysis of the risk of gastric stump cancer: detection of high risk patient subsets for stomach cancer after remote partial gastrectomy for benign conditions. Cancer Res 50, 6486–9.

12. Nakamura T, Nakano G (1985). Histopathological classification and malignant change in gastric polyps. J Clin Pathol 38, 754–64.

13. Drewitz DJ, Sampliner RE, Garewal HS (1997). The incidence of adenocarcinoma in Barrett's oesophagus: a prospective study of 170 patients followed 4.8 years. Am J Gastroenterol 92, 212–5.

14. Arents NL, Thijs JC, Kleibeuker JH (2002). A rational approach to uninvestigated dyspepsia in primary care: review of the literature. Postgrad Med J 78, 707–16.

15. Dicken BJ, Bigam DL, Cass C, Mackey JR, Joy AA, Hamilton SM (2005). Gastric adenocarcinoma: review and considerations for future directions. Ann Surg 241, 27–39.

16. Stephens MR, Lewis WG, White S et al. (2005). Prognostic significance of alarm symptoms in patients with gastric cancer. Br J Surg 92, 840–6.

17. Barr et al. Carcinoma of the stomach. In: Oxford Textbook of Surgery, 2nd ed. Oxford University Press, Oxford.

18. Pieslor PC, Hefter LG (1986). Umbilical metastasis from prostatic carcinoma—Sister Joseph nodule. Urology 27, 558–9.

19. Morgenstern L (1979). The Virchow–Troisier node: a historical note. Am J Surg 138, 703.

20. Gilliland R, Gill PJ (1992). Incidence and prognosis of Krukenberg tumour in Northern Ireland. Br J Surg 79, 1364–6.

21. Winne Burchard BE (1965). Blumer's shelf tumour with primary carcinoma of the lung. A case report. J Int Coll Surg 44, 477–81.

22. Fuchs CS, Mayer RJ (1995). Gastric carcinoma. N Engl J Med 333, 32–41.

23. Mulholland M (2006). Gastric neoplasms. In: Greenfield's surgery: scientific principles and practice, 2nd ed, Lippincott Williams & Wilkins, Philadelphia.

24. Graham DY, Schwartz JT, Cain GD, Gyorkey F (1982). Prospective evaluation of biopsy number in the diagnosis of oesophageal and gastric carcinoma. Gastroenterology 82, 228–31.

25. Karita M, Tada D (1994). Endoscopic and histologic diagnosis of submucosal tumours of the gastrointestinal tract using combined strip biopsy and bite biopsy. Gastrointest Endosc 40, 749–53.

26. Sussman SK, Halvorsen RA Jr, Illescas FF et al. (1988). Gastric adenocarcinoma: CT versus surgical staging. Radiology 167, 335–40.

27. Pollack BJ, Chak A, Sivak MV Jr (1996). Endoscopic ultrasonography. Semin Oncol 23, 336–46.

28. Conlon KC, Karpeh MS Jr (1996). Laparoscopy and laparoscopic ultrasound in the staging of gastric cancer. Semin Oncol 23, 347–51.

29. Yoshida S, Saito D (1996). Gastric pre-malignancy and cancer screening in high-risk patients. Am J Gastroenterol 91, 839–43.

30. National Comprehensive Cancer Network (2007). Clinical practice guidelines in oncology: gastric cancer. Available from: http://www.nccn.org/index.asp.

31. Japanese Research Society for Gastric Cancer (1995). Japanese classification of gastric cancer, 1st English ed, Kanehara & Co Ltd, Tokyo.

32. Cunningham D, Allum WH, Stenning SP *et al.* (2006). Perioperative chemotherapy versus surgery alone for respectable gastroesophageal cancer. *N Engl J Med* 355, 11–20.
33. The Royal College of Surgeons of England (2008). National audit of oesophago-gastric cancer report. Available from: http://www.rcseng.ac.uk/publications/docs/national-audit-of-oesophago-gastric-cancer-report-2008/.
34. National Institute for Health and Clinical Excellence (2008). Laparoscopic gastrectomy of cancer. Available from: http://www.nice.org.uk/Guidance/IPG269.

Neuroendocrine tumours (NETs)*

* The guidelines on this chapter have been sourced and summarized from different UK, Europe, and international government sources, professional organizations, and medical specialty societies. Leading guidelines have been listed in the **Key guidelines** box.

Neuroendocrine tumours (NETs)

Key guidelines

- UKNETwork for neuroendocrine tumours (2005). Guidelines for the management of gastro-enteropancreatic neuroendocrine (including carcinoid) tumours.
- European Neuroendocrine Tumour Society (2007).
- National Comprehensive Cancer Network (2008). Practice guidelines: neuroendocrine tumours.

Basic facts

- **Definition**—neuroendocrine tumours (NETs) originate in the enterochromaffin cells (part of neuroendocrine cell system scattered throughout the body). NETs consist of a heterogeneous group of tumours that share specific 'biological' features and classified into one entity.[1] NETs can be benign or malignant, functional or non-functional, may occur in the pancreas, stomach, small or large bowel, and can be diagnosed based on the function (gastrinoma, insulinoma, etc.) or the mass effect.
- **Incidence**—rare. NETS affect ~2–3 per 100,000 population per year.[1,3,7] Females are more affected, especially in the fifth decade. NETs run in families; the estimated life risk of developing NETs in individuals with one affected first-degree relative is ~4 times compared to the general population, rising to 12 times in the presence of two affected first-degree relatives.[1,7]
- **Pathobiology**—very slow growing malignant tumours with the potential risk of metastasizing to lymph nodes, liver, bone, lungs, and brain (Table 29.1).[1,3]
- **Clinical presentation**—most NETs remain asymptomatic or present with non-specific symptoms due to the local or metabolic effects (Table 29.2).

Recommended investigations

- **General approach**—the diagnosis requires a high index of suspicion and judicious combination of clinical, hormonal, radiological, and other imaging findings.[1,3] Histopathologic confirmation defines the management plan.[1]
- **Baseline tests**—should include chromogranin A (CgA) test and 5-hydroxyindoleacetic acid (5-HIAA) test in the case of carcinoid (of no value in pancreatic NET) [D].[1,3]
  - **Plasma CgA**—large protein produced by all neural crest-derived cells, and in very significant quantities by NET cells.[1,3] CgA role in accurate monitoring of progression remains unclear.[1]
  - **Urine 5-HIAA**—remarkably raised in certain NETs syndrome (70% in midgut tumours, sometimes in foregut tumours, and never in hindgut tumours).
  - **Other tests**—see Table 29.3.
- **Imaging tests**—should be based on clinical suspicion.[1] Imaging tests include USS, CT, endoscopy, MRI, somatostatin receptor scintigraphy (SSRS), EUS, PET, and other selected imaging modalities (e.g. 5H-tryptamine imaging).

Table 29.1 Pathobiology of NETs

- *Frequency of primary NETs*—appendix (35% of total), ileum (15% of total), lung (15% of total), rectum (10% of total), and pancreas (5% of total).[1]

- *Genetics*—most occur sporadically as isolated tumours and few as part of complex familial endocrine cancer syndromes, including multiple endocrine neoplasia (MEN) type 1 and 2, and neurofibromatosis type 1 (NF1). MEN1 incidence varies from 30% in gastrinomas to almost 0% in gut carcinoids. Detailed family history is essential in every case [C]. Further testing should be considered for individuals with a positive family history for carcinoid, NETs, or second endocrine tumour [C].[1]

Table 29.2 Clinical presentation of neuroendocrine tumours

- *Local symptoms*—differ depending on the site and biology of the NET tumour. Gastropancreatic tumours may invoke intense mesenteric desmoplastic reaction (in the case of carcinoid), and lead to shortening and fibrosis of the mesentery, with resultant small bowel obstruction.[1,4] Bronchial carcinoid tumours may present with bronchial obstruction (e.g. obstructive pneumonitis, atelectasis).[1]

- *Carcinoid syndrome*—results from the release of hormones (serotonin, tachykinins, and other vasoactive compounds) directly into the systemic circulation following tumour metastases to the liver. Presents with episodes of intermittent abdominal pain (70% of patients), diarrhoea (50%), flushing (30%), and sometimes episodes of lacrimation, rhinorrhoea, and palpitations.[1,5,6]

- *Other syndromes*—depend on the type, location, and biology of the tumour.
  - *Insulinoma*— dizziness, confusion, and weakness (relieved by eating food).
  - *Gastrinoma*—Zollinger–Ellison syndrome with severe peptic ulceration and diarrhoea.
  - *Glucagonoma*—weight loss, diarrhoea, diabetes mellitus, necrolytic migratory erythema, and stomatitis.
  - *Others*—e.g. VIP hypersecretion in VIPomas (watery diarrhoea, dehydration, lethargy, etc), somatostatin hypersecretion in somatostatinomas (triad of mild diabetes mellitus, steatorrhoea and gallstones).

Table 29.3 Other baseline tests

- Should be considered depending on the clinical and histochemical features of the suspected tumour:
  - Thyroid function tests (TFTs), parathyroid hormone (PTH), α-fetoprotein, carcinoembryonic antigen (CEA), β-human chorionic gonadotrophin (β-HCG), calcium, calcitonin, prolactin [D].[1]

- *Searching for the primary lesion*—might be very challenging, and may require a triple phase CT scan of the thorax and abdomen.
- *SSRS scan*—detects somatostatin receptors subtypes 2 and 5. SSRS scan has a central role in the assessment and localization of the primary in NETs as well as in looking for secondaries. Reported sensitivity achieves ~90%.

- *PET scan*—should be considered as well to increase sensitivity.
- *Intra-arterial calcium infusion*—followed by digital subtraction angiography (for gastrinomas) or hepatic venous sampling (for insulinoma); has high sensitivity (90% sensitivity).

Recommended treatment

- *Main objective*—should be curative (most, if not all, insulinomas are cured) depending on the disease. Maintaining a good quality and symptom-free life for as long as possible may be considered occasionally to be a more realistic goal.
- *Surgical resection.*
  - *Perioperative preparation*—is an essential step to correct abnormal physiologic disturbances relating to NET secretory behaviour and preventing carcinoid crises. If a functioning carcinoid tumour was found preoperatively, octreotide should be administered by constant IV infusion at a dose of 50µg/h for 12h prior to and at least 48h after surgery. Insulinomas require preoperative glucose infusion and sliding scale (glucose infusion should not be required once the insulinoma has been resected). Gastrinomas require PPIs and IV octreotide.
  - *Surgical options*—depends on the site, type, and biologic features of the tumour. In general terms:
    - Stomach NET—can be managed by watchful monitoring, limited endoscopic resection, or major resection with regional lymph node clearance. Selection of the best procedure depends on the type, extent, and potential metastatic profile of the individual tumour.
    - Small bowel NET—should a NET be confirmed histologically post-laparotomy, then re-operation to achieve complete mesenteric lymphadenectomy should be considered.
    - Appendix NET—usually removed during emergency appendicectomy and the diagnosis is made post-operatively. If the size is <1cm and the tumour was completely removed, no further treatment or follow-up would be required. If the tumour size is >2cm, or there is serosal involvement, vascular invasion, or appendix base involvement, radical right hemicolectomy is indicated and 5y follow-up is recommended.[1]
    - Colorectal NET—requires complete resection using the same cancer-type standards (see 📖 Chapter 36, pp.271–280).
    - Pancreatic NETs—localized enucleation of well-defined insulinomas is sometimes possible, but more radical resections may be necessary.
- *Other comments*—somatostatin analogues are the mainstay of treatment for those hormone-secreting tumours. The actual tumour may stabilize or occasionally shrink. PPIs for gastrinomas, diazoxide for some insulinomas, and ondansetron benefits some patients. Interferon-α is suitable for symptomatic carcinoid patients with about 50% symptomatic improvement and 10–15% reduction in size.[1] Limited benefits are seen with platinum-based chemotherapy and patients so treated should be entered into trials. Radionucleotide therapies as well as hepatic artery embolization and tissue ablation technologies are being used in some centres.

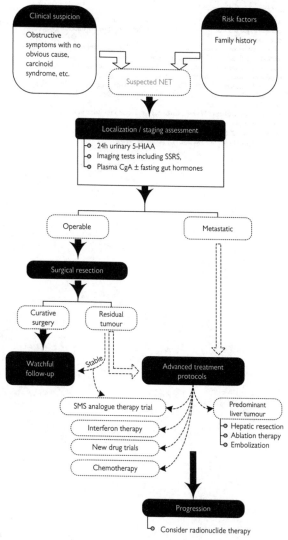

Fig. 29.1 Suggested approach to NETs, based on the UKNET guidelines[1]

Further reading

1. Ramage JK, Davies AH, Ardill J et al.; UKNETwork for neuroendocrine tumours (2005). Guidelines for the management of gastro-enteropancreatic neuroendocrine (including carcinoid) tumours. *Gut* 54 (Suppl 4), iv1–16.
2. European Neuroendocrine Tumour Society (2007). Available from: http://www.library.nhs. uk/guidelinesfinder/ViewResource.aspx?resID=281228.
3. National Comprehensive Cancer Network (2008). Practice guidelines: neuroendocrine tumours. Available from: https://subscriptions.nccn.org/login.aspx.
4. Wareing TH, Sawyers JL (1983). Carcinoids and the carcinoid syndrome. *Am J Surg* 145, 769–72.
5. Kvols LK (1994). Metastatic carcinoid tumours and the malignant carcinoid syndrome. *Ann N Y Acad Sci* 733, 464–70.
6. Soga J, Yakuwa Y, Osaka M (1999). Carcinoid syndrome: a statistical evaluation of 748 reported cases. *J Exp Clin Cancer Res* 18, 133–41.
7. Hemminki K, Li X (2001). Familial carcinoid tumours and subsequent cancers: a nationwide epidemiologic study from Sweden. *Int J Cancer* 94, 444–8.

Surgery for obesity*

* The guidelines on this chapter have been sourced and summarized from different UK, Europe, and international government sources, professional organizations, and medical specialty societies. Leading guidelines have been listed in the Key guidelines box.

Surgery for obesity

Key guidelines
- National Institute for Health and Clinical Excellence (2006). Obesity: guidance on the prevention, identification, assessment, and management of overweight and obesity in adults and children.
- World Health Organization (1997). Obesity: preventing and managing the global epidemic.
- National Obesity Forum. Guidelines on management of adult obesity and overweight in primary care.
- Arterburn DE, DeLaet DE, Schauer DP (2008). Obesity in adults. *BMJ Clin Evid* 1, 604.
- Scottish Intercollegiate Guidelines Network (2003). Management of obesity in children and young people.
- CREST (2005). Guidelines for the management of obesity in secondary care.

Basic facts
- *Definition*—obesity is a condition of excess adipose tissue mass that poses significant effect on the person's health.[1,2,6]
- *Incidence*—serious 'global epidemic'.[1,2] Trebled in the past 20y in the UK, shortening the lives of its sufferers by up to 9y.[1,7] About 22% of men and women are clinically obese (BMI >30kg/m^2), and 43% of men and 34% of women are overweight (BMI 25–29.9kg/m^2).[1,7] The estimated annual cost of care in England is ~£7.4 billion.[1]
- *Comorbidities*—obesity is responsible for ~80% of type 2 diabetes cases, 35% of ischaemic heart disease cases, and 55% of hypertension cases among adult population in Europe (Table 30.1).[9]
- *Classification*—see Table 30.2
  - *BMI*—equals the weight divided by square of the height (weight/ height^2, i.e. kg/m^2).[1] BMI directly correlates with total body fat content (reliable proxy).[1]
  - *Other measures*—waist circumference and ratio of waist-to-hip circumference can identify people at increased risk for cardiovascular event due to excess harmful fat as compared to people with increased muscular compartment without real obesity.[6]
- *Pathogenesis*—complex and multifactorial.[1,3,9]
  - From one aspect, obesity develops simply as a result of 'energy imbalance' due to persistent increased energy intake and/or decreased physical activity.
  - On the other hand, the regulation of energy balance and fat stores requires complex interactions between biological (genetic and epigenetic), social, behavioural, and environmental factors. This makes the process remarkably difficult to accurately quantify all implicated factors involved.

Table 30.1 Comorbidities associated with obesity[1]

- *Common (RR × 3).*
  - *Metabolic*—high insulin resistance, type 2 diabetes, dyslipidaemia, fatty liver, gallstones, hypertension.
  - *Mechanical*—pulmonary complaints, sleep apnoea and daytime sleepiness, difficult mobility and osteoarthritis, social isolation and depression.
- *Fairly common (RR × 2–3).*
  - *Metabolic*—coronary artery disease, stroke, gout.
  - *Mechanical*—hernia, respiratory difficulties, psychosocial disturbances, low self-esteem, and body image disturbances.
- *Slightly increased risk (RR × 1–2).*
  - *Metabolic*—polycystic ovaries, cancer (commonly breast, endometrial, endocrine, and colon), impaired fertility, cataract.
  - *Mechanical*—varicose veins, backache, stress incontinence.

Table 30.2 Obesity classification

BMI (kg/m^2)	Description	Risk of comorbidities
<18.5	Underweight	Low
18.5–24.9	Healthy weight	Average
25–29.9	Pre-obese (overweight)	Mildly increased
30–34.9	Obese class I (moderately obese)	Moderate
35–39.9	Obese class II (severely obese)	Severe
>40	Obese class III (morbidly obese)	Very severe

- In general terms, there is no doubt that environmental factors (food intake and energy expenditure) play a key role in the development of obesity.[1]
- *Clinical presentation*—related to the associated comorbidities (Table 30.1).

Recommended treatment

General approach
- Effective management requires a motivated and well-informed multidisciplinary team.[1,6] All relevant factors should be identified.
  - *Possible manageable aetiology*—should be sought.
  - *Degree of overweight and obesity*—should be estimated (Table 30.2).
  - *Comorbidities*—should be assessed and managed as appropriate.
  - *Willingness and motivation to change*—should be validated.

Initial selection to appropriate management plan
- Should be based on BMI, waist circumference, and the presence of comorbidities (Table 30.3). Recommended initial treatment should be formulated accordingly.

Lifestyle interventions
- Include healthy eating and increased physical activity.
  - *Dietary changes.*
    - Reduced energy intake—diet should contain 600kcal (carbohydrate and/or fat) less than the person's usual needs to stay at the same weight.
    - Low-calorie diets (1,000–1,600kcal/d)—less likely to be nutritionally complete, but may be considered for treatment.
    - Very-low-calorie diets (<1,000kcal/d)—can be used continuously for a maximum of 12wk, or intermittently with a low-calorie diet under close medical supervision.
  - *Physical activity.*
    - Moderate-intensity physical activity—for a minimum of 30min/d for at least 5d/wk.
    - Additional one session or more—with a duration of 10min or more.
    - Regular exercises for 45–60min—may be required to prevent obesity.

Pharmaceutical management[16]
- *General concepts*—drugs should be added to the healthy lifestyle advice (including diet and exercises) and should not be used as the sole element of treatment. Regular monitoring is essential. Stop the drug treatment if the patient regained weight whilst receiving the medications.[16]
- *Formulas*—orlistat, sibutramine, and rimonabant (currently withdrawn). No evidence exists to favour one over the others. Orlistat is recommended for patients on high-fat intake. Sibutramine or rimonabant are recommended for patients unable to control their eating habits. Thyroid hormones, diuretics, or amphetamines have no role in the treatment of obesity.[16]

Table 30.3 Recommended initial treatment for obesity[1]

- *Overweight (BMI <30).*
  - Provide advice on healthy diet and lifestyle.
  - Special advice on lifestyle changes, including diet and exercises ('L advice') should be provided if the waist circumference is high.
  - Drug treatment ('D advice') should be considered in the presence of comorbidities.

- *Mild obesity (BMI <35).*
  - Always provide 'L advice'.
  - Consider 'D advice' if comorbidities exists.

- *Moderate obesity (BMI <40).*
  - Always provide 'L advice'.
  - Always consider 'D advice'.
  - Consider surgery ('S advice') if comorbidities exists.

- *Severe obesity (BMI ≥40).*
  - Always provide 'L advice'.
  - Always consider 'D advice'.
  - Always consider 'S advice'.

L = Lifestyle changes; D = drugs; S = surgery

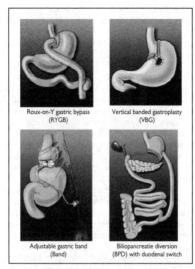

Roux-on-Y gastric bypass (RYGB)

Vertical banded gastroplasty (VBG)

Adjustable gastric band (Band)

Biliopancreatic diversion (BPD) with duodenal switch

Fig. 30.1 Surgical management (bariatric surgery). Reprinted with permission of American Society for Metabolic and Bariatric Surgery, © 2009, all rights reserved

Surgical management (bariatric surgery).
- *Main objectives of preoperative selection*—are to ensure that surgery is being recommended for patients who are expected to get most benefits, lose most weight, and remain safe over the perioperative period.
- *Expected outcome*—in selected patients, bariatric surgery has a better long-term weight loss, improved comorbidities, and quality of life as well as a significant decrease in the overall mortality.[9]
- *Indications.*
  - *First-line option* (before lifestyle interventions or drug treatment) in adults with BMI ≥50kg/m² and acceptable operative risk [C*].[1,4,9,13]
  - *Second-line option*—in patients with BMI ≥40 or 35–39.9kg/m² who have other obesity-related significant diseases (e.g. type 2 diabetes, cardiorespiratory disease, severe joint disease, and obesity-related depression), which put them at a significantly high risk for increased morbidity or premature mortality [C*].[1,4,9,13]
  - Patients should be well-motivated, psychologically fairly stable (stable home life, able to utilize adaptive coping skills, good social support), well-informed of disease management plans and the need for long-term follow-up, and in acceptance of operative risks.
- *Types.*
  - *Vertical banded gastroplasty (VBG).*
    - *Technique*—the stomach size and function are restricted by using vertical staples and an annular band to create a small 15–20mL pouch with a restricted outlet stoma of 4.75–5.0cm. The pouch

limits the amount of food patients can eat at any one time and slows the passage of food to the rest of the stomach and small bowel.

- *Efficiency*—can result in a mean weight loss of 32.2kg at 12mo follow-up (2,080 patients; 21 RCTs), and 32.0kg at and beyond 36mo (1,877 patients; 18 RCTs). The 30d mortality rate is ~0.2–0.3%, morbidity rate is 24%, and re-operation rate is 11%.[15]
- *Laparoscopic-adjusted vertical banded gastroplasty (LA-VBG)*.
  - *Technique*—same principle performed laparoscopically.
  - *Efficiency*—similar outcome to open surgery in reducing weight loss at 12mo. The operating time is significantly longer with the laparoscopic approach (2.10h with laparoscopic vs 1.45h with open), and no significant effect on average hospital stay (4d for both techniques). Complication rate is about the same at 12mo.[4,15] The benefits of laparoscopic surgery still apply.
- *Laparoscopic adjustable gastric banding (LAGB)*.
  - *Technique*—a tight adjustable prosthetic band is placed around the stomach entrance. The band is composed of a soft, locking silicone ring connected to an infusion port placed in the subcutaneous tissue. Injection of saline into the port reduces the band diameter, with resultant increased degree of restriction.
  - *Efficiency*—LAGB has replaced most other bariatric procedures due to its simplicity and relatively low complication rate. LAGB can result in a mean weight loss of 40–55% of excess weight at 12-mo follow-up, and 45–60% of excess weight at and beyond 48mo follow-up.[17]
- *Gastric bypass surgery (GBS)*.
  - *Technique*—the stomach is divided into an upper small pouch (15–30mL) and a lower remnant pouch. Appropriate bypass procedures are then used to ensure adequate drainage of pouches. The procedure restricts the volume of food which can be eaten and reduces weight.
  - *Efficiency*—can result in a mean weight loss of 43.5kg at 12mo follow-up (2,937 patients; 32 RCTs), and 41.5kg at and beyond 36mo follow-up (1,281 patients; 21 RCTs).[4,15] Gastric bypass seems to be more effective at reducing weight compared to gastric banding procedure (18mo follow-up). There is no evidence of this beneficial effect beyond 1–3y follow-up.
  - *Laparoscopic approach*—has a similar effect on weight loss compared to open procedure, but gastric bypass has more side effects, including nutritional and electrolyte abnormalities, gastrointestinal symptoms, surgical complications, and a small risk of perioperative death.[4,15]
- *Biliopancreatic diversion*.
  - *Technique*—complex operation. Rare in use due to side effects. The stomach is resected to create a smaller volume and connected to the ileum to bypass the duodenum and jejunum.

- *Efficiency*—can result in a mean weight loss of 51.9kg at 12mo follow-up (two systematic reviews, but no comparing RCTs), and 53.1kg at and beyond 36mo follow-up.[15] The estimated 30d mortality rate is 0.9 and adverse events are fairly common, including surgical complications (6%), re-operations (4%), and gastrointestinal symptoms (38%).[4,15]

Further reading

1. National Institute for Health and Clinical Excellence (2006). Obesity: guidance on the prevention, identification, assessment, and management of overweight and obesity in adults and children. Available from: http://www.nice.org.uk/nicemedia/pdf/CG43NICEGuideline.pdf.
2. World Health Organization. Obesity: preventing and managing the global epidemic. Report of a WHO consultation on obesity, Geneva, 3-5 June 1997.
3. National Obesity Forum. Guidelines on management of adult obesity and overweight in primary care. Available from: http://nationalobesityforum.org.uk/images/stories/W_M_guidelines/NOF_Adult_Guildelines_Feb_06.pdf; National Obesity Forum. Pharmacotherapy guidelines for obesity management in adults. Available from: http://nationalobesityforum.org.uk/images/stories/W_M_guidelines/NOF_Pharma_Guidelines%284%29.pdf; (iii) An approach to weight management in children and adolescents (2–18 years) in primary care. Available from: http://nationalobesityforum.org.uk/images/stories/W_M_guidelines/Children_and_adolescents.pdf.
4. Arterburn DE, DeLaet DE, Schauer DP (2008). Obesity in adults. *BMJ Clin Evid* 1, 604.
5. Scottish Intercollegiate Guidelines Network (2003). Management of obesity in children and young people. Available from: http://www.sign.ac.uk/pdf/sign69.pdf.
6. CREST (2005). Guidelines for the management of obesity in secondary care. Available from: http://www.crestni.org.uk/obesity-guidelines-report.pdf.
7. Royal Pharmaceutical Society of Great Britain (2005). Practice guidance: obesity. Available from: http://www.rpsgb.org.uk/pdfs/obesityguid.pdf.
8. Clinical Knowledge Summaries (2007). Obesity—management. Available from: http://www.cks.library.nhs.uk/obesity.
9. Tsigosa C, Hainerb V, Basdevant A *et al.* (2008). Management of obesity in adults: European clinical practice guidelines. *Obesity Facts* 1, 106–16.
10. National Institutes of Health, National Heart, Lung, and Blood Institute (1998). Clinical guidelines on the identification, evaluation, and treatment of overweight and obesity in adults. The evidence report. Available from: http://www.nhlbi.nih.gov/guidelines/obesity/ob_gdlns.pdf.
11. Society of American Gastrointestinal Endoscopic Surgeons (2003). Guideline for clinical application of laparoscopic bariatric surgery. Available from: http://guidelines.gov/summary/summary.aspx?doc_id=12384&nbr=006413&string=obesity.
12. Massachussetts Department of Public Health (2004). Expert panel on weight loss surgery. Available from: http://guidelines.gov/summary/summary.aspx?doc_id=12924&nbr=006638&string=expert+AND+panel+AND+weight+AND+loss+AND+surgery.
13. Institute for Clinical Systems Improvement (2004). Prevention and management of obesity (mature adolescents and adults). Available from: http://guidelines.gov/summary/summary.aspx?doc_id=10226&nbr=005389&string=obesity.
14. American Society of Plastic Surgeons (2004). Practice advisory on liposuction. Available from: http://guidelines.gov/summary/summary.aspx?doc_id=6563&nbr=004125&string=obesity.
15. Maggard MA, Shugarman LR, Suttorp M *et al.* (2005). Meta-analysis: surgical treatment of obesity. *Ann Intern Med* 142, 547–59.
16. British National Formulary 57 (2009). Drugs used in the treatment of obesity. Available from: http://www.bnf.org/bnf/bnf/57/3381.htm?q=%22drugs%22%22used%22%22the%22%22treatment%22%22of%22%22obesity%22.
17. Gravante G, Araco A, Araco F, Delogu D, De Lorenzo A, Cervelli V (2007). Laparoscopic adjustable gastric bandings: a prospective randomized study of 400 operations performed with 2 different devices. *Arch Surg* 142, 958–61.

Small bowel
and appendix

Acute appendicitis*

* The guidelines on this chapter have been sourced and summarized from different UK, Europe, and international government sources, professional organizations, and medical specialty societies. Leading guidelines have been listed in the Key guidelines box.

Acute appendicitis

Key guidelines

- Cochrane Library of Systematic Reviews. (i) (2005). Antibiotics versus placebo for the prevention of post-operative infection after appendicectomy; (ii) (2004). Laparoscopic versus open surgery for suspected appendicitis.
- National Guideline Clearinghouse (NGC) (2002). Evidence based clinical practice guideline for emergency appendectomy (US).
- Humes D, Speake W, Simpson J (2007). Appendicitis.

Basic facts

- **Incidence**—the most common surgical emergency in general surgery. General lifetime risk is ~8.5% in men and 6.5% in women.[3] Affects ~35,000 patients every year in England. Male to female ratio is 1.4:1.[4] Most common in second and third decades of life. Peak incidence is age 10–19.[4]
- **Pathogenesis**—most likely related to obstruction of the appendix lumen,[3] mostly due to lymphoid follicular hyperplasia (initiated or exacerbated by viral or bacterial infection) in young patients,[5] and to fibrosis, faecoliths (often due to constipation or fruit stones), or neoplasia (carcinoid or caecal carcinoma) in older population.
- **Natural history**—secreted mucus becomes entrapped by obstruction, resulting in raised intramural pressure and considerably distended appendix distal to obstruction. Small vessels and lymphatic flow becomes occluded, resulting in ischaemic, necrotic, and then (usually in 48h) perforated appendix. This leads to the formation of localized mass, abscess or diffuse peritonitis.[5,6]
- **Bacterial pathogens**—most common (especially in gangrene and perforation) are *Escherichia coli*, *Peptostreptococcus*, *Bacteroides fragilis*, and *Pseudomonas* species.[5]
- **Clinical presentation.**[6,8,9,10]
  - *Initial presentation*—non-specific symptoms (indigestion, feeling unwell, epigastric or periumbilical pain) caused by the luminal obstruction and distension of the appendix, stimulating the visceral autonomic pain nerves. Visceral pain is usually constant, moderate in severity, and poorly localized.
  - *Intermediate period*—venous congestion associated with the inflammatory process stimulates bowel peristalsis, resulting in crampy pain, anorexia (90% of cases), nausea and vomiting (70%), and occasional diarrhoea (10%).
  - *Localized pain*—somatic pain nerves are stimulated once the overlying parietal peritoneum is involved. Symptoms localize to the right iliac fossa (RIF), and become sensitive to movement.
  - *Signs*—initial findings are usually non-specific. Localized signs become prominent once the overlying parietal peritoneum is irritated (Tables 31.1, 31.2, 31.3); a completely soft abdomen is unlikely to harbour acute appendicitis.

Table 31.1 Signs of acute appendicitis

- ***McBurney's point***—two thirds of the distance between the umbilicus and anterior superior iliac spine. Often overlies the base of appendix and is usually not variable with the appendix location.
- ***Rovsing's sign***—tenderness elicited in the RIF on palpation or gentle finger percussion on left iliac fossa (LIF). Indicates a right-sided peritoneal irritation.
- ***Obturator sign***—pain elicited by internal rotation of the hip. Usually associated with pelvic appendix.
- ***Iliopsoas sign***—pain in the RIF elicited by extension of the right hip. Usually indicates a retrocaecal appendix.
- ***Rectal examination***—may reveal tenderness or an inflammatory mass on the right side of the pelvis. Most useful in non-specific cases. Only used if absolutely necessary in children, and after obtaining a proper consent.
- ***Vaginal examination***—may show positive cervical excitation. Indicates acute salpingitis.

Table 31.2 Unusual presentation of acute appendicitis

- ***Retrocaecal appendix***—appendix located far away from the anterior parietal peritoneum. Localized tenderness is usually less remarkable. Patients may complain of diarrhoea, urinary irritation, haematuria, and pyuria.
- ***Pelvic appendix***—may resemble acute gastroenteritis, causing diffuse pain, urinary frequency, dysuria, or rectal symptoms (tenesmus and diarrhoea). Digital rectal examination may raise suspicion of acute appendicitis.
- ***Acute appendicitis during pregnancy***—special challenge (Table 31.3).
- ***Perforated appendix***—suspected in any patient with unusually remarkable high fever (over 39.4°C) or high white cell count.

Recommended investigations

- ***General approach***—a detailed clinical history and repeated physical examination are usually sufficient in making the diagnosis of acute appendicitis in most cases. In suspected situations, hospital admission for 12–24h observation (a wait-and-watch policy) is a safe and effective approach (Fig. 31.1).[8]
- ***Laboratory tests***—no single laboratory test or any combination of tests have been shown to be as effective and accurate as the careful examination and clinical acumen of an experienced surgeon.[1] Nevertheless, laboratory tests are useful adjuncts to the surgeon's clinical impression, particularly in high-risk patients and those with equivocal clinical presentation.[12]
  - *Urinalysis*—helpful in excluding urinary tract infections. Positive results, however, might be confusing as up to a third of acute appendicitis can result in microscopic haematuria and pyuria due to the proximity of the inflamed appendix to the bladder and ureter.[8]
  - *Pregnancy test (urine or blood)*—mandatory in childbearing age to rule out pregnancy (normal or ectopic).[12]

- *White cell count (WCC) test*—leucocytosis is found in 70–92% of cases, with a left shift in 95% of cases. Up to a third of patients with acute appendicitis may have a normal WCC; this does not rule out appendicitis.
- *Serum C-reactive protein (CRP) levels*—have sensitivity of 93%, specificity of 80%, and accuracy of 91%, and are recommended by many authors in all cases.[15]
- *Other tests and investigations*—should be arranged in equivocal cases based on the clinical suspicion and if such investigations will improve outcome.
- *Imaging*—should only be performed in equivocal cases. Imaging is neither cost-effective nor helpful when there is a high or a low probability of acute appendicitis. The best radiological test for acute appendicitis is a CT scan.
  - *Plain abdominal radiograph (AXR)*—usually unhelpful. AXR may show appendicolith or localized right lower quadrant ileus.[10]
  - *Ultrasonography*—in experienced hands, can be useful in diagnosing acute appendicitis in equivocal cases and in detecting pelvic pathologies in women. Acute appendicitis presents as a non-compressible tubular structure at the base of the caecum, thickened wall (>2mm) appendix, luminal distension (diameter >6mm), and free fluid in the pelvis in some cases.[13]
  - *Abdominal CT scan*—can show thickened wall (>2mm) appendix, appendicolith (25% of cases), concentric thickening of inflamed appendiceal wall, fat stranding, phlegmon, abscess, or free fluid. Sensitivity and specificity are >95% and 85%, respectively.

Table 31.3 Acute appendicitis in pregnancy

- *Incidence*—occurs in 1 in 2,000 pregnancies at any trimester. Higher perforation rate at third trimester.
- *Challenges.*
  - *Displaced appendix*—superiorly by the enlarging uterus around the second and third trimesters. The abdominal wall lies away from the appendix being pushed by the gravid uterus.
  - *Masked signs*—skeletal muscles are lax and signs of peritoneal irritation are usually vague.
  - *Physiologic response*—physiologic leukocytosis is normal in pregnant women.
- *Diagnosis*—depends on repeated physical examination, ultrasound scan, and clinical suspicion. Retrocaecal appendix can produce flank pain similar to pyelonephritis.
- *Risks of perforated appendicitis.*
  - *Higher foetal death*—up to 36% of perforated cases vs 1.5% for non-perforated ones. Aggressive but safe approach is justified, and negative laparotomy rates are much more common in pregnant than non-pregnant patients (35% vs 15%).
  - *Pregnancy-related complications (e.g. spontaneous abortion)*—occur frequently when an appendicectomy is performed in the first trimester (33%) as compared to the second (14%) or third trimester (0%).[11]

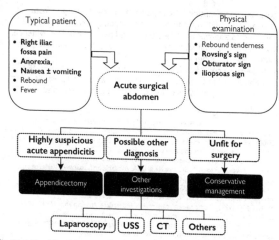

Fig. 31.1 Algorithm for approaching patients with suspected acute appendicitis

- *Diagnostic laparoscopy*—should be viewed as an invasive procedure requiring general anaesthesia. During 'diagnostic' laparoscopy, if no other pathology is identified, (e.g. Crohn's, Meckel's, tubo-ovarian pathology), the appendix should be removed regardless of its gross appearance. This rules out inflammation by pathologic examination and makes the diagnosis of acute appendicitis less likely if the patient complains of similar pain in the future.[16,17]

Recommended treatment

- *Surgery plus perioperative systemic antibiotics*—is the default effective curative treatment, significantly reducing wound infection rate and intra-abdominal abscesses, shortening hospital stay, and enhancing the return to normal activities.[3]
  - *Preoperative preparation*—include adequate hydration, correction of electrolyte abnormalities, and commencement of systemic antibiotics.[8,9]
  - *Choice of antibiotics (type, dose)*—remains to be standardized (see Ch. 17).[5] A perforated appendicitis should be treated therapeutically against enteric Gram negative rods and anaerobes.[10]
  - *Laparoscopic appendicectomy in adults*—can reduce post-operative wound infections, pain, duration of hospital stay, and time off work when compared with open surgery. The risk of intra-abdominal abscesses may increase with this technique.[3] Laparoscopic approach is more likely to benefit women of childbearing age and obese patients requiring larger skin incisions during open appendicectomy.
- *Treatment with antibiotics alone*—although not the standard option, it has been shown by different RCTs to significantly reduce pain and

morphine consumption.[3] Most patients can be discharged from hospital within 48h with no reported mortality if surgery was used when and as appropriate (e.g. generalized peritonitis). The evidence, however, is very limited, and up to a third of those patients require readmission for appendicectomy within 1y.[3]

- **Post-operative complications**—include wound infection (~5–33%),[3] intra-abdominal abscess formation (~2% of cases), and possible effect on female fertility in cases of perforated appendix in childhood.[3]

Further reading

1. Andersen BR, Kallehave FL, Andersen HK (2005). Antibiotics versus placebo for the prevention of post-operative infection after appendicectomy. *Cochrane Database Syst Rev* 20, CD001439; Sauerland S, Lefering R, Neugebauer EA (2004) Laparoscopic versus open surgery for suspected appendicitis. *Cochrane Database Syst Rev* 18, CD001546.
2. National Guideline Clearinghouse (NGC) (2002). Evidence based clinical practice guideline for emergency appendectomy. NGC, Maryland USA. Available at: http://www.guideline.gov.
3. Humes D, Speake W, Simpson J (2007). Appendicitis. *BMJ Clin Evid* 6, 408.
4. Addiss DG, Shaffer N, Fowler BS, Tauxe RV (1990). The epidemiology of appendicitis and appendicectomy in the United States. *Am J Epidemiol* 132, 910–25.
5. Hardin DM Jr (1999). Acute appendicitis: review and update. *Am Fam Physician* 60, 2027–34.
6. Guidry SP, Poole GV (1994). The anatomy of appendicitis. *Am Surg* 60, 68–71.
7. Lau WY, Teoh–Chan CH, Fan ST, Yam WC, Lau KF, Wong SH (1984). The bacteriology and septic complication of patients with appendicitis. *Ann Surg* 200, 576–81.
8. Morris PJ, Wood WC (2000). Chapter 27. In: *Oxford Textbook of Surgery*, 2nd ed. Oxford University Press, Oxford.
9. Mulholland MW (2005). Chapter 54. In: *Greenfield's surgery: scientific principles and practice*, 2nd ed, Lippincott–Raven Publishers.
10. Goldberg JE, Hodin RA (2009). Appendicitis in adults. Available from: http://www.uptodate.com/patients/content/topic.do?topicKey=~MHtFfEZAisADM&selectedTitle=14~21&source=search_result.
11. Andersen B, Nielsen TF (1999). Appendicitis in pregnancy: diagnosis, management and complications. *Acta Obstet Gynecol Scand* 78, 758–62.
12. Longmore M, Wilkinson IB, Turmezei T, Cheung CK (2007). *Oxford Handbook of Clinical Medicine*, 7th ed. Oxford University Press, Oxford.
13. Jeffrey RB Jr, Laing FC, Townsend RR (1988). Acute appendicitis: sonographic criteria based on 250 cases. *Radiology* 167, 327–9.
14. Sivit CJ, Applegate KE, Stallion A et al. (2000). Imaging evaluation of suspected appendicitis in a paediatric population: effectiveness of sonography versus CT. *AJR Am J Roentgenol* 175, 977–80.
15. Eriksson S, Granstrom L, Carlstrom A (1994). The diagnostic value of repetitive preoperative analyses of C-reactive protein and total leucocyte count in patients with suspected acute appendicitis. *Scand J Gastroenterol* 29, 1145–9.
16. Connor TJ, Garcha IS, Ramshaw BJ et al. (1995). Diagnostic laparoscopy for suspected appendicitis. *Am Surg* 61, 187–9.
17. Grunewald B, Keating J (1993). Should the 'normal' appendix be removed at operation for appendicitis? *J R Coll Surg Edinb* 38, 158–60.
18. Kukreja N, Bhan C, Schizas A (2007). An audit of training in laparoscopic appendicectomy in the South Thames Region. *Bulletin of the Royal College of Surgeons of England* 89, 102–4.

Part 6

Colorectal

Constipation in adults*

* The guidelines on this chapter have been sourced and summarized from different UK, Europe, and international government sources, professional organizations, and medical specialty societies. Leading guidelines have been listed in the Key guidelines box.

Constipation in adults

- Bandolier (1997). Constipation.
- American College of Gastroenterology Functional Gastrointestinal Disorders Task Force. (2005). An evidence-based approach to the management of chronic constipation in North America.
- Peppas G, Alexiou VG, Mourtzoukou E, Falagas ME (2008). Epidemiology of constipation in Europe and Oceania: a systematic review.
- British National Formulary 57 (2009). Constipation.

Basic facts

- **Definition**—in simple patient terms, constipation is the passage of hard stool, the infrequent passage of stools, or the need for straining on defecation. The definition and diagnostic criteria (Rome III) have been recommended by the international working committee on functional constipation (Table 32.1).[13]
- **Prevalence**—difficult to estimate (many do not seek medical advice). The average prevalence in Europe is ~22.3%, ranging from 0.7% in paediatric population in Italy to 81% in elderly hospitalized male population.[3]
- **Pathogenesis**—see Tables 32.2 and 32.3.

Recommended investigations (Fig. 32.1)

- **General approach**—the main reason for investigation is to exclude 'serious' disease. Accurate history and physical examination are essential [C].[2]
  - *Clinical history*—patients will often complain about the urge to defecate, and this can be associated with the feeling of rectal fullness and crampy lower abdominal pain. The history should include the pattern of bowel movement (stool features, frequency, usual timing for defecation), general measures used to aid defecation (mobility and daily access to toilets, need for carer to go to toilet, high attention to privacy, laxatives taken and how efficient, dietary habits), nature and duration of constipation (onset, duration, pattern), presence of secondary causes (specific drugs, systemic disorders), presence of ALARM symptoms (e.g. weight loss, rectal bleeding, episodes of diarrhoea, and anaemia).
  - *Physical examination*—may reveal malodorous breath, anal fissures, haemorrhoids (more likely effect rather than cause), and solid faeces on digital rectal examination. Some of these findings may be causative and some consequential upon the constipation. A change of bowel habit to constipation is not a high-risk symptom for colorectal cancer.

Table 32.1 Rome III criteria for constipation*

- *Diagnostic requirements*—the presence of two or more main complaints over the last year for a period of 12wk or more (not necessarily consecutive).

- *Main complaints.*
  - *Lumpy or hard stool*—for >25% of bowel movements.
  - *Decreased bowel movements*—to <3 per wk.
  - *Straining*—during more than 25% of bowel movements.
  - *Sensation of anorectal blockage*—for >25% of bowel movements.
  - *Sensation of incomplete evacuation*—for >25% of bowel movements.
  - *The need for manual evacuation (digital or other techniques)*—for >25% of bowel movements.
  - *The absence of*—loose stools or irritable bowel syndrome (diagnosed by full criteria).

* The Rome process is an international effort to define and categorize the functional gastrointestinal disorders.[13]

Table 32.2 Causes of constipation[8,11]

- *Physiologic changes.*
  - Pregnancy, irritable bowel syndrome.

- *Medications.*
  - See Table 32.4.

- *Underlying medical disorder.*
  - *Neurologic disorder.*
    - Multiple sclerosis, spinal cord injury, Parkinson's disease, myotonic dystrophy.
    - Peripheral neuropathy, diabetes mellitus, pseudo-obstruction, Hirschprung's disease, autonomic neuropathy.
  - *Metabolic disorder.*
    - Hypokalaemia, hypercalcaemia, hypothyroidism, panhypopituitarism, anorexia nervosa.

- *Idiopathic.*
  - *Normal transit constipation*—about 60% of cases. Stools transverse the colon at normal speed and evacuate at similar frequency to average population, but the patient believes he/she is constipated.
  - *Defecatory disorders*—about 25% of idiopathic cases. The rectum fails to effectively empty from stool. More common in:
    - Fear of defecation—due to pain associated with anal fissures, complicated haemorrhoids, or large hard stool.
    - Structural abnormalities—rectocoele, rectal intussusception, and excessive perineal descent.
    - Lack of coordination—between abdominal, rectoanal, and pelvic floor muscles during defecation.
  - *Slow transit constipation*—occurs less frequently (13%) and is associated with delayed emptying of the colon, especially the proximal end.

- *Diagnostic tests*—not required when ALARM features are absent and the patient is under the age of 45 [C].[2,7]
  - *AXR*—may reveal faecal loading in the colon, and/or features of megacolon. Useful for regular monitoring of the bowel during treatment.
  - *Bowel visualization*—indicated in patients with ALARM symptoms. Colonoscopy can reliably exclude underlying organic pathology (cancer, stricture, extrinsic compression). CT colonography and barium enema also have a place. Flexible sigmoidoscopy is the first-line investigation in younger patients [C].[7]
- *Physiologic studies*—indicated in selected patients according to their response (or lack of response) to treatment in the absence of any justifying reason.
  - *Colonic transit studies*—useful in evaluating patients whose major complaint is infrequent defecation.
    - *Technique*—patients need to swallow radio-opaque markers and undergo regular abdominal radiographs to monitor the passage throughout the colon.
    - *Outcome*—colonic inertia is diagnosed if the transit is delayed in the right colon. Outlet delay is diagnosed when the markers reach and accumulate in the rectum.
  - *Defecography*—useful in diagnosing defecatory disorders.
  - *Motility studies*—useful in some patients with severe constipation.

Recommended treatment (Fig. 32.1)

- *General approach*—effective management requires a thorough approach that extends well beyond the simple use of laxatives. Attention to simple details is essential (associated pain, dietary habits, fluid intake, mobility, toileting).
- *Patient education*—includes appropriate reassurance, proper explana-tion of normal bowel habits, encouragement to reduce excessive use of laxatives, and advice on good toileting practice (consistent toileting each day, use of patient's own triggering factor like meal or morning call) [C].[2,10]
- *Toileting education/support*—visual and auditory privacy should be safeguarded. Squat position is recommended for a good and effective defecation and should be achieved or, in the case of bedbound patients, simulated by left-side lying position [C].[2,10]
- *Dietary changes*—high-fibre diet and adequate fluid intake should be encouraged [C].[5,6] Fibre intake should be increased to 25–30g/d with increased fluid intake (1.5–2L/d).
  - *Efficiency*—stool frequency is expected to increase significantly from a mean baseline of 1.8/wk to 4.2/wk with an improvement in stool consistency.[1,5,6]
  - *Side effects*—may be associated in the first week with some gastrointestinal disturbance (flatulence and abdominal bloating), but disappears usually by the third week.[5]

Table 32.3 Medications causing constipation

- ***Common surgical acute medications***—analgesics, opiates, antispasmodics, antihistamines, 5HT3 antagonists.

- ***Chronic disease medications***—antidepressants, antipsychotics, antihypertensives, calcium channel blockers.

- ***Supplements***—iron supplements, antacids, sucralfate.

- ***Preparations***—unprocessed wheat and oat bran, taken with food or fruit juice, is the most effective bulk-forming preparation.[4] Table 32.4 shows some examples of dietary fibre contents.
- ***Daily exercises***—effective in reducing the prevalence of constipation when compared with a sedentary lifestyle in adults (OR × 0.70) and should be encouraged [D].[2,5]
  - *Walking*—highly recommended for mobile individuals, 15–20min once or twice a day, 3–5 times a week [D].[2,5]
  - *Patients unable to walk or bedbound*—should be offered specific exercises such as pelvic tilt, low trunk rotation, and single leg lifts [D].[2,5]
- **Bulk-forming laxatives.**
  - *Mechanism of action*—increase the volume of faecal mass which stimulates peristalsis.
  - *Efficiency*—increase the average mean frequency of bowel movements by 1.4 per wk.[5]
  - *Preparations*—ispaghula (Fybogel® 1 sachet or 2 level 5mL spoonfuls in water twice daily, preferably after meals)[4], sterculia (Normacol® 1–2 heaped 5mL spoonfuls, or the contents of 1–2 sachets, washed down without chewing with plenty of liquid once or twice daily after meals)[4], and methylcellulose.
- **Osmotic laxatives.**
  - *Mechanism of action*—increase the water content within the large bowel by attracting fluid from the body into bowel lumen or by retaining water in colon, lowering the pH, and increasing colonic peristalsis.
  - *Macrogols* (polyethylene glycols—Movicol®)
    - *Efficiency*—effective and reliable in treating chronic constipation and faecal impaction [A].[5,11,12] Can increase the number of bowel movements to 4.5 per wk (compared to 2.7 in placebo) at 2wk of use, and can achieve a return to normal bowel habits (3 or more bowel movements per wk, no straining at defecation) in up to 70% of patients (compared to 30% in placebo) at 20wk of use.
    - *Harm*—can cause abdominal pain and diarrhoea. Not significantly different from placebo in the overall frequency of adverse effects.
    - *Dose*—Movicol® is given as 1–3 sachets daily in divided doses usually for up to 2wk for chronic constipation; as 8 sachets daily dissolved in 1L of water and drunk within 6h, usually for maximum of 3d for faecal impaction.[4]

Table 32.4 Estimated food fibre contents

Food	Each serving	Fibre content
Fruit		
Apple (with skin)	Medium-sized	●●●●
Apricots (dried)	1 cup	●●●●●●●●●●
Dates	1 cup (chopped)	●●●●●●●●●●●●
Grapes	10	●●●
Orange	1	●●●
Peach (with skin)	1	●●●
Pear (with skin)	1	●●●●●
Pineapple	1 cup (diced)	●●●
Raspberries	1 cup	●●●●●●●
Strawberries	1 cup	●●●
Juice		
Apple	1 cup	●
Grape	1 cup	●●
Orange	1 cup	●
Cooked vegetables		
Bean (string, green)	1 cup	●●●●
Broccoli	1 stalk	●●●●●
Brussels sprout	7–8	●●●●●
Carrot	1 cup	●●●●●
Cauliflower	1 cup	●●●
Corn (canned)	1 cup	●●●●●
Parsnip	1 cup (cooked)	●●●●●●
Peas	1 cup (cooked)	●●●●●●●
Potato (without skin)	1 boiled	●●
Spinach	1 cup (raw)	●●●●●
Tomato	1	●●
Legumes		
Baked beans, tomato sauce	1 cup	●●●●●●●●●●●●●●●●●●●●
Dried peas (cooked)	½ cup	●●●●●

Bread, pasta, flour		
Bran muffin	1	⊙⊙⊙⊙⊙⊙
Mixed grains		⊙⊙⊙⊙
Oatmeal	1 cup	⊙⊙⊙⊙⊙⊙
White bread	1 slice	⊙
Wholewheat bread	1 slice	⊙⊙

* ⊙ = about 1g/serving

- *Lactulose.*
  - *Efficiency*—effective and reliable in treating chronic constipation and faecal impaction [B].[5,11,12]
  - *Benefits*—(30mL, 4 times/d) can significantly reduce the cramping, flatulence, tenesmus, and bloating sensation associated with the constipation. Lactulose does not increase the number of weekly bowel movements significantly (0.9 per week), but does achieve a good overall patient satisfaction at 1mo (satisfaction scores 5.2 on a score of 10 where 10 is 'excellent').[5,12]
  - *Harm*—no serious side effects.
  - *Dose*—initially 15mL twice daily, adjusted according to patient's needs.[4]
- *Other laxatives*—many available but little evidence to support one over the others.
  - *Stimulant laxatives*—act on the intestinal mucosa or nerve plexus and alter water and electrolyte secretion.
    - *Common preparations*—bisacodyl and senna.
    - *Harm*—often cause abdominal cramp and should be avoided in intestinal obstruction. Excessive use can cause diarrhoea and related effects such as hypokalaemia.
  - *Glycerol suppositories*—mild rectal stimulant.
  - *Arachis oil enemas*—contains ground nut oil and peanut oil. Act by lubricating and softening impacted faeces, and promoting bowel movement.[4]
- *Surgery for constipation*—indicated occasionally to correct specific anatomical deformities (e.g. rectocoele) or for the very occasional longstanding debilitating symptoms refractory to conservative management. Total abdominal colectomy with anastomosis or ileostomy may be indicated.

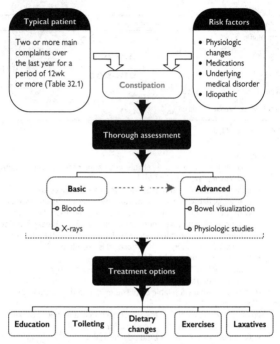

Fig. 32.1 Approaching patients with constipation

Further reading

1. Bandolier (1997). Constipation. Available from: http://www.medicine.ox.ac.uk/bandolier/band46/b46-3.html.
2. Brandt L, Schoenfeld P, Prather C, Quigley E, Schiller L, Talley N; American College of Gastroenterology Functional Gastrointestinal Disorders Task Force. (2005). An evidence-based approach to the management of chronic constipation in North America. *Am J Gastroenterol* 100, S1–21.
3. Peppas G, Alexiou VG, Mourtzoukou E, Falagas ME (2008). Epidemiology of constipation in Europe and Oceania: a systematic review. *BMC Gastroenterol* 8, 5.
4. British National Formulary 57 (2009). Constipation. Available from: http://www.bnf.org/bnf/bnf/57/2190.htm.
5. Frizelle F, Barclay M (2007). Constipation in adults. *BMJ Clin Evid* 12, 413.
6. Registered Nurses' Association of Ontario (2005). Prevention of constipation in the older adult population. Available from: http://www.rnao.org/bestpractices/PDF/BPG_Prevent_constipation_rev05.pdf.
7. American Society for Gastrointestinal Endoscopy (2005). Guideline on the use of endoscopy in the management of constipation. Available from: http://www.guideline.gov/summary/summary.aspx?doc_id=7780&nbr=4485&ss=6&xl=999.
8. Hsieh C (2005). Treatment of constipation in older adults. *Am Fam Physician* 72, 2277–84.
9. Fallon M, O'Neill B (1997). ABC of palliative care. Constipation and diarrhoea. *BMJ* 315, 1293–6.

10. Locke GR 3rd, Pemberton JH, Phillips SF (2000). American Gastroenterological Association medical position statement: guidelines on constipation. *Gastroenterology* 119, 1761–6.
11. Ramkumar D, Rao SS (2005). Efficacy and safety of traditional medical therapies for chronic constipation: a systematic review. *Am J Gastroenterol* 100, 936–71.
12. Longstreth GF, Thompson WG, Chey WD, Houghton LA, Mearin F, Spiller RC (2006). Functional bowel disorders. *Gastroenterology* 130, 1480–91.
13. The Association of Coloproctology of Great Britain and Ireland (2007). Guidelines for the management of colorectal cancer. Available from: http://www.acpgbi.org.uk/assets/documents/COLO_guides.pdf.

Diverticular disease*

* The guidelines on this chapter have been sourced and summarized from different UK, Europe, and international government sources, professional organizations, and medical specialty societies. Leading guidelines have been listed in the Key guidelines box.

Diverticular disease

Key guidelines
- Clinical Knowledge Summaries (2008) Diverticular disease and diverticulitis.
- World Gastroenterology Organization (2007) Diverticular disease.

Basic facts
- **Definitions**—diverticula of the colon are small, blind, narrow-necked pouches formed by mucosal herniation through the muscle layer of the bowel wall (Table 33.1).[1]
- **Prevalence**—difficult to estimate. Ranges from ~4% at age 40 to ~65% at age 65. More common in western countries and has been increasing over the years.[1] Evidence to correlate diverticular disease with specific risk factors are insufficient to draw solid conclusions (Table 33.2). The sigmoid colon is mostly affected.
- **Pathogenesis**—results from the formation of false or pulsion diverticulum where the bowel mucosa and submucosa protrude through weakest areas of the muscular layer (where the vasa recta pass through) and form several outpouchings covered only by serosa.[3,6,8]
  - *Acute diverticulitis*—results from the inflammation of the diverticula, caused by stasis or obstruction with subsequent bacterial overgrowth and local tissue ischaemia. This results in a micro- or macroscopic perforation of the wall and confined or complicated pericolic infection.[8]
  - *Diverticular bleeding*—occurs when the vasa recta is exposed to injury and ruptures into the lumen.
- **Clinical presentation.**
  - *Uncomplicated diverticular disease*—may be associated with non-specific lower abdominal pain, bloating, and constipation. About 10–25% of asymptomatic cases will develop symptoms with time.[3] Diverticular colitis is now a recognized entity.
  - *Diverticulitis*—most cases (75–95%) are simple (Table 33.3).[3] Hinchey classification scheme can be used for staging purposes.[8]
  - *Diverticular bleeding*—painless maroon or bright red rectal bleeding, usually self-limiting. Rare to coexist with acute diverticulitis.[15] Frequent or small PR bleeding is unlikely to be caused by diverticulosis and requires further investigations.[1]

Recommended investigations (Fig. 33.1)
- **Uncomplicated diverticular disease**—symptomatic patients require investigation to exclude coexistent lesions such as polyps or carcinoma (see 📖 Chapter 36, pp.271–80), and confirm the presence of diverticular disease.
  - *Recommended investigations*—colon visualization includes full colonoscopy, flexible sigmoidoscopy with double contrast barium enema, or CT colonography.[1]

Table 33.1 Definitions

- **Diverticula**—small, blind, narrow-necked pouches formed by mucosal herniation through the muscle layer of the bowel wall.
- **Diverticulosis**—incidental finding of asymptomatic diverticula in the colon.
- **Diverticular disease**—a term used when diverticula cause symptoms.
- **Diverticulitis**—a term used when diverticula are associated with inflammation.

Table 33.2 Risk factors

- **Low fibre intake**—inversely correlates to the incidence of diverticular disease.[8,9,10] RR is 0.58 for highest vs lowest fibre intake (a 47,000 men study).[10]
- **Western diet**—high fat, red meat, and low fibre. RR × 2.35–3.32.[10]
- **Smoking, caffeine, or alcohol**—no specific correlation exists.[11]
- **Physical activity**—lack of physical activity increases the risk of developing symptomatic diverticular disease (RR × 0.63 for highest vs lowest extremes) after adjustment for age and dietary habits.[12] The effect of moderate exercise remains unclear.[1]

Table 33.3 Types and classification of diverticulitis

- **Simple diverticulitis (stage 1)**—small, confined pericolic or mesenteric abscesses.
  - Presentation—LIF pain (70% of cases), few days' history; previous similar episode (>50% of cases); nausea and vomiting (20–60%), constipation (50%), diarrhoea (25–35%) and urinary symptoms (10–15%).[13] Right colon diverticulitis occurs in 1.5% of cases, mimicking appendicitis.[14]
- **Pelvic abscess (stage 2)**—abscesses are larger, but often confined to the pelvis. Mortality rate is <5%.[8]
- **Perforated purulent diverticulitis (stage 3)**—ruptured peridiverticular abscess, causing purulent peritonitis. Mortality rate is ~15%.[8]
- **Perforated faecal diverticulitis (stage 4)**—rupture into the free peritoneal cavity, causing faecal contamination. Mortality rate is ~45%.[8]

- **Acute diverticulitis.**
  - *Abdominal and pelvis CT scan*—the first-line investigation of choice when indicated [A].[1,2,8] Oral, IV, and rectal contrasts are useful to enhance accuracy.[2]
    - *Accuracy*—very high. Sensitivity, specificity, positive and negative predictive values (with contrast) are all well over 97%.[3]
    - *Findings*—colonic diverticula (84% of cases), increased soft tissue density within the pericolic fat (98% of cases), thickening of bowel wall (70%), and soft tissue masses (pericolic fluid collections, abscess, or phlegmon) in 35% of cases.[2]
  - *Other investigations*—include single contrast enema (preferably water-soluble), compression ultrasound scan, cystography, and possible limited and gentle flexible sigmoidoscopy in selected cases where the risk of perforation is minimal [B].[1,2,8]

- *Diverticular bleeding.*
  - *General approach*—following active resuscitation, investigation choices depend on available resources and expertise.
  - *Early colonoscopy* (for diagnosis and treatment)—the first-line investigation of choice when experience and facilities are available [A].[17]
    - *Efficiency*—in dedicated centres, early colonoscopy can reduce the length of hospital stay (from 5 to 2d).[17,18,20]
    - *Preparation*—stop aspirin, warfarin, and NSAIDs if possible [C].[17,18,20] Consider upper GI endoscopy for severe bleeding as possible upper GI source, or if negative colonoscopy [A].[17,18,20] Bowel preparation using polyethylene glycol-based solutions when colonoscopy is indicated can improve visualization, therapeutic yield, and patient safety,[17] providing the patient is fit enough.[17,18,20]
  - *Other investigations*—angiography and/or tagged red blood cell scanning can be used with high identification rate (~75%) in active persistent bleeding (0.1mL/min for tagged red blood cell scanning and 1mL/min for angiography) or in cases of non-diagnostic endoscopic findings.[17]
  - *Control of bleeding*—by superselective arterial embolization can be achieved in ~45–90% of cases,[17] and may be required for diagnostic and therapeutic purposes in severe unstable cases (e.g. >6 units of blood transfusion in 24h).[17] Colonoscopy with thermal, laser, injection, or clip modalities may be possible. Preoperative localization of bleeding site should always be attempted to allow for limited segmental colonic resection rather than 'blind' colectomy, with resultant high morbidity and mortality.[17]

Recommended treatment (Fig. 33.1)
- Good quality randomized trials are few.
- *Asymptomatic incidental diverticulosis*—no further investigations are required.[1] Encourage a healthy diet and an active lifestyle.[1] Despite usual practice, there is little evidence to support the use of added fibre (bran or ispaghula husk) or laxatives (lactulose, methylcellulose) to prevent complications in diverticulosis (no significant difference from placebo in long-term follow-up).[3]
- *Symptomatic uncomplicated diverticular disease*—following appropriate investigations, a healthy diet and an active lifestyle are advised.[1] Simple analgesia may be required.[1]
  - *Added fibre or laxatives*—little evidence to support the efficiency of this practice compared to placebo.[3]
  - *Dietary fibre supplements + antibiotics (US practice: rifaximin 400mg bd for 12mo)*—may relieve symptoms at 12mo more than fibre alone (~70% with rifaximin vs 40% with placebo alone), but may cause side effects (nausea, headache, and weakness).[3] The place of mesalazine, pre- and probiotics is not clear. More evidence is required to draw solid recommendations.[3]
  - *Elective open or laparoscopic surgery*—no evidence to recommend preventive surgery in uncomplicated diverticular disease.[3]
- *Diverticulitis*—treatment options depend on the severity of the case and the individual patient circumstances (Table 33.4).

- *Recurrent attacks*—a later second attack of diverticulitis occurs in
~10–35% of cases, and a further third of patients will have a third
attack.[2,8,16,19] Recurrent diverticulitis is more likely in patients who
already had recurrent attacks (the risk doubles in each subsequent
hospital admission), young patients (<50y), and patients with other
coexisting conditions (e.g. obesity).[8,19] Recommendation for elective
surgery should be tailored according to the individual patient risk-
benefit assessment [B].[2,8,16] Patients willing to avoid a second severe
attack of diverticulitis or recurrent attacks, who have acceptable operative risk and understands the implication of surgery, should be offered
sigmoid resection. This can be performed 6wk after the acute attack.
- **Diverticular bleeding**—see 📖 OHCS Chapter 11.

Table 33.4 Treatment of diverticulitis

- *Primary or secondary care.*
  - **Treat as outpatient**—for uncomplicated mild cases where patient can
  tolerate oral fluid and be followed up. Patients not improving after 48h
  of treatment require hospitalization.[1]
  - **Treat as inpatient**—if patient is unable to tolerate oral fluid and in
  more severe cases (fever, peritoneal irritation), elderly patients, and
  immunosuppressed patients [B].[1,2]
- *Medical treatment.*
  - **Oral intake**—clear fluid (or NBM with IV hydration) is commonly
  recommended initially.[1,8] Solid food can be gradually introduced thereafter.[1]
  - **Broad spectrum antibiotics**—to cover both aerobic and anaerobic
  bacteria [B].[1,2]
    - **Recommended antibiotics**—co-amoxiclav (500mg/125mg tablets tds)
    or ciprofloxacin (500mg bd) and metronidazole (400mg tds).[1]
    - **Duration**—minimum 7d
  - **Analgesia**—paracetamol is safe and effective.[1] NSAIDs and long-term
  opioids should be used with caution as they have been identified as risk
  factors for diverticular perforation.[1]
  - **Treatment outcome**—most cases (75–100%) respond to conservative
  management within 48–72h.[2,8,16] Severe unresolving cases should be
  approached as complicated cases (see above) and treated accordingly.
  Other causes should be considered.
  - **Follow-up**—confirmation of diagnosis is recommended following resolution
  of the acute attack [D],[2] usually within 4–6wk.
- *Percutaneous drainage of abscess*—the recommended best treatment for
large (>2–4cm) diverticular abscesses [B].[2] This approach reduces the need
for emergency surgery and improves overall patient outcome.[2]
- *Emergency surgery*—required for severe unresponsive cases or for patients
with significant complications (peritonitis, bowel obstruction) [B].[2] Options
include Hartmann's procedure (sigmoid colectomy with end colostomy) and
sigmoid colectomy with primary anastomosis (± proximal colonic washout and
diverting ileostomy).[2]
- *Elective surgery*—after resolution of an acute episode should be recommended
in individual cases based on the risk-benefit assessment [B].[2,8,16]

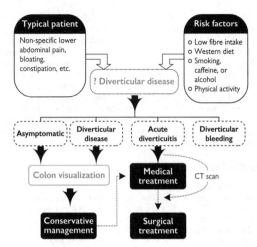

Fig. 33.1 Approaching patients with diverticular disease

Further reading

1. Clinical Knowledge Summaries (2008). Diverticular disease and diverticulitis. Available from: http://www.cks.library.nhs.uk/diverticular_disease/view_whole_topic#.
2. Rafferty J, Shellito P, Hyman NH, Buie WD (2006). Practice parameters for sigmoid diverticulitis. *Dis Colon Rectum* 49, 939–44.
3. BMJ Clinical Evidence. Available from: http://clinicalevidence.bmj.com/ceweb/conditions/dsd/0405/0405.jsp. Accessed May 2009 (via ovid)
4. The Society for Surgery of the Alimentary Tract (1996). Surgical treatment of diverticulitis. Available from: http://www.ssat.com/cgi-bin/divert.cgi.
5. World Gastroenterology Organization (2007). Diverticular disease. Available from: http://www.worldgastroenterology.org/assets/downloads/en/pdf/guidelines/07_diverticular_disease.pdf.
6. Meyers MA, Alonso DR, Gray GF, Baer JW (1976). Pathogenesis of bleeding colonic diverticulosis, *Gastroenterology* 71, 577–83.
7. Painter NS, Truelove SC, Ardran GM, Tuckey M (1965). Segmentation and the localization of intraluminal pressures in the human colon, with special reference to the pathogenesis of colonic diverticula. *Gastroenterology* 49, 169–77.
8. Jacobs DO (2007). Clinical practice. Diverticulitis. *N Engl J Med* 357, 2057–66.
9. Painter NS, Burkitt DP (1971). Diverticular disease of the colon: a deficiency disease of Western civilization. *Br Med J* 2, 450–4.
10. Aldoori WH, Giovannucci EL, Rimm EB, Wing AL, Trichopoulos DV, Willett WC (1994). A prospective study of diet and the risk of symptomatic diverticular disease in men. *Am J Clin Nutr* 60, 757–64.
11. Aldoori WH, Giovannucci EL, Rimm EB, Wing AL, Trichopoulos DV, Willett WC (1995). A prospective study of alcohol, smoking, caffeine, and the risk of symptomatic diverticular disease in men. *Ann Epidemiol* 5, 221–8.
12. Aldoori WH, Giovannucci EL, Rimm EB *et al.* (1995). Prospective study of physical activity and the risk of symptomatic diverticular disease in men. *Gut* 36, 276–82.
13. Konvolinka CW (1994). Acute diverticulitis under age forty. *Am J Surg* 167, 562–5.
14. Ngoi SS, Chia J, Goh MY, Sim E, Rauff A (1992). Surgical management of right colon diverticulitis. *Dis Colon Rectum* 35, 799–802.
15. Meyers MA, Alonso DR, Gray GF, Baer JW (1976). Pathogenesis of bleeding colonic diverticulosis. *Gastroenterology* 71, 577–83.

16. Janes SE, Meagher A, Frizelle FA (2006). Management of diverticulitis. *BMJ* 332, 271–5.
17. American Society for Gastrointestinal Endoscopy (2005). The role of endoscopy in the patient with lower GI bleeding. Available from: http://www.guideline.gov/summary/summary. aspx?doc_id=8209&nbr=4584&ss=6&xl=999.
18. Jensen DM, Machicado GA, Jutabha R, Kovacs TO (2000). Urgent colonoscopy for the diagnosis and treatment of severe diverticular haemorrhage. *N Engl J Med* 342, 78–82.
19. Sarin S, Boulos PB (1994). Long-term outcome of patients presenting with acute complications of diverticular disease. *Ann R Coll Surg Engl* 76, 117–20.
20. State LL, Syngal S (2003). Timing of colonoscopy: impact on length of hospital stay in patients with acute lower intestinal bleeding. *Am J Gastroenterol* 98, 317–22.

Anal fissures*

* The guidelines on this chapter have been sourced and summarized from different UK, Europe, and international government sources, professional organizations, and medical specialty societies. Leading guidelines have been listed in the **Key guidelines** box.

Anal fissures

Key guidelines
- Clinical Knowledge Summaries (2008). Anal fissure: management.
- American Society of Colon and Rectal Surgeons (2004). Practice parameters for the management of anal fissures.
- BMJ Clinical Evidence (2007). Anal fissure (chronic).

Basic facts
- *Definition*—tears or splits in the squamous lining of the anal canal distal to the dentate line (Table 34.1).
- *Incidence*—common condition.[1,3] Exact prevalence difficult to estimate as many people attribute any anorectal discomfort to piles, and many do not seek medical attention.[7] Anal fissures affect both genders equally at any age.[1] Anterior fissures are more common in females.[1]
- *Pathogenesis*—no simple or unified theory to explain pathogenesis. Increased anal tone is a common pathway for all primary anal fissures. Elevated internal sphincter pressures (due to repeated trauma or other unidentified mechanism) causes severe anal pain, local ischaemia, initiates or keeps the fissure edges apart, and impairs the wound healing.[1,5] Impaired healing with associated pain increases the spasm and maintains the vicious cycle.
  - *Anatomic location*—about 90% of primary anal fissures occur posteriorly, possibly due to the distinctive distribution of blood flow into the anoderm, where blood supply is less than one half that in other parts of the anal canal.[8]
  - *Secondary causes of anal fissures*—see Table 34.2.[1]
- *Clinical presentation*—severe anal pain, spontaneously or during the passage of stool, lasting from a few minutes to a few hours, and accompanied commonly by rectal bleeding. Rectal bleeding presents with small amounts of bright red blood, on the toilet paper or the surface of the stool (typically separated from stool). Other symptoms may include perianal discharge; itching and skin irritation can be prominent. Multiple fissures occurring away from the midline and large funny-shaped fissures may hide some serious underlying disease, including Crohn's, sexually transmitted diseases, tuberculosis, or malignancies. (Table 34.3).

Table 34.1 Anal fissure—definitions[1,4]

- *Acute anal fissures*—fissures presenting for <6wk.
- *Chronic anal fissures*—fissures presenting for >6wk with morphologic signs of chronicity.
- *Primary anal fissures*—fissures associated with increased anal tone or posterior ischaemia, but no identifiable underlying cause can be found.
- *Secondary anal fissures*—fissures associated with an identifiable underlying cause, not with increased anal tone or posterior ischaemia.

Table 34.2 Secondary causes of anal fissures[1,4]

- **Severe constipation.**
- **Inflammatory bowel disease**—associated inflammatory process causes ulceration of mucosa.
- **Pregnancy (especially third trimester) and childbirth**—commonly located anteriorly and often associated with low anal sphincter pressures.
- **Sexually transmitted disease**—the infectious process may result in tissue breakdown.
- **Rectal cancer.**

Table 34.3 Physical examination for anal fissures[1,4]

- **Acute anal fissure.**
  - **Technique**—best performed by spreading the buttocks apart gently and looking carefully at the posterior midline. Inspection of the entire anal canal is essential.
  - **Appearance**—fresh laceration in the anoderm, with sharply demarcated edges.
  - **Other findings**—involuntary spasm of the anus may indicate the presence of anal fissure, perianal abscess.
  - **Digital rectal examination and proctoscopy**—often too uncomfortable and best to avoid.
- **Chronic anal fissure.**
  - **Appearance**—linear or pear-shaped split with raised edges and exposed white, horizontally oriented fibres (internal anal sphincter) at the base.
  - **Secondary features**—include external (sentinel) skin tags, hypertrophied anal papillae at the proximal end, and induration of the edges.

Recommended treatment

- **Conservative measures**—can eventually reach a healing rate of ~35% without any other intervention and is the first treatment of choice [B] (Table 34.4).[1,2,3]
- **Medical management.**
  - *Indications*—persistent symptoms (>1wk) despite conservative management in the absence of contraindications (e.g. pregnancy, breastfeeding).[1]
  - *Objectives*—to reduce the internal sphincter spasm, decrease the pressure in the anal canal, and enhance blood flow to the anoderm with subsequent healing of the fissure.
  - *Topical glyceryl trinitrate (GTN)*—first-line treatment for chronic anal fissures [A].[1,2]
    - *Mechanism*—increases local blood flow in the anal canal and reduces pressure in the internal anal sphincter, which may further facilitate healing.[6]
    - *Application*—apply as a 0.2–0.6% topical ointment (a pea-sized amount) to the anal margin twice a day. This should be continued until complete healing of the anal mucosa.
    - *Risks and benefits*—see Table 34.5.

- *Topical diltiazem.*
  - *Mechanism*—calcium antagonist that inhibits calcium ion entry through voltage-sensitive areas of vascular smooth muscles, causing relaxation and dilatation.[5]
  - *Application*—topical diltiazem 2% gel to the anal margin twice a day (not widely available or licensed).
  - *Risks and benefits*—see Table 34.5.
- *Botulinum toxin injection.*
  - *Mechanism*—potent inhibitor of acetylcholine release from nerve endings. Historically been used in treating certain spastic disorders of skeletal muscles.
  - *Application*—inadequate consensus on dosage, precise site of administration, number of injections, or efficacy.[2]
  - *Risk and benefits*—see Table 34.5.
- **Surgical management.**
  - *Objectives*—to reduce the internal sphincter tone and enhance blood flow to the anoderm with subsequent healing of the fissure.
  - *Indications*—usually reserved as a backup treatment for refractory cases not responding to medical therapy, but is considered a completely acceptable first-line treatment (after failed conservative measures) for some patients following informed decision on risks and benefits [A].[2,3]
  - *Anal stretch*—Lord's or four finger dilatation (healing rate 75–90%) is no longer recommended due to the risk of anal sphincter injury and consequent risk of incontinence (0–25%).[3,6]

Table 34.4 Conservative measures in managing anal fissures

- **Patient education**—essential to achieve compliance.

- **Ensure soft and easily passed stool**—advise patients on increasing fluid (1.5–2L/d) and fibre (18–30g/d) intake, add laxatives if necessary (osmotic laxatives for children, and bran or bulk-forming laxatives for adults), and manage constipation as appropriate (see 📖 Chapter 32, pp.239–248).[3,9]

- **Warm sitz baths**—using salted warm water for 10 or 15min after each bowel movement. This traditional measure, although shown previously to be safe and effective in reducing anal sphincter tone,[6] is not anymore recommended by expert reviewers.[3]

- **Pain relief and soothing.**
  - **Topical lubricants (Petroleum jelly)**—instilled before opening the bowel.[3,9]
  - **Topical anaesthetic creams**—useful and effective [D].[3] Long-term use is not recommended.[3]

Table 34.5 Medical treatment for anal fissures

- *Topical GTN.*
  - *Benefits*—healing rate is ~50–70%, which is marginally but significantly better than the best supportive conservative treatment. The median time to heal is 6wk (range 4–8wk).[6] The relapsing rate is ~25–40% and may require further prescription of GTN.[3]
  - *Risks*—main side effect is headache, which occurs in 20–50% of patients and causes up to 20% of patients to stop therapy.[2,3]
- *Topical diltiazem.*
  - *Benefits*—healing rate comparable to GTN ointment.[3] Few studies showed better response rate in cases unresponsive to GTN.[5] Similar indications to GTN if available and licensed [A].[1,2]
  - *Risks*—fewer side effects than GTN.[2,5] May cause headache (33%).
- *Botulinum toxin.*
  - *Benefits*—acceptable alternative to GTN in 'failed to responding' cases [B].[2] Short-term healing rate is >90%, but similar to GTN in the long term.[3] The relapsing rate is ~40% and may require further injections.[3]
  - *Risks*—invasive and expensive. The main side effect is the occasional transient incontinence to flatus.[3]

- *Lateral sphincterotomy.*
  - *Technique*—divide the internal anal sphincter linearly from the distal external end up to the dentate line or to a distance equal to that of the fissure, using closed or open technique. Sphincterotomy healing is better if performed on the right or left lateral positions (compared to posterior or anterior midline). No surgical repair of the fissure itself is required. Biopsy may be warranted for fissures with atypical appearance.[4,5]
  - *Benefits*—highest healing rate (>95%) at 8wk compared to GTN (OR × 6.6) or other modalities.[3]
  - *Risks*—some degree of flatus and faecal incontinence may occur quite often in the immediate post-operative period (25–40%), and therefore, it is imperative to err on the side of doing too little rather than too much. It is always possible to go back and do more.[3]
- *Anal advancement flap*—this operation avoids disruption to the anal sphincter by using a triangular or square-shaped sliding graft skin flap.[5] It was shown to be as effective as an internal anal sphincterotomy in fissure healing rates at 3mo, but further studies are required to draw solid conclusions.[2,3]

Further reading

1. Clinical Knowledge Summaries (2008). Anal fissure: management. Available from: http://cks.library.nhs.uk/anal_fissure#.
2. American Society of Colon and Rectal Surgeons (2004). Practice parameters for the management of anal fissures. Available from: http://www.guideline.gov/summary/summary.aspx?doc_id=6506&nbr=004075&string=anal+AND+fissure.
3. Nelson R (2007). Anal fissure (chronic). *BMJ Clin Evid* 12, 407
4. Lindsey I, Jones OM, Cunningham C, Mortensen NJ (2004). Chronic anal fissure. *Br J Surg* 91, 270–9.

5. Bhardwaj R, Parker MC (2007). Modern perspectives in the treatment of chronic anal fissure. *Ann R Coll Surg Engl* 89, 472–8.
6. Dodi G, Bogoni F, Infantino A, Pianon P, Mortellaro LM, Lise M (1986). Hot or cold in anal pain? A study of the changes in internal anal sphincter pressure profiles. *Dis Colon Rectum* 29, 248–51.
7. Nelson RL, Abcarian H, Davis FG, Persky V (1995). Prevalence of benign anorectal disease in a randomly selected population. *Dis Colon Rectum* 38, 341–4.
8. Schouten WR, Briel JW, Auwerda JJ (1994). Relationship between anal pressure and anodermal blood flow. The vascular pathogenesis of anal fissures. *Dis Colon Rectum* 37, 664–9.
9. British National Formulary 57 (2009). Management of anal fissures. Available from: http://www.bnf.org/bnf/bnf/57/129346.htm?q=%22management%22%22of%22%22anal%22%22fissures%22.

Haemorrhoid disease*

* The guidelines on this chapter have been sourced and summarized from different UK, Europe, and international government sources, professional organizations, and medical specialty societies. Leading guidelines have been listed in the Key guidelines box.

Haemorrhoid disease

Key guidelines
- Clinical Knowledge Summaries (2008). Haemorrhoids: management.
- American Society of Colon and Rectal Surgeons (2005). Practice parameters for the management of haemorrhoids.
- National Institute for Health and Clinical Excellence. (i) (2007). Haemorrhoid—stapled haemorrhoidopexy; (ii) (2003). Circular stapled haemorrhoidectomy.

Basic facts

- *Definition*—chronic engorgement of the haemorrhoidal physiologic complex, causing enlargement and displacement of the vascular cushions within the anal canal, with resultant bleeding, prolapse, and pain.[1,4]
- *Incidence*—common condition.[1,4] Estimated prevalence in Europe and US is ~4% of the population.[1] Affects both genders equally (men report their complaint more commonly to GPs), peaking between 45–65y of age to decline thereafter.[1]
- *Pathogenesis*—normal haemorrhoids are physiologic vascular and connective tissue structures in the anal canal, contributing to the anal continence mechanism by providing compressible spongy cushions that allow for complete closure of the anus.[1] Risk factors include advancing age, prolonged sitting and straining, pregnancy and pelvic tumours, diarrhoea and chronic constipation. Different pathogenesis theories exist (Table 35.1).
- *Clinical presentation*—often presents with painless bleeding (bright red, on toilet paper, or drips into toilet bowel), prolapsing piles (reducible initially), mucus discharge, and pruritus.[1,4] Pain is rarely significant in internal haemorrhoids (see below), but may be so prominent in thrombosed external piles to warrant hospitalization.[1] Other causes of perianal pain should be investigated.
- *Classification*—see Table 35.2.

Recommended investigations

- *Thorough history and physical examination*—the mainstay of diagnosis. Laboratory tests are not usually required [B].[1,2,4]
  - *Focused clinical history*—should include the nature, severity, duration and progression of symptoms, usual bowel habits and dietary fibre intake, and any relevant family history, including bowel cancer [B].[2]
  - *Physical examination*—should include inspection of the anus, digital rectal examination, and proctoscopic examination of the anal canal and distal rectum.[2,4]
  - *High-risk patients*—should be investigated with colonoscopy or barium enema and flexible sigmoidoscopy (see Ch. 36) [B].[2]

Table 35.1 Pathogenesis of haemorrhoids

- *Aging theory*—advancing age or other aggravating conditions cause weakness in the connective tissue anchoring haemorrhoidal tissue to the underlying sphincter, with resultant sliding into the anal canal.[1,5]

- *Straining theory*—abnormally increased tone of internal anal sphincter causes solid faecal material to forcefully squeeze haemorrhoidal plexus against the firm internal sphincter, with resultant congested and enlarged haemorrhoids.[1,5,6]

- *Abnormal cushions' theory*—haemorrhoidal cushions with its erectile properties become abnormally swollen, accompanied by possible congenital weakness in venous plexus walls, causing enlarged haemorrhoids.[1,7]

Table 35.2 Classification of haemorrhoids

- *Internal vs external.*
  - *Internal haemorrhoids*—arise from superior haemorrhoidal cushions above the dentate line. Located in the left lateral, right anterior, and right posterior positions. The overlying mucosa has visceral innervation.
  - *External haemorrhoids*—arise from the inferior haemorrhoidal plexus beneath the dentate line. Overlying squamous epithelium contains somatic pain receptors.
    - *Skin tags*—residual excess skin (remnant external thrombosed piles) and not haemorrhoidal tissue.
    - *Acutely thrombosed piles*—present with severely tender, tense, and oedematous mass.
- *Internal haemorrhoid severity classification.*[3,4]
  - *First degree*—painless bleeding with no prolapse.
  - *Second degree*—bleeding associated with prolapse (with Valsalva manoeuvres) and spontaneous reduction.
  - *Third degree*—bleeding with associated prolapse which requires manual reduction.
  - *Fourth degree*—chronically prolapsed and is irreducible.

Recommended treatment

- *Natural history*—untreated haemorrhoids heal spontaneously (25%), progress into recurrent condition (66%), or develop complications (ulceration, maceration, thrombosis, sepsis, and anaemia).[1,9] Most patients use over-the-counter preparations and only seek medical advice for relatively severe disease.
- *Conservative management*—the first-line treatment of choice [B].[1,2,10] Successful for most patients with mildly symptomatic haemorrhoids.
  - *Main objectives*—to relieve symptoms as quick as possible and maintain remission.
  - *Options*—include topical agents, high-fibre diet, and behavioural modifications (Table 35.3).

Table 35.3 Conservative management of haemorrhoids

- **Topical agents.**
  - **Action**—reduce symptoms by applying local anaesthetic or anti-inflammatory effects.[1,2,10] No effect on haemorrhoids cure rate.[1]
  - **Efficiency**—quite efficient as short-term first-line measures [C].[1,10]
  - **Options**—no clinical trials to support one product over the others. Options include simple analgesia, sitz bath, soothing (astringent) preparations, anaesthetic preparations, and topical corticosteroids.
  - **Harm**—avoid using opioids (risk of constipation) or NSAIDs (in rectal bleeding). Long-term use of local steroids can produce perianal dermatitis [B].[10]

- **High-fibre diet.**
  - **Method**—ensure adequate fluid and fibre dietary intake (see 🕮 Chapter 32, pp.239–248), with bulk-forming agents if necessary [B].[1,2,10]
  - **Efficiency**—relief of constipation occurs usually in a few days and relief of haemorrhoidal symptoms in a few weeks. Fibre supplement for 6wk can reduce haemorrhoidal bleeding in 95% of patients (compared to 56% in placebo). NNT is 3 (need to treat three patients to achieve one significant response).[10]

- **Behavioural modifications**—include avoiding reading in toilet, excessive straining, and encourage to lose weight and to maintain good anal hygiene.

- **Non-surgical management**—include:
  - *Rubber band ligation (RBL).*
    - *Indications*—common choice for first, second, and selected third grade haemorrhoids in conjunction with conservative management [B].[10]
    - *Technique*—using anoscope to identify diseased haemorrhoids, a special machine with suction is used to place a special rubber ring on the base of the selected haemorrhoid.
    - *Benefits and risks*—see Table 35.4. All patients should be formally consented before using this procedure due to the serious, but rare, possible side effects.
  - *Injection sclerotherapy.*
    - *Indications*—alternative therapy for first and second degree haemorrhoids [B].[10]
    - *Technique*—a total of 3mL of 5% phenol (an irritant chemical solution) is injected into the submucosa of each pile. Sclerosants induce intense inflammatory reaction, provoke fibrosis, destroy redundant haemorrhoidal tissue, and ultimately fix the haemorrhoidal cushion.[10]
    - *Benefits and risks*—see Table 35.5.
  - *Other options.*
    - *Bipolar, infrared, and laser coagulation*—bipolar current, infrared, or laser light is applied to induce coagulation and necrosis, with resultant fibrosis in the submucosal layer. May be as effective as RBL with few side effects, but more frequent recurrences.[2,4]

Table 35.4 Rubber band ligation—benefits and risks

- *Efficacy*—effective in treating haemorrhoidal bleeding or prolapse in ~75–95% of cases at 1y follow-up. About 10% of patients require repeated therapy over this period. A 4y recurrence of bleeding and/or prolapse occurs in 61% and 12% of patients, respectively.[2,4,10]

- *Harm.*
  - *Pain*—occurs in ~13% of patients.
  - *Anal stenosis*—requires anal dilatation, occurs rarely.

- *Cryosurgery*—special probes cooled with liquid nitrogen are used to induce freezing and necrosis, with resultant fixation of the haemorrhoidal cushion. Has higher rate of complication and decreased patient satisfaction.[2]
- **Surgical haemorrhoidectomy.**
  - *Indications*—usually reserved for refractory cases, patients who are unable to tolerate minor procedures, large external haemorrhoids, and combined internal and external haemorrhoids with significant prolapse [B].[2]
  - *Options*—see Table 35.6.
  - *Complications.*
    - *Urinary retention*—can be up to 30% of patients. Some patients require urinary catheterization.
    - *Urinary tract infection*—about 5% of cases, possibly secondary to urinary retention.
    - *Delayed haemorrhage*—in 1–2% within 7–16d. Possibly results from sloughing of primary clot.
    - *Faecal impaction*—associated with post-operative pain and opiate use.
    - *Local infection*—is very uncommon. Submucosal abscess affects <1% of cases.
    - *Pain*—nearly universal and may in part be due to spasm of the internal sphincter. Topical diltiazem ointment (2%) can be applied three times daily for 7d post-operatively.
    - *Other complications*—include delayed healing, sphincter damage, and stricture formation.

Table 35.5 Injection sclerotherapy—benefits and risks

• **Efficacy**—effective in treating haemorrhoidal bleeding or prolapse in ~60–90% of cases at 1y follow-up. About 30% of patients require repeated therapy over this period. A 4y recurrence of bleeding and/or prolapse occurs in 81% and 36% of patients, respectively.[2,4,10]

• **Harm**—uncommon, but serious side effects include septic complications and chemical prostatitis (therefore, injecting anteriorly should not be performed).

Table 35.6 Surgical options

• **Closed haemorrhoidectomy.[4]**
  • **Technique**—a narrow incision is made around the external haemorrhoidal tissue and extended across the dentate line to the superior base of the haemorrhoidal column; the defect is closed with a continuous suture.
  • **Efficiency**—effective in relieving symptoms (>95%). Recurrence rate at 1y ranges from 4% for small haemorrhoids to 22% for large ones.
  • **Harm**—associated with more post-operative complications than stapled haemorrhoidopexy.

• **Open haemorrhoidectomy.[4]**
  • **Technique**—the excision and ligation are left open without mucosal closure.
  • **Efficiency**—effective in relieving symptoms (>95%) in first to fourth degree haemorrhoids. Patient usually returns home in 2–3d. Recurrence rate at 1y is 3.8% for small haemorrhoids and 15.4% for large ones.
  • **Harm**—similar to closed procedure.

• **Stapled haemorrhoidopexy.[4,11]**
  • **Technique**—a special device is used to excise a circumferential column of mucosa and submucosa from the upper anal canal. This brings protruding haemorrhoids back and fixes the lining in position.
  • **Efficiency**—effective where the operative treatment of haemorrhoids is indicated. Have shorter length of hospital stay (1d), less post-operative pain, but no significant difference in recurrence rates from traditional methods.
  • **Harm**—this procedure should only be performed by a fully trained colorectal surgeon.
  • **Recommendations**—NICE recommends this procedure as an alternative option to traditional surgery where appropriate skills and clinical governance setting exist.

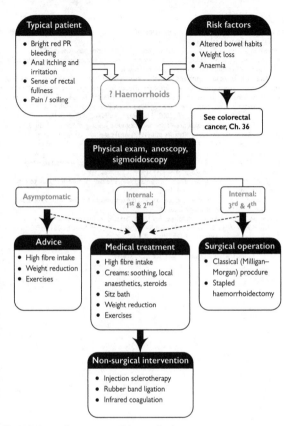

Fig. 35.1 Approaching patients with haemorrhoids

Further reading

1. Clinical Knowledge Summaries (2008). Haemorrhoids: management. Available from: http://cks. library.nhs.uk/haemorrhoids#.
2. American Society of Colon and Rectal Surgeons (2005). Practice parameters for the management of haemorrhoids. Available from: http://www.guidelines.gov/summary/summary. aspx?doc_id=7284&nbr=004337&string=hemorrhoids.
3. (i) National Institute for Health and Clinical Excellence (2007). Haemorrhoid—stapled haemorrhoidopexy. Available from: http://www.nice.org.uk/guidance/index.jsp?action=byID&o=11835; (ii) National Institute for Health and Clinical Excellence (2003) Circular stapled haemorrhoidectomy. Available from: http://www.nice.org.uk/guidance/index.jsp?action=byID&o=11075.
4. Reese GE, von Roon AC, Tekkis PP (2009). Haemorrhoids. *BMJ Clin Evid* 1, 415.
5. Studd P (2005). Haemorrhoids: prevention and treatment. *Nursing in Practice* 25, 50–3.
6. Arabi Y, Alexander–Williams J, Keighley MR (1977). Anal pressures in haemorrhoids and anal fissure. *Am J Surg* 134, 608–10.
7. Thomson WH (1975). The nature of haemorrhoids. *Br J Surg* 62, 542–52
8. Kluiber RM, Wolff BG (1994). Evaluation of anaemia caused by haemorrhoidal bleeding. *Dis Colon Rectum* 37, 1006–7.
9. Jensen SL, Harling H, Arseth–hansen P, Tange G (1989). The natural history of symptomatic haemorrhoids. *Int J Colorectal Dis* 4, 41–4.
10. Johanson JF (2002). Evidence-based approach to the treatment of haemorrhoidal disease. *Evidence-based Gastroenterology* 3, 26–31.
11. Jayaraman S, Colquhoun PH, Malthaner RA (2006). Stapled versus conventional surgery for haemorrhoids. *Cochrane Database Syst Rev* 2006, Issue 4, Art. No. CD005393. DOI: 10.1002/14651858. CD005393 Pub 2
12. Alonso–Coello P, Guyatt G, Heels–Ansdell D et al. (2005). Laxatives for the treatment of haemorrhoids. *Cochrane Database Syst Rev* 4, CD004649.

Colorectal cancer (CRC)

Colorectal cancer (CRC)

Key guidelines

- The Association of Coloproctology of Great Britain and Ireland (2007). Guidelines for the management of colorectal cancer.
- National Institute for Health and Clinical Excellence (2004). Improving outcomes in colorectal cancer.
- Scottish Intercollegiate Guidelines Network (2003). Management of colorectal cancer.
- Cancer Research UK (2008). Bowel (colorectal) cancer.
- NHS Cancer Services Collaborative (2006). Bowel cancer.

Basic facts

- **Incidence**—third most common cancer in the UK after breast and lung. Incidence has increased in the UK (by 1% per year) up till 1999, when a slight decrease has been noticed since.[4] The lifetime risk for developing CRC is ~1 in 18–20. The male to female ratio is 1.2:1.[4]
- **Pathogenesis**—the attributes of malignancy (genetic damage, invasiveness, lack of normal differentiation, increased rate of growth, ability for local invasion, and distant spread) are acquired in a stepwise fashion, a process known as tumour progression. This correlates at the genetic level with the accumulation of successive mutations.[5] Most risk factors are related to environmental and genetic factors (Table 36.1).
- **Natural history**—most CRCs result from malignant changes in polyps (adenomas) that developed at least a decade earlier.[2] CRC growth usually follows an exponential curve, with a doubling time of about 40mo for early cancer to 4mo or less for advanced cancer.[7] Patients with hepatic metastases, diagnosed at the time of surgery, have a median survival period of only 4.5mo.[8]
- **Cancer distribution**—caecum: 13%; ascending colon, hepatic flexure, transverse colon, and splenic flexure: 13%; descending and sigmoid colon: 20%; rectosigmoid and rectum: 36%; anus 2%; unspecified: 15%.[4]
- **Clinical presentation**—see Table 36.2. Commonly presents with abdominal pain (~45%), change in bowel habits (~45%), rectal bleeding of short duration or blood mixed with stool (~40%), and/or iron deficiency anaemia (~10%).[1,9,10] Advanced cancer is the initial presentation in about one fifth of patients. Cancer can present initially with bowel obstruction or perforation causing peritonitis.[4] Distant metastasis is found in 15–20% of cases at initial presentation.[1]

Recommended investigations

- **Endoscopy**—using colonoscopy or sigmoidoscopy (rigid or flexible) with double contrast barium enema (in distal cancers) are the recommended investigations of choice **[B]**.[1,2] Colonoscopy is currently considered the 'gold standard'.[1]

Table 36.1 Risk factors

- **Age**—major risk factor. Risk increases dramatically after the age of 40. Most cases (95%) occur after the age of 50.[4]
- **Dietary factors**—promotional or protective role.
  - **Red and processed meat consumption**—risk increase × 0.55; **high consumption of fish**—RR × 0.3; **high-fibre diet**—RR × 0.2 **high intake of fruit and vegetables**—correlation is modest;[4] **folic acid**—RR × 0.25;[6] **alcohol**—risk increase × 1.5[4]
  - **Smoking**—has been linked with increased polyp formation. The link to cancer formation remains unclear.[4]
- **Medications.**
  - **NSAIDs**—the long-term (>10y) regular use of NSAIDs can significantly reduce the risk of bowel cancer, possibly due to the inhibition of cyclooxygenase-2, with resultant increased apoptosis and impairment of tumour cells.[4]
  - **Statins (HMG-CoA reductase inhibitors) for over 5y**—may reduce the risk of bowel cancer according to preliminary evidence from case-control studies.[4]
  - **HRT**—may reduce the risk of CRC by 20–50% with 5–10y of use.[4]
  - **Oral contraceptives**—may reduce the risk of CRC by 11–18%.[4]
- **Medical conditions.**
  - **Type 2 diabetes mellitus**—increases the risk of CRC by ~30%. One possible reason is the hyperinsulinaemia status as insulin is an important growth factor for colonic mucosal cells and can stimulate colonic tumour cells.[4]
  - **Gall bladder disease or cholecystectomy**—have been linked with significant increase in the risk of right-sided colon cancer (up to 50% in some meta-analyses) when followed up to 33y after surgery.[4]
  - **Inflammatory bowel disease.**[4]
- **Familial predisposition**—has a strong link to colon cancer (Table 36.6).[4]

Table 36.2 CRC dynamics

- **Right colon tumours**—usually become fairly large before giving any obstructive symptoms or causing significant change in bowel habits. This results from the liquid nature of faecal material passing through the ileocaecal valve. Right colon cancers usually ulcerate and cause chronic, sub-clinical intermittent blood loss with no change in the colour of stool. Patients often present with iron deficiency anaemia with related symptoms.
- **Transverse and left colon tumours**—the water content of stool passing through the transverse and descending colon reduces dramatically. Stool becomes concentrated and tumours block the passage of stool, giving rise to crampy abdominal pain and occasional obstruction. Rectal and sigmoid cancers commonly present with rectal bleeding, abdominal discomfort, change in bowel habit to looser and more frequent motions, and tenesmus. Iron deficiency anaemia is uncommon as the initial presentation.
- **Rectal cancers**—are defined as cancers where the distal margin lies at 15cm or less from the anal verge using a rigid sigmoidoscope.[1]

- *Referral guidelines*—all high-risk patients (Table 36.3) should be referred urgently for further investigations [C] .[1,2] Patients referred for a specialist opinion should normally be referred for a diagnostic test in the first instance.[14] Options include routine flexible sigmoidoscopy (Belfry plan), abdominal examination and FBC (Portsmouth), patients directed to specific diagnostic tests according to their symptoms (Leicester), and patients complete a detailed questionnaire leading to a risk score predicting the likelihood of cancer and guiding the choice of a specific test (Cheshire).[14]
- *CT colonography*—is an acceptable alternative to barium enema when available [B].[1] Accuracy depends on lesion size, with highly variable results ranging from 45–97% sensitivity (26–97% specificity) for polyps <6mm to 93% sensitivity (97% specificity) for polyps ≥1cm.[1]
- **Histologic confirmation**—essential in rectal tumours, and optional in highly suspicious lesions on double contrast barium enema or CT colonography in patients with iron deficiency anaemia and/or symptoms suggestive of cancer.[1]

Recommended initial staging

- **Basic investigations**—chest, liver, and pelvis imaging is essential prior to any elective treatment of CRC [B].[1,2]
  - *CXR*—can identify most pulmonary metastases. Less sensitive than CT scan and can miss significant numbers of lung metastases in recurrent cases.[1]
  - *Liver USS*—is sensitive in detecting metastases in ~55–80% of cases.[11] LFTs may not be deranged in small hepatic metastases.[11]
- **Thoracic, abdominal, and pelvic CT scan**—should be performed on all patients with CRC [B].[1,2]
  - *Accuracy*—CT scan can demonstrate transmural invasion of tumour in ~50% of cases, regional lymph nodal involvement in ~45–75% of cases, and distant metastases in ~75–90% of cases.[12,13]
  - *Special cases*—complete staging is not necessary if no influence on management is expected. The 18-fluoro-2-deoxyglucose (18-FDG) PET-CT can be used to accurately detect hepatic and extra-hepatic disease.[1] It is used to help difficult interpretation of CT scans.
- **MDT discussion**—essential requirement prior to commencing any definitive staging or treatment [G].[1] Decisions are taken in the context of predicted prognosis and expected effect of any investigation or treatment intervention on quality of life.[1]
- **Breaking bad news**—essential step to ensure adequate compliance. Should be done in a professional and effective way. The role of the cancer care nurse is essential [G].[1]

Table 36.3 High-risk patients[1]

- *All patients >40y old.*
  - With rectal bleeding associated with change in bowel habits (looseness or increased bowel frequency) for ≥6wk.
- *All patients >60y old.*
  - With change in bowel habits (looseness or increased bowel frequency) for ≥6wk and no PR bleeding.
  - With rectal bleeding for ≥6wk and no anal complaints (pain, itching, or lumps) or change in bowel habits.
- *All patients (any age).*
  - With palpable right lower abdominal mass.
  - With palpable rectal mass (intraluminal and not pelvic).
  - With iron deficiency anaemia and Hb <11 (any male) or Hb <10 (any non-menstruating female).

Table 36.4 Preoperative preparation in CRC

- ***Preparation for possible stoma formation***—should be done by a specialist stoma nurse, or in the case of an emergency, by an experienced surgeon who should mark the stoma site [C].[1,2]
- ***Blood cross-matching***—is recommended in rectal cancer operations and other extensive procedures. Right hemicolectomy requires 'group and save' only [C].[1] Blood transfusion has no significant effect on cancer recurrence and is indicated where necessary (see 📖 Chapter 13, pp.91–6) [C].[1,2]
- ***Bowel preparation***—is not recommended routinely before CRC operations [B].[1,2] Mechanical bowel preparation, polyethylene glycol (PEG) preparation, and phosphate enema have potential harm on anastomotic leak and outcome. Picolax® preparation has no influence (compared to no preparation) on outcome.[1]
- ***Thromboembolism prophylaxis***—using mechanical and pharmaceutical measures is recommended (see 📖 Chapter 11, pp.81–6) [A].[1,2]
- ***Antibiotic prophylaxis***—is recommended before any CRC surgery [A].[1,2] The exact regime of antibiotics for best prophylaxis remains unclear. Post-operative surgical site infection rate should not exceed 10% [A].[1,2]
- ***Enhanced recovery programme (ERP)***—has gained wide acceptance. The programme requires a dedicated team to ensure smooth preoperative planning, appropriate bowel preparation if indicated, proper application of preoperative preparations, good and effective pain control, proper post-operative enhanced mobility, and special diet regime perioperatively (high-calorie preoperatively and rapid diet-and-fluid build-up on d1 post-operatively).

- *Advanced staging*—only required if the patient is a candidate for surgical resection.[1]
  - *MRI*—should be performed in patients with rectal cancer to accurately assess tumour invasion and extension into adjacent organs [B].[1]
  - *Endorectal USS*—should be performed in all patients with rectal cancer where local excision is being considered [B].[1]
  - *Complete visualization of the colon*—should be achieved in all CRC patients, preferably preoperatively if possible, but within a few months post-operatively if unable to do so (e.g. obstructive lesion). The incidence of synchronous lesions is ~4–5%.[1]
- *TNM staging*—see Table 36.5.

Recommended treatment

General approach

- Complete surgical resection of CRC in suitable patients with or without adjuvant/neo-adjuvant therapy represents the best opportunity for long-term survival.[1,2]
- In general, ~70% of CRC patients presents with a resectable-for-cure cancer. Primary resection ± adjuvant/neo-adjuvant therapy is the only treatment required for 64% of this group. The other 36% experience recurrent disease, usually within the first 24mo. Therefore, advanced disease is found in a total of 55%, presenting either initially (30%) or developing as a post-operative recurrence (25%).[4]
- Complete curative resection is expected to be ~60% overall.[1]

Standards for surgical resection

- *Perioperative preparation*—see Table 36.4.
- *Extent of cancer resection.*
  - *Cancers in the right and transverse colon*—best treated using right or extended right hemicolectomy rather than segmental resection.[1] Involved extracolonic organs should be carefully resected (partially or totally) to achieve clear margins as appropriate.[1,2]
  - *Rectal cancer*—requires total mesorectal excision (TME) for all tumours in the lower two thirds. Rectal cancers in the upper third require a minimum of 5cm mesorectal excision below the lower margin of cancer while preserving the pelvic autonomic nerves [B].[1,2]
  - *Abdominal perineal resection (APR)*—should be considered in operations expected to fail in achieving ≥1cm clearance from the lower limit of the tumour. The APR rate should not exceed 30% of all rectal cancer resections [G].[1] Hartmann's procedure (see below) is appropriate is some older patients with poor sphincter control.
  - *Other issues*—the no-touch isolation technique (vascular control before manipulating the tumour) has no significant effect on outcome.[1,2] Tumour perforation during surgical manipulation adversely affects the local recurrence rate independent from preoperative cancer stage.[1]

- *Anastomosis.*
  - *Technique*—the lowest anastomotic leak rate can be achieved using interrupted sero-submucosal method [B].[1] Stapling techniques are used for low pelvic anastomoses [B].[1]
  - *Rectal stump washout*—is highly recommended using cytocidal solution prior to anastomosis [G].[1]
- **Defunctioning stoma**—should be judiciously considered in low rectal anastomosis [B].[1,2]
- **Local excision of rectal cancers**—is appropriate for (pathologic staging) T1 tumours, <3cm in diameter, and with well or moderately well differentiated histology [B].[1] Benefits and risks of local recurrence should be fully discussed with patient.[2]
- **Laparoscopic approach**—that maintains operative standards should be performed by properly trained surgeons [C].[1,2] These procedures are becoming the standard procedure in some units.
- **Emergency surgery for obstructing CRC**—should be preceded by CT scanning to exclude pseudo-obstruction, and is preferably performed during daytime by the colorectal team [C].[1,2] Immediate cancer resection (segmental or subtotal colectomy) with defunctioning colostomy (Hartmann's) or primary anastomosis (with possible temporary defunctioning ileostomy) are safe and appropriate options [C].[1,2] Insertion of an expanding stent for palliation or bridging to definitive surgery is acceptable where experience exists [B].[1,2]

Chemo/radiotherapy in CRC
- **Radiotherapy**—should be considered for all patients with resectable rectal cancer. Preoperative short-course radiotherapy (25Gy in 5 fractions in 1wk) is preferable, and surgical resection can be performed within 1wk of completion of radiation [A].[1,2]
  - *Long-course radiotherapy (45Gy in 25 fractions over weeks with a planned boost dose)*—is used to downstage more extensive rectal tumours and surgery is postponed for ~2mo after finishing the treatment. This is now often combined with synchronous chemotherapy.
  - *Post-operative radiotherapy*—should be considered for patients who have not received preoperative radiotherapy and have histologic risk factors for local recurrence (e.g. tumour at circumferential resection margins).[1]
- **Chemotherapy**—should be considered for patients with node-positive cancers. Choices to be jointly made with the patient taking into account contraindications and side effects.[5] Benefits and risks should also be extensively discussed with patients who have node-negative, but high-risk cancers, i.e. with adverse features (peritoneal involvement, vascular invasion, etc.) [A].[1]
  - *Timing*—should start within 6wk of surgery, and standard treatments with 6mo of 5-fluorouracil (5-FU) and folinic acid (FA)[2] have been updated with capecitabine as monotherapy or oxaliplatin in combination with 5-FU/FA.[5] Where possible, patients should be entered into RCTs as this is a fast developing field with new agents and combinations becoming available.

Follow-up

- Remains controversial. Limited evidence exists for intensive follow-up following CRC resection.[15,16]
  - 2002 guidelines—patients below the age of 70 would benefit from a CT scan for liver secondaries [A] and colonoscopy 5-yearly up to the age of 70 [B].[16] Routine CEA remains questionable.[16]
  - 2007 guidelines—recommend one CT scan in the first 2y post-operatively and 5-yearly 'clean' (i.e. no polyps) colonoscopy.
  - Meta-analyses have shown benefits for intensive follow-up and American guidelines advise more intensive follow-up with, for instance, 3-yearly colonoscopies, no age limits, and with the routine use of CEA.[15,17]

Table 36.5 Rectal cancer—recommended approach

- ***Basic facts***—diagnosed in ~850 patients in the UK each year.[4] A total of 80% of patients have evidence of HPV infection (commonly types 16 and 18), the same that causes cervical cancer, and the disease is more often found in women. Diminished immunity, larger numbers of sexual partners, and smoking are also relevant.

- ***Clinical presentation***—fresh bleeding, perianal lump, discharge, pain, and sometimes minimal symptoms. Induration on examination is an important predictor of disease. Lymph drainage is to the groins and they must be examined.

- ***Diagnosis***—awareness (complicated haemorrhoids are more common) and biopsy (may require general anaesthesia).

- ***Staging***—EUA, sigmoidoscopy, rectal USS, pelvic MRI. CT scans as for colon cancer.

- ***Treatment***—best performed within a multidisciplinary anal cancer teams. Well-differentiated anal margin lesions <2cm can be locally excised [C].[1] Anal canal lesions should usually be treated with concurrent chemotherapy (5-FU and mitomycin C or cisplatin) and radiotherapy.[1] Entry into trials is encouraged as optimal treatment is uncertain. Radical surgery is sometimes required as is multimodality palliative care.

- ***Prognosis***—about 60% of men and 70% of women will be alive at 5y following treatment when taking all stages of anal cancer into account.[4]

Table 36.6 Familial predisposition in CRC—facts and figures

- **Estimated risk**—one member of the family who has had bowel cancer (4–10% of all presentations) doubles the risk to other members. The advice of regional genetic services is strongly recommended in patients with significant family history.[1,18,19]

- **FAP surveillance.**
  - With negative mutations (minority)—annual flexible sigmoidoscopy is indicated for age 13–30 and 3–5 yearly until 60.[1]
  - Patients identified as having FAP should be encouraged to undergo proctocolectomy and ileoanal pouch between the ages of 16–20 [B].[1] The anastomosis and anorectal cuff must be checked subsequently on a yearly basis. Patients with FAP have a significant risk of upper GI cancer and should have 3-yearly OGDs, or more frequently if extensive duodenal polyposis [B].[1,18]

- **HNPCC surveillance**—should be biennial from the age of 25 or 5y younger than the incidence in the youngest family member.
  - **Total colonoscopy**—is the investigation of choice and should be continued to the age of 75 if the mutation abnormality is not identified [B].[1,18]
  - At present, there is insufficient data to recommend prophylactic colectomy in patients with known mutations, but total colectomy should be offered for patients who develop a curative colonic carcinoma,[18] and continue with regular surveillance of remaining bowel.
  - OGDs should be advised for patients in families with known gastric cancers from the age of 50 or 5y earlier than the youngest reported case in the family [C].[18]

- **High–moderate risk**—three or more affected relatives, none aged <50y, should be offered 5-yearly colonoscopy (or 3-yearly if adenomas found) aged 55–75.[1]

- **Moderate risk**—one first-degree relative aged <45 or two affected first-degree relatives should be offered a single colonoscopy at the age of 55 and continued surveillance if adenomas are found.[1] Earlier guidance had suggested that consideration for surveillance should be at age 35–40;[19] this was a relative recommendation, but took into consideration the anxiety of a patient having to wait until the age of 55.

- **Low risk**—patients should be reassured and advised to be involved in population screening (FOB test).[1]

- **US guidelines**—differ. A family history of CRC or adenomas in a first-degree relative aged <60 or in two or more relatives of any age, then colonoscopy from age 40 or 10y before the youngest case in the immediate family every 5y.[20]

Further reading

1. The Association of Coloproctology of Great Britain and Ireland (2007). Guidelines for the management of colorectal cancer. Available from: http://www.acpgbi.org.uk/assets/documents/COLO_guides.pdf.
2. National Institute for Health and Clinical Excellence (2004). Improving outcomes in colorectal cancer. Available from: http://www.nice.org.uk/guidance/CSGCC.
3. Scottish Intercollegiate Guidelines Network (2003). Management of colorectal cancer. Available from: http://www.sign.ac.uk/pdf/sign67.pdf.

4. Cancer Research UK (2008). Bowel (colorectal) cancer. Available from: http://info. cancerresearchuk.org/cancerstats/types/bowel/?a=5441.

5. NHS Cancer Services Collaborative (2006). Bowel Cancer. Available from: http://www.ebc-indevelopment.co.uk/nhs/colorectal/index.html. Accessed May 2009.

6. Giovannucci E, Stampfer MJ, Colditz GA et al. (1998). Multivitamin use, folate, and colon cancer in women in the Nurses' Health Study. Ann Intern Med 129, 517–24.

7. Matsui T, Yao T, Yao K et al. (1996). Natural history of superficial depressed colorectal cancer: retrospective radiographic and histologic analysis. Radiology 201, 226–32.

8. Bengtsson G, Carlsson G, Hafström L, Jönsson PE (1981). Natural history of patients with untreated liver metastases from colorectal cancer. Am J Surg 141, 586–9.

9. Speights VO, Johnson MW, Stoltenberg PH, Rappaport ES, Helbert B, Riggs M (1991). Colorectal cancer: current trends in initial clinical manifestations. South Med J 84, 575–8.

10. Steinberg SM, Barkin JS, Kaplan RS, Stablein DM (1986). Prognostic indicators of colon tumours. The Gastrointestinal Tumour Study Group experience. Cancer 57, 1866–70.

11. Niederhuber JE (1993). Colon and rectum cancer: patterns of spread and implications for workup. Cancer 71 (12 Suppl), 4187–92.

12. Hundt W, Braunschweig R, Reiser M (1999). Evaluation of spiral CT in staging of colon and rectum carcinoma. Eur Radiol 9, 78–84.

13. Isbister WH, al-Sanea O (1996). The utility of preoperative abdominal computerized tomography scanning in colorectal surgery. J R Coll Surg Edinb 41, 232–4.

14. Selvachandran SN, Hodder RJ, Ballal MS, Jones P, Cade D (2002). Prediction of colorectal cancer by a patient consultation questionnaire and scoring system: a prospective study. Lancet 360, 278–83.

15. Renehan AG, Egger M, Saunders MP, O'Dwyer ST (2002). Impact on survival of intensive follow-up after curative resection for colorectal cancer: systematic review and meta-analysis of randomized trials. BMJ 324, 813.

16. Scholefield JH, Steele RJ, British Society for Gastroenterology, Association of Coloproctology for Great Britain and Ireland (2002). Guidelines for follow-up after resection of colorectal cancer. Gut 51 (Suppl 5), V3–5.

17. Anthony T, Simmang C, Hyman N et al. (2004). Practice parameters for the surveillance and follow-up of patients with colon and rectal cancer. Dis Colon Rectum 47, 807–17.

18. Dunlop MG, British Society for Gastroenterology, Association of Coloproctology for Great Britain and Ireland (2002). Guidance on gastrointestinal surveillance for hereditary non-polyposis colorectal cancer, familial adenomatous polyposis, juvenile polyposis, and Peutz–Jeghers syndrome. Gut 51 (Suppl 5), V21–7.

19. Dunlop MG, British Society for Gastroenterology, Association of Coloproctology for Great Britain and Ireland (2002). Guidance on large bowel surveillance for people with two first-degree relatives with colorectal cancer or one first-degree relative diagnosed with colorectal cancer under 45 years. Gut 51 (Suppl 5), V17–20.

20. Levin B, Lieberman DA, McFarland B (2008). Screening and surveillance for the early detection of colorectal cancer and adenomatous polyps, 2008: a joint guideline from the American Cancer Society, the US Multi-Society Task Force on Colorectal Cancer, and the American College of Radiology. Gastroenterology 134, 1570–95.

Pancreas

Paradiso

Acute pancreatitis*

* The guidelines on this chapter have been sourced and summarized from different UK, Europe, and international government sources, professional organizations, and medical specialty societies. Leading guidelines have been listed in the Key guidelines box.

Acute pancreatitis

Key guidelines

- Working Party of the British Society of Gastroenterology, Association of Surgeons of Great Britain and Ireland, Pancreatic Society of Great Britain and Ireland, Association of Upper GI Surgeons of Great Britain and Ireland (2005). UK guidelines for the management of acute pancreatitis.
- National Institute for Health and Clinical Excellence (2003). Percutaneous pancreatic necrostomy.
- AGA Institute Clinical Practice and Economics Committee, AGA Institute Governing Board (2007). Technical review on acute pancreatitis.
- International Association of Pancreatology (2002). Guidelines for the surgical management of acute pancreatitis.

Basic facts

- *Incidence*—affects ~15–45 persons per 100,000 population and appears to be rising.[1]
- *Pathogenesis*—inflammatory process resulting from autodigestion of pancreatic substance by inappropriately activated pancreatic enzymes.[1,3] Most common causes are obstructing gallstone and alcohol abuse (Table 37.1).
- *Clinical presentation*—typically presents with severe and persistent epigastric or upper abdominal pain radiating through to the back (40–70% of cases),[3] often following the consumption of a large meal, and is associated with nausea, vomiting, and retching. Systemic signs may be prominent in severe cases (Table 37.2).

Recommended investigations

- *Immediate assessment*—should include evaluation of cardiovascular, respiratory, and renal functions, BMI, LFTs, and CXR.[1]
- *Diagnosis confirmation*—is usually made by the combination of raised pancreatic enzymes and associated clinical picture.[1]
  - *Serum amylase*—the usual cornerstone of diagnosis. Values of 3 or 4 times greater than normal have been used historically although the interpretation should be careful (amylase may not rise in mild attacks, falsely rise in non-pancreatitis conditions, or drops down by the time of blood collection).[1,3] Raised amylase values (within appropriate clinical context) has moderate sensitivity (45–85%) and high specificity (91–99%).[3]
  - *Plasma lipase*—has slightly superior sensitivity and specificity, and greater overall accuracy than amylase (still requires careful interpretation).[3] Serum lipase, where available, is the preferred method to support the diagnosis as it remains elevated in the serum longer than amylase (lipase has a longer half-life) [A].[1]
- *Abdominal USS*—can demonstrate gallstones and dilatation of the common bile duct (CBD), and exclude other pathologies unrelated to the pancreas such as abdominal aortic aneurysm.[1] Classical findings include a diffusely enlarged, hypoechoic pancreas.
- *Abdominal CT scan*—the gold standard investigation where the diagnosis is unclear [C].[1]

Table 37.1 Acute pancreatitis—aetiology

● **Gallstone disease.**
  • Accounts for ~35–40% of cases (only 3–7% of patients with gallstone develop acute pancreatitis).[1,3]
  • Small stones (<5mm) and male gender increases the risk of developing acute pancreatitis.[5,6]
  • Raised ALT and/or AST (but not bilirubin or alkaline phosphatase) are strong predictive laboratory tests for gallstone-related pancreatitis (positive predictive value >95%).[6]
  • **Other obstructive lesions**—periampullary tumours, ascariasis, and periampullary diverticula.

● **Alcohol**—accounts for ~20–25% of cases (about 10% of chronic alcoholics develop attacks of acute pancreatitis).[1,3,8]
  • **Other toxic aetiologies**—scorpion venom and organophosphate poisoning.

● **Other causes**—include **metabolic** (serum triglycerides >11mmol/L, hypercalcaemia), **drug-induced** (e.g. furosemide, thiazides, azathioprine, valproic acid), **infection-related** (e.g. mumps, CMV, HIV, salmonella, aspergillus, toxoplasma, ascaris), **trauma-induced** (blunt or penetrating, surgery, ERCP), **congenital** (pancreas divisum), **vascular** (ischaemia, vasculitis), **genetic** (CFTR), other **miscellaneous** reasons (pregnancy, renal transplantation), and **idiopathic** (only after vigorous search for underlying cause. Should not exceed 20–25% of cases [B]).[1,3]

Table 37.2 Acute pancreatitis—possible physical findings

● **Local features**—epigastric tenderness, flank discoloration (Grey–Turner's sign) or the periumbilical region (Cullen's sign) (<1% of cases, non-diagnostic), epigastric mass (pancreatic pseudocyst).

● **Systemic features**—fever, multiorgan failure, jaundice (gallstone-related or alcoholic liver disease), subcutaneous nodular fat necrosis (panniculitis), thrombophlebitis in the legs, and polyarthritis.

● **Objective scoring of severity**—should support the clinical assessment to formulate appropriate management plan [A].[1]
  • *Definitions*—severe acute pancreatitis (potentially lethal pancreatitis) is defined as the presence of organ(s) failure and/or local pancreatic complications, complemented by the presence of unfavourable prognostic signs (using Ranson's criteria and Acute Physiology and Chronic Health Evaluation [APACHE] II) (Atlanta Criteria).[1,3,4,11]
  • *Benefits of objective scoring*—early prediction of severe cases allows appropriate admission to higher level of care (see 📖 Chapter 15, pp.101–6), aggressive fluid management, timely correction of metabolic abnormalities, and possible institution of severity reduction procedures.[3,4]
  • *First 24h*—severity is best predicted by experienced clinical judgement (initial low accuracy, but equivalent to APACHE II prediction power by 48h),[3] APACHE II score >8 (sensitivity and specificity ~70%) (Table 37.3),[3] and obesity [B].[1,3]

- *At 48h*—severity is best assessed using Glasgow score ≥3 (Table 37.3), CRP >150mg/L, and persistent organ failure [B].[1]
- *Other scoring systems*—have also been developed and used (APACHE III, APACHE IV, SAPS II, etc.).[3]

Recommended treatment

- **Level of care**—all patients with severe acute pancreatitis should be treated in a level 2/3 care (HDU or ICU; see 📖 Chapter 15, pp.101–6).[1]
- **General supportive treatment**—should follow the care of critically ill surgical patient principles (Table 37.4) (see also 📖 Chapter 15).
- **Pain management**—should be effective and multimodal (see 📖 Chapter 19, pp.133–140).
- **Prophylactic antibiotics**—remain of unproven benefits and specific recommendations cannot be made.[1]
  - The decreased mortality (though a similar rate of pancreatic necrosis infection) suggested by a Cochrane systematic review[12] is consistent with the AGA recommendations of using antibiotics in patients who are at reasonable risk of developing infected pancreatic necrosis.[3] This may correlate well with pancreatic necrosis of over 30%.[3]
  - The maximum duration of prophylactic antibiotics should not exceed 14d [B].[1]
  - Selective gut decontamination is not recommended as there is no clear benefit and no statistically significant reduction in mortality.[1,16]
- **Nutritional support**—not recommended for mild acute pancreatitis (no restriction on diet and fluid).[1] UK guidelines have made no specific recommendations on nutritional support for severe acute pancreatitis.[1] Nevertheless, a more recent meta-analysis and systematic review, as well as the fact that most patients with severe cases are unable to eat or drink within 5–7d (due to nausea, ileus, and abdominal pain), are in consistence with the AGA recommendations of using nutritional support (preferably enteral [A])[1] to reduce the infection rate (RR × 0.46), length of hospital stay (4d) and possible mortality (RR × 0.26).[3,13,14]
- **Treatment of gallstone-related pancreatitis.**
  - *Urgent therapeutic ERCP (within 72h)*—is recommended for all gallstone-related pancreatitis patients who have signs of obstructed bile duct or cholangitis [A].[1,3,4] ERCP is best performed within 72h of the onset of pain, and sphincterotomy should be performed on all those patients regardless of finding a stone [C].[1] Urgent ERCP for severe (or predicted severe) pancreatitis is more controversial (recommended in the UK and Hong Kong).[1,3,4]
  - *Early laparoscopic cholecystectomy (in the same hospital admission and no more than 2–4wk)*—should be recommended for all fit patients [B].[1,3,4]
- **Treatment of complications.**
  - *Pancreatic necrosis*—requires fine needle aspiration (FNA) for culture and sensitivity if the necrosis is over 30% [B].[1,4] This should be performed in 1–2wk from the onset of pancreatitis [B].[1]

- *Sterile necrosis*—should be managed conservatively if possible [B].[3] Surgical intervention should be reserved for individual cases [B].[3]
- *Septic necrosis*—requires radiological and/or surgical drainage depending on available experience and the individual case [B].[1,3,4]
- *Current surgical options*—should aim at an 'organ-preserving approach'.[4] Options include open necrosectomy with closed continuous lavage of the pancreatic bed, open necrosectomy with planned re-laparotomy and drainage, and open necrosectomy with packing and planned re-laparotomies.[4]
- *Pancreatic fluid collection and pseudocyst*—can be treated conservatively if remains small (<6cm) and symptom-free. Larger symptomatic cysts require endoscopic, radiologic, or surgical intervention, depending on the anatomic location and available experience.[1,3,4]

Table 37.3 Severity scoring systems

APACHE II—Score
- check the following parameters:
  - –General: Age, Presence of chronic organ insufficiency
  - –Vital signs: Temperature, Heart rate, respiratory rate
  - –Basic Tests: WCC, Hct, Na, K, Cr
  - –ABG: PH, A-a Gradient, PO_2
- Calculate APACHE II score using appropriate online tool:
  - –www.mdcalc.com/apache-ii-score-for-icu-mortality
  - –www.medicalcriteria.com/sitei/apache II.jpg

Glasgow scoring

Source: OHCM. 2001. p.467:
- Modified Glasgow Criteria

• Age >55y	• LDH >600 U/l
• WCC >15 × 10⁹/L	• Alb <32 g/L
• Urea >16 mmol/l	• PaO₂ <8 kPa
• Glucose (Blood) >10 mmol/L	• Ca <2 mmol/L

Score ≥ 3 within 48h is consistent with severe disease

Table 37.4 Supportive management—special considerations

- ***Oxygen management***—usually required as hypoxia is common.[3] Pleural effusion can be treated conservatively unless affecting pulmonary function.[3]

- ***Fluid management***—crystalloids are preferred over colloids. Aggressive fluid resuscitation (even for mild cases) is preferable if no contraindications exist (better outcome).[3] A CVP line may be required if fluid management is compromised by poor cardiac function.[3]

- ***Hypocalcaemia***—is common (due to hypoalbuminaemia) and does not require treatment (unless severe or symptomatic).[3]

- ***Hypomagnesaemia***—is common.

- ***Hypo- or hyperglycaemia***—are common as well.

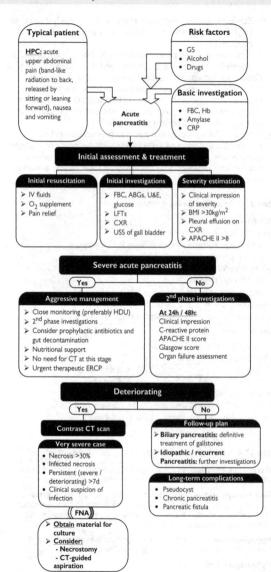

Fig. 37.1 Recommended approach to patients with acute pancreatitis

Further reading

1. Working Party of the British Society of Gastroenterology, Association of Surgeons of Great Britain and Ireland, Pancreatic Society of Great Britain and Ireland, Association of Upper GI Surgeons of Great Britain and Ireland (2005). UK guidelines for the management of acute pancreatitis. *Gut* 54 (Suppl 3:iii), 1–9.

2. National Institute for Health and Clinical Excellence (2003). Percutaneous pancreatic necrostomy. Available from; http://www.nice.org.uk/nicemedia/pdf/ip/IPG033guidance.pdf.

3. Forsmark CE, Baillie J; AGA Institute Clinical Practice and Economics Committee, AGA Institute Governing Board (2007). AGA Institute technical review on acute pancreatitis. *Gastroenterology* 132, 2022–44.

4. Uhl W, Warshaw A, Imrie C et al. (2002). IAP guidelines for the surgical management of acute pancreatitis. *Pancreatology* 2, 565–73.

5. Sanders G, Kingsnorth AN (2007). Gallstones. *BMJ* 335, 295–9.

6. Venneman NG, Buskens E, Besselink MG et al. (2005). Small gallstones are associated with increased risk of acute pancreatitis: potential benefits of prophylactic cholecystectomy? *Am J Gastroenterol* 100, 2540–50.

7. Tenner S, Dubner H, Steinberg W (1994). Predicting gallstone pancreatitis with laboratory parameters: a meta-analysis. *Am J Gastroenterol* 89, 1863–6.

8. Ammann RW, Heitz PU, Klöppel G (1996). Course of alcoholic chronic pancreatitis: a prospective clinicomorphological long term study. *Gastroenterology* 111, 224–31.

9. Fortson MR, Freedman SN, Webster PD 3rd (1995). Clinical assessment of hyperlipidaemic pancreatitis. *Am J Gastroenterol* 90, 2134–9.

10. Balthazar EJ, Freeny PC, van Sonnenberg E (1994). Imaging and intervention in acute pancreatitis. *Radiology* 193, 297–306.

11. Bradley EL 3rd (1993). A clinically based classification system for acute pancreatitis. Summary of the International Symposium on Acute Pancreatitis, Atlanta GA, September 11 through 13, 1992. *Arch Surg* 128, 586–590.

12. Villatoro E, Bassi C, Larvin M (2006). Antibiotic therapy for prophylaxis against infection of pancreatic necrosis in acute pancreatitis. *Cochrane database Syst Rev* 4, CD002941.

13. Marik PE, Zaloga GP (2004). Meta-analysis of parenteral nutrition versus enteral nutrition in patients with acute pancreatitis. *BMJ* 328, 1407.

14. McClave SA, Chang WK, Dhaliwal R, Heyland DK (2006). Nutrition support in acute pancreatitis: a systematic review of the literature. *JPEN J Parenter Enteral Nutr* 30, 143–56.

15. Banks PA, Freeman ML, the Practice Parameters Committee of the American College of Gastroenterology (2006). Practice guidelines in acute pancreatitis. *Am J Gastroenterol* 101, 2379–400.

16. Luiten EJ, Hop WC, Lange JF, Bruining HA (1995). Controlled clinical trial of selective decontamination for the treatment of severe acute pancreatitis. *Ann Surg* 222, 57–65.

Chronic pancreatitis*

---

* The guidelines on this chapter have been sourced and summarized from different UK, Europe, and international government sources, professional organizations, and medical specialty societies. Leading guidelines have been listed in the Key guidelines box.

Chronic pancreatitis

Key guidelines
- Whitcomb DC, Yadav D, Adam S et al. (2008). Multicentre approach to recurrent acute and chronic pancreatitis in the United States: the North American Pancreatitis Study 2 (NAPS2).
- Ihse I, Andersson R, Albiin N (2003). Guidelines for management of patients with chronic pancreatitis. Report from a consensus conference.
- BMJ ABC of diseases (2001). ABC of diseases of liver, pancreas, and biliary system: chronic pancreatitis.
- Etemad B, Whitcomb DC (2001). Chronic pancreatitis: diagnosis, classification, and new genetic developments.
- Society for Surgery of the Alimentary Tract (2004). Operative treatment for chronic pancreatitis.

Basic facts
- **Definition**—syndrome characterized by progressive long-standing inflammatory changes in the pancreas with consequent permanent structural damage and resultant impairment of exocrine and endocrine functions.[1,3,4]
- **Incidence**—affects ~3–9 persons per 100,000 population.[3,6]
- **Risk factors**—see Table 38.1.
- **Clinical manifestations**—commonly presents with abdominal pain (Table 38.2) and pancreatic insufficiency (fat malabsorption, vitamin deficiency, and pancreatic diabetes) at a later stage.[2,3,6,8]
- **Complications**—include pseudocyst formation (10% of cases), bile duct or duodenal obstruction (5–10% of cases), pancreatic ascites or pleural effusion (due to pancreatic fistula or rupture of pseudocyst), splenic vein thrombosis, and pancreatic cancer.

Recommended investigations (Fig 38.1)
- **Confirmation of diagnosis**—can be challenging. Clinical manifestations may be atypical, laboratory tests may be normal, and imaging investigations might be inconclusive. A proper combination of clinical, functional, histologic, or morphologic criteria can be helpful (Table 38.3). The diagnosis has often to be made on the exclusion of other diseases.

Recommended treatment (Fig 38.1)
As a general rule, a multidisciplinary approach is required to treat chronic pancreatitis, preferably in specialist centres.
- **Objectives**—management of excessive alcohol consumption, pain relief, correction of pancreatic insufficiency, and management of complications.
- **Alcohol consumption**—should be avoided as a first step (consensus opinion).[6] Stopping alcohol consumption has clear benefits and can prevent further injury to the pancreas and other organs.[2,3,6,8]

Table 38.1 Risk factors for chronic pancreatitis

- *Alcohol abuse*—accounts for most cases (70–80%).[1,3] Other factors play important role in alcohol-induced chronic pancreatitis, e.g. only ~5–10% of alcoholics will suffer from chronic pancreatitis. Cigarette smoking and genetic factors might predispose alcoholics to serious hyper-reaction to alcohol.[7]

- *Other risk factors*—include hereditary pancreatitis (autosomal dominant trait affecting younger ages and increasing the risk of pancreatic adenocarcinoma), persistent pancreatic ductal obstruction (trauma, pseudocysts, stones, or tumours), tropical pancreatitis (In a few tropical areas, most notably Kerala in southern India, malnutrition and ingestion of large quantities of cassava root are implicated in the aetiology. The disease affects men and women equally, with an incidence of up to 50/1,000 population)[3], systemic diseases (hypertriglyceridemia, hyperparathyroidism, cystic fibrosis, and systemic lupus erythematosus), and idiopathic pancreatitis (majority of cases not related to alcohol abuse). Work on genetic and molecular factors is progressing.[1,2,8]

Table 38.2 Pain types in chronic pancreatitis[8]

- *Type A pain*—short episodes of <10d separated by long pain-free intervals. Predominant pattern in idiopathic senile or late onset chronic pancreatitis (ISCP) and hereditary pancreatitis. Can successfully be managed without invasive procedures.

- *Type B pain*—≥1–2mo intermittent intervals. Occurs in ~60% of idiopathic juvenile or early onset chronic pancreatitis (IJCP). Usually requires surgery and is commonly associated with local complications (e.g. pseudocysts and obstructive cholestasis). This has a major implication on the widespread recommendation of endoscopic therapy in chronic pancreatitis.

Table 38.3 Diagnosis of chronic pancreatitis[9]

- *Confirmed chronic pancreatitis* (within appropriate clinical setting)— presence of pancreatic stones on screening KUB, USS, or CT scan; scattered irregular dilatation of pancreatic duct branches (or main duct with proximal obstruction) on ERCP/MRCP; decreased pancreatic enzyme and bicarbonate output on secretin test; irregular fibrosis and loss of exocrine parenchyma on histologic examination; and/or the presence of protein plugs or cyst formation.

- *Probably chronic pancreatitis*—coarse hyper-reflectivity on USS; pancreatic deformity on CT scan; irregular isolated dilatation on ERCP; decreased pancreatic enzyme or bicarbonate output on secretin test; and atypical chronic changes on histologic specimens.

- *Pain management*—follow a stepwise approach with judicious use of analgesics. (See Ch. 19). Placebo effect has significant role in those patients (effective in up to 30% of cases).[10]
  - *Tramadol*—more effective than morphine at reducing pain within 4d, but is associated with more adverse gastrointestinal effects.[6]
  - *Coeliac plexus block/ablation*—reserved for patients with refractory pain to opioid analgesics. Supportive evidence of consistent efficiency is weak. Best performed on patients with small duct pancreatitis (large duct patients may benefit more from surgical

drainage as a last option). Using endoscopic ultrasound-guided plexus block/ablation may be more effective in managing the pain at 4wk compared with CT-guided nerve blocks.[6,11]

- **Dietary changes.**
  - *Low-fat diet*—there is no supporting evidence of any significant beneficial effect on pain management or progression of chronic pancreatitis.[3,6] A low-fat diet may help in alleviating steatorrhoea by decreasing the overall amount of ingested fat.
  - *Pancreatic enzyme supplement*—not been shown to be more effective when compared with placebo in reducing the pain at 2–32wk of follow-up.[6] Pancreatic enzyme supplements have a significant effect in reducing steatorrhoea.[3,6]
  - *Oral citrate*—is less effective than placebo in reducing pain at 18mo.[6] However, it is more effective at reducing the calcification within the same time period.

- **Endoscopic procedures.**
  - *Endoscopic pancreatic duct decompression*—has been shown to be effective in reducing pain in two thirds of patients when done selectively.[12] It has a relatively quick recovery, but has slightly lower results compared to surgery in controlling the pain and helping in gaining weight. However, views have been expressed that the quality of studies has been limited and the benefits limited,[8] with further evidence from a recent randomized trial showing better results with surgical procedures.[13]
  - *Endoscopic biliary duct decompression*—may be required in 5–10% of patients to treat jaundice and prevent cholangitis.

- **Surgical interventions.**[2,3,5,6]
  - *Indications*—usually reserved for patients with complications, patient who failed to control symptoms with adequate analgesia and/or endoscopic measures, and patients who would prefer to avoid the risk of addiction to opioid analgesia.
  - *Benefits*—with careful selection, can control the pain in ~35% of patients who failed endoscopic procedures and increase the body weight at 5y follow-up.
  - *Harm*—no significant difference in complication rates compared to endoscopic procedures.
  - *Technique*—most commonly are the duodenal preserving resection of the pancreatic head (Beger's procedure) and Frey's ductal decompression (pancreatico-jejunostomy). There is no significant difference in outcome between the two procedures. Occasionally total and subtotal pancreatectomies are necessary. NICE have supported laparoscopic distal pancreatectomy under careful clinical governance conditions.

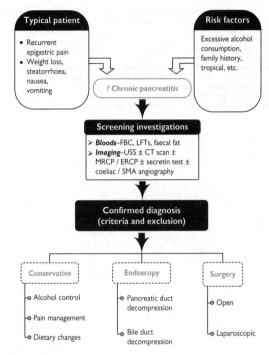

Fig. 38.1 Approaching chronic pancreatitis

Further reading

1. Whitcomb DC, Yadav D, Adam S et al. (2008). Multicentre approach to recurrent acute and chronic pancreatitis in the United States: the North American Pancreatitis Study 2 (NAPS2). Pancreatology 8, 520–31.
2. Ihse I, Andersson R, Albiin N (2003). Guidelines for management of patients with chronic pancreatitis. Report from a consensus conference. [Article in Swedish.] Lakartidningen 100, 2518–25.
3. Bornman PC, Beckingham IJ (2001). ABC of diseases of liver, pancreas, and biliary system: chronic pancreatitis. BMJ 322, 660–3.
4. Etemad B, Whitcomb DC (2001). Chronic pancreatitis: diagnosis, classification, and new genetic developments. Gastroenterology 120, 682–707.
5. Society for Surgery of the Alimentary Tract (2004). Operative treatment for chronic pancreatitis. Available from: http://www.guideline.gov/summary/summary.aspx?ss=15&doc_id=5506&nbr=3749.
6. Kocher HM, Froeling FE (2008). Chronic pancreatitis. BMJ Clin Evid 12, 417.
7. Maisonneuve P, Lowenfels AB, Mullhaupt B et al. (2005). Cigarette smoking accelerates progression of alcoholic chronic pancreatitis. Gut 54, 510–4.
8. DiMagno MJ, DiMagno EP (2006). Chronic pancreatitis. Curr Opin Gastroenterol 22, 487–97.
9. Homma T, Harada H, Koizumi M (1997). Diagnostic criteria for chronic pancreatitis by the Japan Pancreas Society. Pancreas 15, 14–5.

10. Warshaw AL, Banks PA, Fernández-Del Castillo C (1998). AGA technical review: treatment of pain in chronic pancreatitis. *Gastroenterology* 115, 765–76.
11. Gress F, Schmitt C, Sherman S, Ikenberry S, Lehman G (1999). A prospective randomized comparison of endoscopic ultrasound and computed tomography-guided coeliac plexus block for managing chronic pancreatitis pain. *Am J Gastroenterol* 94, 900–5.
12. Rösch T, Daniel S, Scholz M *et al.* (2002). Endoscopic treatment of chronic pancreatitis: a multicentre study of 1,000 patients with long-term follow-up. *Endoscopy* 34, 765–71.
13. Cahen DL, Gouma DJ, Nio Y *et al.* (2007). Endoscopic versus surgical drainage of the pancreatic duct in chronic pancreatitis. *N Engl J Med* 356, 676–84.
14. National Institute for Health and Clinical Excellence (2007). Laparoscopic distal pancreatectomy. Available from: http://www.nice.org.uk/nicemedia/pdf/IPG204guidance.pdf.

Pancreatic cancer*

* The guidelines on this chapter have been sourced and summarized from different UK, Europe, and international government sources, professional organizations, and medical specialty societies. Leading guidelines have been listed in the Key guidelines box.

Pancreatic cancer

Key guidelines

- Pancreatic Section of the British Society of Gastroenterology, Pancreatic Society of Great Britain and Ireland, Association of Upper Gastrointestinal Surgeons of Great Britain and Ireland, Royal College of Pathologists, Special Interest Group for Gastrointestinal Radiology (2005). Guidelines for the management of patients with pancreatic cancer periampullary and ampullary carcinomas.
- Society for Surgery of the Alimentary Tract (2004). Surgical treatment of pancreatic cancer.
- Cancer Research UK (2008). Pancreatic cancer.
- National Institute for Health and Clinical Excellence (2007). Laparoscopic distal pancreatectomy.

Basic facts

- **Incidence**—the tenth most common cancer in the UK and fourth most common cause of cancer death in developed countries.[1,3,5] Most cases occur in the 60–80y age group (85% cases affect patients over the age of 60).[3] The incidence has been declining steadily in men (most likely due to decreased smoking behaviour), but remained fairly steady in females since the late 1970s.[3] Periampullary carcinomas (e.g. lower CBD and duodenal) are less common, but present with the same symptoms. Neuroendocrine tumours of the pancreas are not considered in this chapter (see 📖 Chapter 29, pp.215–220).
- **Risk factors**—smoking accounts for 1 in every 5 cases of pancreatic cancer.[3] Other risk factors include chronic pancreatitis, type 1 or 2 diabetes, obesity, and familial cancers (Table 39.1).[1,3,5] Underlying pancreatic cancer should be excluded in adult onset of non-familial diabetes and in unexplained attack of pancreatitis (5% of pancreatic cancer presentations).[1]
- **Pathology**—most pancreatic cancers are of ductal origin.
- **Clinical presentation**—initial presentation varies depending on the tumour size and location. Symptoms are caused primarily by mass effect rather than exocrine or endocrine dysfunction. Over 50% of patients have metastatic disease at the time of diagnosis. Only 8% of cancer remain localized (Table 39.2).

Recommended investigations

- **Abdominal USS**—liver, bile duct, and pancreatic USS are the initial investigation of choice [B].[1] USS has a sensitivity of ~80% and specificity of 90% in detecting the pancreatic cancer (larger than 2cm) and/or liver metastasis.[1,3] USS is less sensitive in detecting pancreatic body or tail cancers.
- **CT and/or MR scan**—the gold standard imaging modality, but only indicated in patients with highly suspicious signs of pancreatic malignancy [B].[1,3] The selective use of CT scan, MRI scan (including MRCP and occasionally MRA), and other supporting modalities can

accurately delineate tumour size, infiltration, resectability, and the presence of metastatic disease in >95–97% of cases.[1,3]

Table 39.1 Risk factors for pancreatic cancer

- **Smoking**—very important risk factor (RR × 1.5–2.5). Smoking accounts for ~25–30% of cases, and risk reduces by 48% within 2y of stopping smoking.[8]
- **Genetic susceptibility**—have a role in ~10% of patients.[3,9] Risk increases in families with hereditary pancreatitis (RR × 50–70), familial pancreatic cancer (OR × 1.5–5.25),[10] and other familial-related cancers (familial atypical multiple mole melanoma, Peutz–Jeghers syndrome, hereditary non-polyposis colorectal carcinoma (HNPCC), familial breast-ovarian cancer syndromes, and familial adenomatous polyposis (FAP)).[1,3]
- **Medical diseases**—include chronic pancreatitis (RR × 5–15) and adult onset diabetes of <2y duration (RR × 2.1).[11,12]
- **Other factors**—of unproven correlation, includes diet (high fat and protein, low fruit and vegetable intake), coffee and alcohol consumption, and occupation.[1,3]
- **Primary prevention**—includes educational programmes in smoking cessation, secondary screening for high-risk patients, and pre-emptive surgery if appropriate [B].[1]

Table 39.2 Symptoms and signs of pancreatic cancer

- **Main symptoms**—weight loss (~90–100% of cases at presentation), abdominal pain (~70–85% of cases), and jaundice (82% of cancers in the head and 7% of cancers in the body and tail).[1,3,13]
  - **Other symptoms**—include nausea (45%), anorexia (33–66%), malaise (40%), and vomiting (35%).[7]
  - **Advanced disease**—may present with back pain, marked and rapid weight loss, abdominal mass, migratory thrombophlebitis, ascites, and supraclavicular lymphadenopathy.[1,13]
- **Physical examination**—may be non-specific.
  - **Courvoisier's sign**—distended, palpable, but non-tender gall bladder in a jaundiced patient. Has ~85% specificity, but only 26–55% sensitivity for malignant obstruction of the bile duct.[7]
  - **Lymphadenopathies**—left supraclavicular (Virchow's node) or umbilical (Sister Mary Joseph's nodule), and recurring superficial thrombophlebitis (Trousseau's sign).[7]
  - **Other findings**—tender enlarged liver, ascites, palmar erythema, and spider angioma.

- **Serum markers**—several has been introduced, the most useful of them is the carbohydrate antigen 19-9 (CA 19-9). Conditions that can raise CA 19-9 levels are obstructive jaundice, chronic pancreatitis, and biliary or gastrointestinal cancers. Therefore, CA 19-9 is not recommended as a screening test for pancreatic cancer.[3,15]
- **ERCP**—is indicated when other modalities are inconclusive and suspicion for malignancy is still high.[1] It might also be used when delineation of the biliary tree is crucial or for placing a stent to relieve

biliary obstruction when necessary. ERCP has the advantage of providing the facility for cytologic or histologic sampling.

- **Tissue diagnosis**—should be attempted during the endoscopic procedure [C].[1,3] Failure to obtain histological confirmation in highly suspicious imaging-detected lesion has no significant effect on final outcome, and the plan for surgical resection in appropriate patients should proceed ahead [C].[1] This situation occurs in ~5% of cases and is considered acceptable.
  - *Transperitoneal techniques*—should be avoided in potentially resectable cancers [C].[1,3,14]
  - *End stage patients*—would benefit from tissue diagnosis to guide the palliative care drug selection [C].[1]

Recommended initial assessment (Fig 39.1)

- **Assessment of health fitness**—only those patients with appropriate ASA score should be considered for surgery.
- **MDT discussion**—an essential requirement prior to commencing any definitive staging or treatment. Decisions are taken in the context of predicted prognosis and expected effect of any investigation or treatment intervention on quality of life.[1] The MDT team should typically include physicians, surgeons, oncologists, radiologists, histopathologists, specialist nurses, research personnel (for clinical trials), and representatives from intensive care, palliative care, and nutritional services.[1]
- **Breaking bad news**—an essential step to ensure adequate compliance. Should be done in a professional and effective way. The role of the cancer care nurse is essential.
  - *Recommended points to discuss*—confirmation of diagnosis, available treatment options, expected perioperative period experience, contact details, and sources for further information (including patient support groups). Discussion should be documented and communicated to other members of the team (e.g. GP, oncologists, and cancer care nurses).
- **Advanced staging**—only required if the cancer is found localized enough for curative resection (resectability) and the patient is a good candidate for surgical resection (operability).[1]

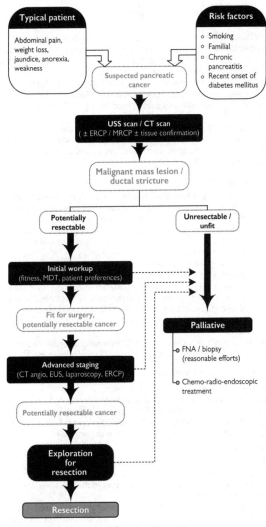

Fig. 39.1 Recommended approach for pancreatic cancer

Recommended advanced staging

- *EUS.*
  - *Indications*—in selected cases to confirm diagnosis and assess resectability [B].[1,3] Results vary between centres, reflecting in part the differences in gold standards against which EUS is compared and the available local expertise.[16]
  - *Benefits*—ideal for the assessment of small tumours (<2cm in diameter), lymph node metastases, and involvement of the portal venous system, with an accuracy reaching 94–100% in some series.[1,16]
- *Laparoscopy*—including laparoscopic ultrasound, can detect occult metastatic lesions in the liver and peritoneal cavity which have not been identified by other imaging modalities. This should be used selectively where available [B].[1]
- *ERCP.*
  - *Indications.*
    - *Delayed operation*—little evidence that relieving jaundice prior to resection is beneficial [A].[1] However, if definitive surgery must be delayed for more than 10d, biliary drainage should be performed and the operation should be delayed for 3–6wk to allow the jaundice to resolve [C].[1] If a stent is placed prior to surgery, this is recommended to be plastic [C].[1]
    - *Surgical incurable cases*—this includes tumours invading the critical peripancreatic vascular structures, distant organs, or distant nodes at the time of attempted resection. Plastic stents can relieve the symptoms of obstructive jaundice effectively in advanced cancer cases and is the recommended practice [A].[1] Palliative limited surgery should be considered for duodenal obstruction [C].[1]
- *Cancer staging*—is based on the 2002 International Union Against Cancer (UICC) tumour node metastasis (TNM) classification.[17]

Recommended treatment

General approach

- **Resection with intent to cure**—should be recommended for patients with localized tumors, who are fit enough to tolerate major surgery [B].[1] This should be undertaken in a specialist centre with appropriate workload to maximize benefits and minimize harm [B].[1]

Standards for surgical resection

- **Options**—include proximal pancreatico-duodenectomy with antrectomy (Whipple procedure), proximal pancreatico-duodenectomy with pylorus preservation, total pancreatico-duodenectomy, and left (distal) pancreatectomy.[1]
  - *Whipple procedure*—involves resection of the pancreatic head, duodenum, first part of the jejunum, common bile duct, and gall bladder (with partial gastrectomy). Anastomoses are performed between the pancreas, biliary tree (bile duct bypass is preferable to gall bladder bypass [B]),[1] and the gastrointestinal tract. Portal vein involvement usually indicates unresectable tumour, and extended resection should be performed in selected cases only (survival does

not increase significantly in extended resections) [C].[1] In contrary, involvement of the splenic vein or artery is not considered a contraindication for extended resections [B].[1]

- Laparoscopic distal pancreatectomy.[4]
  - *Indications*—mainly for malignant cystic tumours. Adenocarcinomas rarely present at the tail of pancreas. Large tumours usually require open surgery.
  - *Efficacy*—shorter hospital stay (~1wk) and shorter return to work (median 3wk). Tumour procedure-related recurrence rate is ~6% at 27mo follow-up.
  - *Safety*—conversion rate, re-operation rate, and fistula formation rate is ~14%, 8%, and 13%, respectively. The 30d mortality rate is ~0.5%.
  - *Current recommendations*—evidence is adequate to support the use of this procedure within appropriate clinical governance framework.[4]

Recommendation for palliative treatment

- **General approach**—an appropriate palliative treatment plan should be formulated at the MDT meeting for patients with inoperable cancers. A direct involvement of the palliative care team is recommended.
- **Options.**
  - *Palliative duodenal bypass surgery*—should be considered to relieve symptoms of duodenal obstruction [A].[1,3]
  - *Endoscopic stent placement*—is indicated to relieve obstructive jaundice and is preferable over percutaneous stenting, and also can be used to stent duodenal obstruction [A].[1]
  - *Chemotherapy*—adjuvant and neo-adjuvant in conjunction with surgery should be given as part of a clinical trial [A].[1,3] Gemcitabine and capecitabine have shown encouraging results in phase II trials and have been adopted as standard first-line treatment.[3,18]
  - *Other measures*—include nutrition and pancreatic supplements, support for pain management, and involvement of palliative care physicians.[1,3]

Further reading

1. Pancreatic Section of the British Society of Gastroenterology, Pancreatic Society of Great Britain and Ireland, Association of Upper Gastrointestinal Surgeons of Great Britain and Ireland, Royal College of Pathologists, Special Interest Group for Gastrointestinal Radiology (2005). Guidelines for the management of patients with pancreatic cancer periampullary and ampullary carcinomas. Gut 54, v1–16.
2. Society for Surgery of the Alimentary Tract (2004). Surgical treatment of pancreatic cancer. Available from: http://www.guideline.gov/summary/summary.aspx?doc_id=5510&nbr=003753&string=pancreatic+AND+cancer.
3. Cancer Research UK (2008). Pancreatic cancer. Available from: http://info.cancerresearchuk.org/cancerstats/types/pancreas/?a=5441.
4. National Institute for Health and Clinical Excellence (2007). Laparoscopic distal pancreatectomy. Available from: http://www.nice.org.uk/guidance/IPG204.
5. O'Sullivan A, Kocher HM (2008). Pancreatic cancer. BMJ Clin Evid 1, 409.
6. Holly EA, Chaliha I, Bracci PM, Gautam M (2004). Signs and symptoms of pancreatic cancer: a population-based case-control study in the San Francisco Bay area. Clin Gastroenterol Hepatol 2, 510–7.
7. Freelove R, Walling AD (2006). Pancreatic cancer: diagnosis and management. Am Fam Physician 73, 485–92.

8. Fuchs CS, Colditz GA, Stampfer MJ et al. (1996). A prospective study of cigarette smoking and the risk of pancreatic cancer. *Arch Intern Med* 156, 2255–60.

9. McWilliams RR, Rabe KG, Olswold C, De Andrade M, Petersen GM (2005). Risk of malignancy in first-degree relatives of patients with pancreatic carcinoma. *Cancer* 104, 388-94.

10. Klein AP, Hruban RH, Brune KA, Petersen GM, Goggins M et al. (2001). Familial pancreatic cancer. *Cancer J* 7, 266–73.

11. Ekbom A, McLaughlin JK, Karlsson BM et al. (1994). Pancreatitis and pancreatic cancer: a population-based study. *J Natl Cancer Inst* 86, 625–7.

12. Everhart J, Wright D (1995). Diabetes mellitus as a risk factor for pancreatic cancer. A meta-analysis. *JAMA* 273, 1605–9.

13. Kalser MH, Barkin J, MacIntyre JM (1985). Pancreatic cancer. Assessment of prognosis by clinical presentation. *Cancer* 56, 397–402.

14. Kosugi C, Furuse J, Ishii H et al. (2004). Needle tract implantation of hepatocellular carcinoma and pancreatic carcinoma after ultrasound-guided percutaneous puncture: clinical and pathologic characteristics and the treatment of needle tract implantation. *World J Surg* 28, 29–32.

15. Locker GY, Hamilton S, Harris J et al. (2006). ASCO 2006 update of recommendations for the use of tumour markers in gastrointestinal cancer. *J Clin Oncol* 24, 5313–27.

16. Dewitt J, Devereaux BM, Lehman GA, Sherman S, Imperiale TF et al. (2006). Comparison of endoscopic ultrasound and computed tomography for the preoperative evaluation of pancreatic cancer: a systematic review. *Clin Gastroenterol Hepatol* 4, 717–25.

17. Sobin LH, Wittekind C, eds. (2002). *TNM classification of malignant tumours*, 6th ed. John Wiley & Sons, New York.

18. Cartwright TH, Cohn A, Varkey JA et al. (2002). Phase II study of oral capecitabine in patients with advanced or metastatic pancreatic cancer. *J Clin Oncol* 20, 160–4.

Hepatobiliary

Gallstone disease*

* The guidelines on this chapter have been sourced and summarized from different UK, Europe, and international government sources, professional organizations, and medical specialty societies. Leading guidelines have been listed in the Key guidelines box.

Gallstone disease

Key guidelines
- BMJ Clinical Review (2007). Gallstones.
- BMJ ABC of diseases (2001). ABC of diseases of liver, pancreas, and biliary system. Gallstone disease.
- BMJ Clinical Evidence (2008). Acute cholecystitis.
- Bellows CF, Berger DH, Crass RA (2005). Management of gallstones.
- The Society for Surgery of the Alimentary Tract (2006). Treatment of gallstone and gall bladder disease.

Basic facts

- **Incidence**—very common and costly medical condition in developed countries. The estimated prevalence is 10–15% of adults.[1,27] Over 5 million people have gallstones in the UK, resulting in over 50,000 cholecystectomy operations performed each year.[1,2]
- **Pathogenesis**—failure to maintain biliary solutes, primarily cholesterol, and calcium salts in a solubilized state (Table 40.1).
- **Clinical presentation.**
  - *Incidental (asymptomatic) gallstones*—can be found unexpectedly on USS during evaluation for abdominal pain, pelvic diseases, or abnormal LFTs.
  - *Biliary colic*—usually results from a stone or sludge being forced against the gall bladder outlet (or cystic duct) during contraction of the gall bladder (Table 40.2).
  - *Atypical symptoms*—uncommon presentation. May present with non-specific abdominal pain, fat intolerance, nausea, and early satiety. These symptoms may be due to chronic dysfunction of the gall bladder (chronic cholecystitis). However, in the majority, such symptoms are unlikely to be due to gall bladder disease, even in the presence of gall bladder stones. The less consistent the symptoms are with biliary colic, the higher the likelihood that they will not respond to cholecystectomy.[2,9]
  - *Complications*—the initial presentation may be with a complication. Examples include acute pancreatitis due to small stones, cholangitis or obstructive jaundice in the elderly due to a large bile duct stone

Recommended investigations

- **USS**—the initial investigation of choice in clinically suspected gallstone disease [C].[4] USS is a non-invasive, relatively inexpensive, and safe modality (Table 40.3).
- **Other imaging modalities (such as MRCP scan)**—may be required in some occasions, where no objective evidence of gallstones is found despite the presence of classic biliary pain.

Table 40.1 Risk factors

- *Patient demographics.*
  - *Age*—major risk factor. The incidence increases significantly after the age of 40.[10]
  - *Females*—much more affected than males. The female to male ratio is 2.9:1 in patients younger than 40, and 1.2:1 in patients over the age of 50.[19]

- *Reproductive factors.*
  - *Pregnancy*—established risk factor for cholesterol gallstones. More common in multiparous patients (12%) compared to nulliparous (1.3%). Following delivery, over 30% of small gallstones (<10mm) found during pregnancy disappear completely.[20]
  - *Oestrogen replacement therapy*—increases the risk of developing symptomatic gallstone disease by about 3.7 times compared to non-users. Cholecystectomy rate in HRT is significantly higher (RR × 2.1).
  - *Oral contraceptives*—increase slightly the risk of gallstone formation at the beginning of its use.[21]

- *Medical conditions.*
  - *Obesity (BMI >30)*—established risk factor for cholesterol gallstones (up to 3-fold increase in risk).
  - *Rapid weight loss*—gallstones occur in ~35% of patients after proximal gastric bypass, and other types of bariatric surgery.

Table 40.2 Clinical features of biliary colic

- Dull pressure-like discomfort.
- Sudden onset in epigastrium or right upper quadrant. May radiate round to the back and right shoulder blade.
- Persists from 15min up to 24h, and subsides spontaneously or with opioid analgesics.
- Accompanied by nausea or vomiting.
- Classically occurs 1–2h following the ingestion of fatty meals, and occurs in a characteristic pattern and timing known to the individual patient.
- Pain does not usually change with movement, squatting, passing of flatus or faeces.

Recommended treatment

General approach
- The pure finding of gallstones on USS does not confirm the diagnosis of gallstone-related pain unless it has been associated with a proper clinical scenario (see Fig 40.1).

Asymptomatic gallstones
- *General approach*—can be safely managed conservatively. Surgical removal is not recommended [C].[1–6]
- *Natural history*—the majority of patients remain asymptomatic over the years. The risk of developing symptoms is ~1–4% per year, and when symptoms occur, they usually present with a self-limiting biliary colic rather than a life-threatening major complication.[1,2,4]

- *Prophylactic cholecystectomy*—may be considered in patients with asymptomatic gallstones who are at increased risk of complications. This includes patients with small stones less than 5mm (independent risk factor for the development of acute pancreatitis)[1,8] and very young patients. Diabetic patients have a higher risk of developing severe complications,[25] but no data support the benefits of prophylactic cholecystectomy in this group.[1,2,6] However, prompt surgery is recommended if symptoms develop.[26] Prophylactic cholecystectomy is practised in patients living in endemic regions to reduce the gall bladder cancer risk (e.g. Peru).
- *Gall bladder cancer*—the risk in the presence of gallstones is <0.01%.[2] The risk is higher in certain cases such as the presence of porcelain gall bladder (25% risk),[26] gall bladder adenoma (larger polyps are more likely to contain foci of invasive cancer),[28] gallstones over 3cm in size,[7] and in certain ethnic groups and endemic regions. Prophylactic cholecystectomy is recommended in such individual cases for this reason.

Symptomatic gallstones

- *Biliary colic*—the management is mainly directed at relieving pain (Table 40.4).
- *Medical curative treatment of gallstones*—can be used in carefully selected patients with a functioning gall bladder and radiolucent stones <10mm in diameter. Complete dissolution occurs in ~50% of such patients within 6mo to 2y with ursodeoxycholic acid (UDCA) [B].[4]
- *Laparoscopic cholecystectomy*—the most effective and optimal treatment for the majority of patients with symptomatic disease [B].[1–6]
  - *Natural history*—about 70% of patients with symptomatic gallstones are expected to develop further symptoms or complications within 2y of initial presentation.[7,14] Life-threatening complications are very uncommon in mildly symptomatic patients, and ~30% of patients may not experience any more episodes of biliary colic or complications in the long term.[16]
  - *Benefits*—laparoscopic cholecystectomy is a cost-effective treatment option for patients with symptomatic gallstones who are willing to prevent another episode of pain in the future. The procedure has a low rate of complication (2–4%), bile duct injury (0.2–0.5%), and mortality (<0.1%), and it is effective in completely relieving the biliary colic in over 90% of patients.[3,4,15] Laparoscopic cholecystectomy is now increasingly performed as a day case procedure.
  - *Side effects*—commonly accepted to have no long-lasting physiologic effects, but can cause increased frequency of less formed stool in ~50% of patients in some studies; 10–15% of them had to seek medical attention.[17]
  - *Decision-making*—the decision between immediate intervention and expectant management in patients not keen on taking the risk of surgery to prevent another pain attack may become a matter of personal choice or convenience.[7]
- *Open cholecystectomy*—Open surgery has been shown to have no significant difference in terms of long-term complications and mortality rate compared to the laparoscopic approach.[15] Open cholecystectomy is only indicated as a conversion procedure for difficult laparoscopic procedure or in certain individual cases (e.g. repair of a fistula from the gall bladder into the bile duct or intestine, and perforation and abscess formation).[3,15]

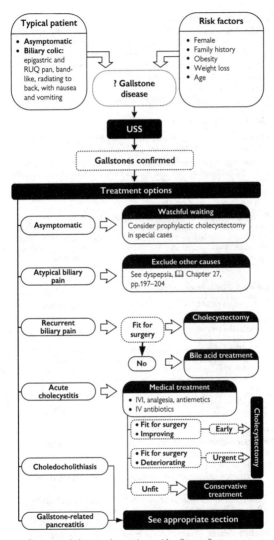

Fig. 40.1 Recommended approach to patients with gallstone disease

Other issues to consider:
- *Biliary dyskinesia*—attributed to the sphincter of Oddi dysfunction, is defined as a gall bladder ejection fraction of <50% on cholecystokinin hepatobiliary imino-diacetic acid scintigraphy scan, associated with typical biliary colic. Most patients with dyskinesia associated with microlithiasis or sludge can be successfully treated with cholecystectomy.[24]
- *Management of bile duct stones*—will be considered later in this chapter.

Table 40.3 USS for gallstones

- *Accuracy*—can identify gallstones with a sensitivity ranging from 76 to 99% (average 84%) and specificity of 99% (95% CI 97–100%).[1,22]
- *Findings*—gallstones present with acoustic 'shadowing' of opacities lying within the gall bladder lumen and typically change with the patient's position (gravitational dependency). Gall bladder sludge is an echogenic shadow that has no acoustic shadow, more viscous than surrounding bile, and does not move with the change in a patient's position.[23]
- *Preparation*—patients should keep fasting (ideally >8h) to allow the gall bladder to be at its maximum distension. The examiner should use both sagittal and axial planes to visualize the gall bladder, and should look specifically at Hartmann's pouch as well as at the cystic duct down to the porta hepatis. CBD and peri-gall bladder spaces should all be examined thoroughly.

Table 40.4 Management of biliary colic

- *Nil by mouth (NBM)*—to reduce the secretion of cholecystokinin.
- *Analgesia*—best achieved by:
  - *Pethidine (IV)*—has fewer adverse effects on the motility of the sphincter of Oddi.[11,12]
  - *NSAIDs*—also effective with expected complete pain relief in >75% of cases.[13] NSAIDs can also reduce the progression of biliary colic to cholecystitis, possibly due to its effect on prostaglandins and the role of the latter in the pathogenesis of acute cholecystitis.[13]
- *IV fluids*—should be considered in the presence of nausea, vomiting, or in the need for long fasting.

Acute cholecystitis
- *Definition*—acute inflammation of the gall bladder wall, usually following obstruction of the cystic duct by a stone.
- *Mechanisms*—three factors invoke the inflammatory response:
  - Mechanical inflammation produced by increased intraluminal pressure.
  - Chemical inflammation caused by the release of lysolecithin.
  - Bacterial inflammation in 50–85% of patients.
- *Organisms*—most frequently isolated organisms are *Escherichia coli*, *Klebsiella* species, *Streptococcus* species, and *Clostridium* species.[6,7]
- *Clinically*—prolonged, more generalized biliary colic with low-grade fever, chills and rigors, late jaundice, nausea, and vomiting.[6,7]
- *Diagnosis*—usually made on the basis of characteristic history and physical examination.[6,7] USS is required to confirm the diagnosis.
- *Management.*

- *Conservative management*—usually the first-line treatment.[6,7]
  If admission to hospital is necessary, patients require IV fluids, analgesia, and suspension of oral intake. NGT may be required when vomiting is excessive. IV antibiotics should be started if the patient fails to respond.
- *Surgery*—most patients should be offered cholecystectomy, ideally on the next convenient operating list.[6]

Management of common bile duct stones (CBDS)[29]

Basic facts

- CBDS originate mainly in the gall bladder and migrate. *De novo* CBDS (those arising primarily in the CBD) have a different composition and may result from infection or stasis.
- The prevalence of CBDS in symptomatic gallstone patients ranges from 10 to 20%. CBDS is less common (<5%) with normal LFTs and non-dilated duct on USS.
- CBDS can pass spontaneously to the duodenum and cause no symptoms. CBDS that are able to cause symptoms have a high risk of causing further complications, and therefore should be extracted when possible [B].

Recommended investigations

- *Transabdominal USS*—is the primary investigation of choice [B].
  No one test can be relied upon to exclude the presence of CBDS. The combination of relevant clinical, biochemical and/or imaging tests should be used to identify high risk patients for CBDS [B], e.g. the presence of age >55, bilirubin >30, and dilated CBD on USS in patients with known gallstones correlate with a 70% chance of finding CBDS on ERCP. The absence of all of these factors decreases the risk of CBDS to <5%.
- *MRCP*—has a high accuracy in detecting (and excluding) the presence of CBDS. Different studies have shown an MRCP accuracy of >90% when compared to ERCP, with decreasing accuracy in small (<5mm) CBD stones.
- *Other tests*—include CT cholangiography (sensitivity of 65–95% and specificity of 85–100%), and EUS (comparable accuracy to ERCP and comparable, and sometimes superior accuracy to MRCP).
- *Intra-operative cholangiography (IOC)*—is recommended for patients with medium to high risk of CBDS where other diagnostic tests have failed to confirm this [B].
- *ERCP*—should NOT be used as a purely diagnostic tool, but only on patients who are likely to require intervention [B].

Recommended management.

- *ERCP*—is the gold standard non-operative treatment for CBDS.
  - *Selection of patients*—should be based on the clinical, biochemical, and non-invasive imaging tests. ERCP should not be used as a purely diagnostic tool [B], e.g. dilated CBD on USS with normal LFTs should be investigated with MR first before proceeding to ERCP. Patients should be properly consented, and FBC and clotting screen should be checked no more than 72h prior to the procedure [B]. Aspirin and LMWH are not contraindications to ERCP and/or sphincterotomy [B].

- *High-risk patients for complications*—include younger ages (<60), female gender, the presence of comorbidities (coagulopathy, cirrhosis, etc.), and where the indication for ERCP is less clear (e.g. normal CBD diameter).
- *Sphincterectomy (using pure cut)*—in patients with high risk for ERCP-induced pancreatitis (who have low risk of bleeding) may be preferable [A].
- *Achieving adequate biliary drainage*—is essential [B]. Using biliary stents (temporarily or permanently in high-risk end-of-life patients) is advisable where appropriate, but not as a routine management for CBDS [A]. Short-term pancreatic stenting for patients at high risk for post-ERCP pancreatitis is advisable as well [A].
- **Surgical extraction of CBDS**—usually takes place during laparoscopic cholecystectomy.
  - *Laparoscopic common bile duct exploration (LCBDE)*—is a technically demanding procedure and yet to be widely available in the UK. However, open bile duct exploration requires blind instrumentation of the bile duct and increases the risk of stricture formation. The use of choledochoscopes facilitates direct vision and should be taken into consideration where experience exists.
  - *Patient selection*—for common bile duct exploration should be based on a clear risk-benefit balance. LCBDE has reached a comparable morbidity (2–17%) and mortality (1–5%) rate to that for ERCP in many centres, and both approaches are deemed acceptable. ERCP is preferable where the surgical risk (due to technical difficulties or lack of resources) is considered higher [B].

Beyond the guidelines and the future

Laparoscopic cholecystectomy has revolutionised the management of symptomatic gallstone disease. The indications for laparoscopic cholecystectomy have broadened. At present disseminated intravascular coagulation is regarded as the only absolute contraindication for laparoscopic cholecystectomy. Laparoscopic bile duct exploration is increasingly practised and in centres with expertise a 'one stop approach' has become the first line treatment for patients with gallbladder stones and concomitant bile duct stones. Intraoperative ultrasound is practiced as a complementary procedure to laparoscopic cholangiography to facilitate the detection of bile duct stones.

The technological advancements have resulted in the development of newer laparoscopes with superb resolution and illumination that produce excellent three-dimensional images. Miniaturization of laparoscopes and production of miniature instruments which are sturdy has refined the dexterity and precision of the technique of laparoscopic cholecystectomy. The traditional four part technique is giving way to three and two port techniques. The 12mm ports have been replaced with 2mm ports. The bile duct injury rate following laparoscopic approach is still approximately twice that of the open procedure and this issue continues to be a concern.

Beyond the guidelines and the future (*continued*)

Tele-robotic laparoscopic cholecystectomy and computer assisted surgery (CAS) is practiced in some centres but there is no evidence that such developments offer real advantages over conventional laparoscopic cholecystectomy. However the availability of digitalized data and the ability to transmit over a distance may open a new era of surgical practice in the future. Minimal access endoscopic surgery has now become the first line of treatment for bile duct stones. The operation of endoscopic sphincterotomy (ES) first performed in 1974 to facilitate the access to the bile duct and has revolutionised the management of bile duct stones. The newer modalities such as extra-corporeal shock wave lithotripsy (ESWL), electro-hydraulic lithotripsy and laser mechanical stone crushing/extraction and other accessory tools have increased the success rates of endoscopic stone extraction almost to 100%.

Natural orifice trans-luminal endoscopic surgery (NOTES) is a technique where in the future gall-bladder surgery may be performed without an incision. The principle is to enter the peritoneal cavity using the endoscope creating a controlled perforation of the gastrointestinal tract, to gain access to perform cholecystectomy. The technique has already been performed on animal models. Newer bowel closing methods such as glues and staples coupled with the advancement of endoscopic technology and accessories is keenly awaited by the enthusiasts of this novel technique. The benefits of this approach are hotly debated and the ability to perform incisionless trans luminanal endoscopic gall bladder surgery with minimal risk in the future, and the patient perceptions of such advancements remains to be seen.

Prof. Mohan De Selva

Further reading

1. Sanders G, Kingsnorth AN (2007). Gallstones. *BMJ* 335, 295–9.
2. Beckingham IJ (2001). ABC of diseases of liver, pancreas, and biliary system. Gallstone disease. *BMJ* 322, 91–4.
3. Fialkowski E, Halpin V, Whinney R (2008). Acute cholecystitis. *BMJ Clin Evid* 12, 411.
4. Bellows CF, Berger DH, Crass RA (2005). Management of gallstones. *Am Fam Physician* 15, 637–42.
5. The Society for Surgery of the Alimentary Tract (2006). Treatment of gallstone and gall bladder disease. Available from: http://www.ssat.com/cgi-bin/chole7.cgi.
6. British Columbia Guidelines and Protocols (2007). Gallstones—treatment in adults. Available from: http://www.bcguidelines.ca/gpac/pdf/gallstones.pdf.
7. American College of Physicians (1993). Guidelines for the treatment of gallstones. *Ann Intern Med* 119, 620–2.
8. Venneman NG, Buskens E, Besselink MG et al. (2005). Small gallstones are associated with increased risk of acute pancreatitis: potential benefits of prophylactic cholecystectomy? *Am J Gastroenterol* 100, 2540–50.
9. Kraag N, Thijs C, Knipschild P (1995). Dyspepsia—how noisy are gallstones? A meta-analysis of epidemiologic studies of biliary pain, dyspeptic symptoms, and food intolerance. *Scand J Gastroenterol* 30, 411–21.
10. Davide Festi, Ada Dormi, Simona Capodicasa, Tommaso Staniscia, Adolfo F Attili, Paola Loria, Paolo Pazzi, Giuseppe Mazzella, Claudia Sama, Enrico Roda, Antonio Colecchia. Incidence of gallstone disease in Italy: Results from a multicenter, population-based Italian study (the MICOL project). *World J Gastroenterol* 2008 September 14; 14(34): 5282–5289. URL: http://www.wjgnet.com/1007-9327/14/5282.pdf

11. Thompson DR (2001). Narcotic analgesic effects on the sphincter of Oddi: a review of the data and therapeutic implications in treating pancreatitis. *Am J Gastroenterol* 96, 1266–72.

12. Thune A, Baker RA, Saccone GT, Owen H, Toouli J (1990). Differing effects of pethidine and morphine on human sphincter of Oddi motility. *Br J Surg* 77, 992–5.

13. Akriviadis EA, Hatzigavriel M, Kapnias D, Kirimlidis J, Markantas A, Garyfallos A (1997). Treatment of biliary colic with diclofenac: A randomized double-blind, placebo-controlled study. *Gastroenterology* 113, 225–31.

14. Thistle JL, Cleary PA, Lachin JM, Tyor MP, Hersh T (1984). The natural history of cholelithiasis: the National Cooperative Gallstone Study. *Ann Intern Med* 101, 171–5.

15. Keus F, de Jong JA, Gooszen HG, van Laarhoven CJ (2006). Laparoscopic versus open cholecystectomy for patients with symptomatic cholecystolithiasis. *Cochrane Database Syst Rev* 4, CD006231.

16. Vetrhus M, Soreide O, Solhaug JH, Nesvik I, Sondenaa K (2002). Symptomatic, non-complicated gall bladder stone disease. Operation or observation? A randomized clinical study. *Scand J Gastroenterol* 37, 834–9.

17. Zakko SF, Guttermuth MC, Jamali SH et al. (1999). A population study of gallstone composition, symptoms, and outcomes after cholecystectomy. *Gastroenterology* 116, A43.

18. Bateson MC (2000). Gallstones and cholecystectomy in modern Britain. *Postgrad Med J* 76, 700–3.

19. The Rome Group for Epidemiology and Prevention of Cholelithiasis (GREPCO) (1988). The epidemiology of gallstone disease in Rome, Italy. Part I. Prevalence data in men. *Hepatology* 8, 904–6.

20. Maringhini A, Ciambra M, Baccelliere P et al. (1993). Biliary sludge and gallstones in pregnancy: Incidence, risk factors, and natural history. *Ann Intern Med* 119, 116–20.

21. Grodstein F, Colditz GA, Stampfer MJ (1994). Postmenopausal hormone use and cholecystectomy in a large prospective study. *Obstet Gynecol* 83, 5–11.

22. Kalimi R, Gecelter GR, Caplin D et al. (2001). Diagnosis of acute cholecystitis: sensitivity of sonography, cholecintigraphy, and combined sonography-cholecintigraphy. *J Am Coll Surg* 193, 609–13.

23. Brink JA, Simeone JF, Mueller PR, Richter JM, Prien EL, Ferrucci JT (1988). Physical characteristics of gallstones removed at cholecystectomy: implications for extracorporeal shock-wave lithotripsy. *AJR Am J Roentgenol* 151, 927–31.

24. Dill JE, Hill S, Callis J et al. (1995). Combined endoscopic ultrasound and stimulated biliary drainage in cholecystitis and microlithiasis—diagnoses and outcomes. *Endoscopy* 27, 424–7.

25. Reiss R. Nudelman I. Gutman C. Deutsch AA (1990). Changing trends in surgery for acute cholecystitis. *World J Surg* 14, 567–70.

26. Vollmer C, Strasberg S (2002). Biliary surgery. In: *Washington manual of Surgery*, 3rd ed. Lippicott Williams & Wilkins, Philadelphia.

27. Bateson MC (2000). Gallstones and cholecystectomy in modern Britain. *Postgrad Med J* 76, 700–3.

28. Okamoto M, Okamoto H, Kitahara F, Kobayashi K (1999). Ultrasonographic evidence of association of polyps and stones with gall bladder cancer. *Am J Gastroenterol* 94, 446–50.

29. Williams EJ, Green J, Beckingham I, Parks, R, Martin D, Lombard M; British Society of Gastroenterology (2008). Guidelines on the management of common bile duct stones (CBDS). *Gut* 57, 1004–21.

Surgical management of liver metastasis*

* The guidelines on this chapter have been sourced and summarized from different UK, Europe, and international government sources, professional organizations, and medical specialty societies. Leading guidelines have been listed in the Key guidelines box.

Surgical management of liver metastasis

Key guidelines
- Garden OJ, Rees M, Poston GJ et al. (2006). Guidelines for resection of colorectal cancer liver metastases.
- National Cancer Institute. Liver Metastasis. 1998 (US)
- Society for Surgery of the Alimentary Tract (2004). Surgery for hepatic colorectal metastases.

Basic facts
- **Incidence**—over 20 times more common than primary hepatocellular carcinoma. The liver is the most common site for cancer metastasis, and over 50% of patients who die from cancer have liver metastasis.
- **Pathophysiology**—metastatic lesions tend to be more aggressive than its extrahepatic primary. Most common primary cancer sites are colorectal, bronchial, pancreas, breast, stomach, and cancers of unknown origin.
- **Clinical presentation**—most patients with liver metastasis are asymptomatic initially. Metastases are usually found either incidentally during the staging period, in patients with raised carcinoembryonic antigen (CEA) or abnormal LFTs during the follow-up period, or in advanced end-stage disease. Advanced liver metastasis is usually accompanied by fatigue, anorexia, dull pain, dyspepsia, jaundice, fever, weight loss, palpable intra-abdominal mass and/or hepatomegaly.

Recommended investigations
- **Careful preoperative staging**—essential in any cancer patient. PET scan, laparoscopy, and other modalities should be considered for high-risk primary cancers (e.g. T4 perforated disease, C2 with involved apical node) [C].[1,2]
- **Detection of liver metastasis**—best achieved by combining a thorough history and physical examination, LFTs, and CEA in the case of colorectal cancer.
  - *LFTs*—found raised in ~65% of patients with liver metastasis and 80% of those with advanced liver metastasis.
  - *Raised CEA* (>5ng/mL) has an overall sensitivity of >78% in detecting disease relapse in patients with completely resected colorectal cancer. Patients undergoing serial CEA monitoring and liver imaging may have better survival than patients not undergoing this surveillance.[5] However, the benefits of routine serial CEA measurements remain unproven [C].[1]
  - *Abdominal and pelvis CT scan*—should be performed in maximum 2y following completion of treatment for the primary disease [C].[1]
  - Finding liver metastasis requires further staging investigations with chest, abdomen, and pelvis CT scan. The imaging protocols should be agreed with the liver unit which will ultimately deal with the case [C].[1,2]

Recommended treatment

- ***General approach***—surgical resection offers the greatest likelihood and the only chance of cure for patients with liver metastasis.
  - Average 5y survival rates—after resection of colorectal cancer liver metastasis is ~40% compared to only 5–9% with the most active systemic chemotherapy regimens.[3,4]
- ***Recommended patient selection***—multidisciplinary decision, involving surgeons, radiologists, anaesthetists, and other staff with experience in the management of liver metastases is necessary [B].
  - *Contraindications*—a consensus statement by OncoSurge therapeutic decision model defined absolute unresectability as the existence of untreatable extrahepatic disease, unfitness for surgery, or the involvement of more than 70% of the liver or six of the liver segments.[6]
  - *Indications*—patients with solitary, multiple, or bilobar disease who have had radical treatment for their primary colorectal cancer and have no absolute contraindication (see above) should always be considered candidates for liver resection [C].
- ***Radiofrequency (RF)-assisted liver resection***—aims at transecting the liver with minimum blood loss. Evidence of efficiency and safety supports its use as one optional technique for liver resection (within appropriate training and clinical governance setting).[7] However, evidence is inadequate to support any significant advantages of RF-assessed liver resection over traditional methods.[7]

Further reading

1. Garden OJ, Rees M, Poston GJ *et al.* (2006). Guidelines for resection of colorectal cancer liver metastases. *Gut* 55 (Suppl 3), iii1–8.
2. Society for Surgery of the Alimentary Tract (2004). Surgery for hepatic colorectal metastases. Available from: http://www.guideline.gov/summary/summary.aspx?ss=15&doc_id=5699&nbr=3837.
3. Al-Asfoor A, Fedorowicz Z, Lodge M (2008). Resection versus no intervention or other surgical interventions for colorectal cancer liver metastases. *Cochrane Database Syst Rev* 16, CD006039.
4. McLoughlin JM, Jensen EH, Malafa M (2006). Resection of colorectal liver metastases: current perspectives. *Cancer Control* 13, 32–41.
5. BMJ Clinical Evidence. Available from: http://clinicalevidence.bmj.com/ceweb/conditions/dsd/0401/0401_I3.jsp. Accessed May 2009 (via ovid)
6. Poston GJ, Adam R, Alberts S *et al.* (2005). OncoSurge: a strategy for improving resectability with curative intent in metastatic colorectal cancer. *J Clin Oncol* 23, 7125–34.
7. National Institute for Health and Clinical Excellence (2007). Radiofrequency-assisted liver resection. Available from: http://www.nice.org.uk/nicemedia/pdf/IPG211guidance.pdf.

Hepatocellular carcinoma (HCC)*

* The guidelines on this chapter have been sourced and summarized from different UK, Europe, and international government sources, professional organizations, and medical specialty societies. Leading guidelines have been listed in the Key guidelines box.

Hepatocellular carcinoma (HCC)

Key guidelines
- British Society of Gastroenterology (2003). Guidelines for the diagnosis and treatment of hepatocellular carcinoma (HCC) in adults.
- American Association for the Study of Liver Diseases (2005). Management of hepatocellular carcinoma.
- National Institute for Health and Clinical Excellence (2007). Microwave ablation of hepatocellular carcinoma.

Basic facts
- *Incidence*—wide geographical variation. Affects 2–4 per 100,000 population in western countries (and >60 per 100,000 population in some areas of Africa and Asia) and accounts for ~1,500 death per year in the UK. The overall incidence has been rising over the years.[1,2]
- *Pathogenesis*—strongly associated with cirrhosis. High-risk groups include patients with cirrhosis due to hepatitis B (HBV) or C (HCV) virus (annual risk of 3–5%), cirrhosis due to genetic haemochromatosis (annual risk of 7–9%), and patients with primary biliary cirrhosis.[1,2]
- *Surveillance programmes*—should be considered in high-risk patients using 6-monthly abdominal USS combined with serum alpha (α)-fetoprotein (AFP) estimations [B].[1,2]
- *Clinical manifestations*—vague and usually related to the underlying liver disease. HCC should be suspected in patients with previously compensated liver cirrhosis who develop symptoms and signs of decompensation such as jaundice, ascites, encephalopathy, or variceal bleeding.[1,2]

Recommended investigations (Fig 42.1)
- *Imaging tests*—nodules >2cm in diameter found on USS surveillance in cirrhotic patients, which are not clearly haemangiomas, have >95% risk of being HCC.[1,2]
- *Diagnosis*—can be confirmed using spiral chest and abdominal CT scan if the lesion appearance proved typical to HCC (i.e. hypervascular with washout in the portal/venous phase) [B].
  - *Raised AFP (>200ng/mL)*—within this context, can confirm the diagnosis with enough confidence to require no further biopsies [B].[1,2]
  - *Other imaging modalities (MRI with contrast, contrast ultrasound or angiography)*—can support the diagnosis in suspicious cases.[1,2]
- *Indefinite cases*—lesions <2cm in diameter has a probability of 75% to be HCC. If the diagnosis cannot be made using appropriate scanning techniques and/or the titration of AFP, a repeated examination can be performed in 3–6 monthly intervals to detect any suspicious changes [C].[1,2]

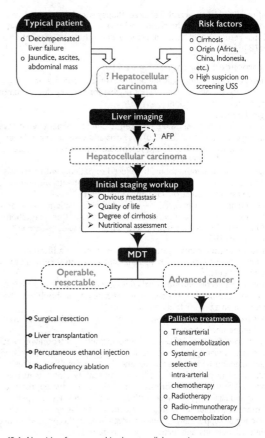

Fig. 42.1 Algorithm for approaching hepatocellular carcinoma

- *Confirmation biopsy*—rarely required. Biopsy should be considered if diagnostic imaging results are inconclusive, but still suspicious, and if biopsy results would have a direct impact on the management plan [B].[1,2]

Recommended treatment (Fig 42.1)

- *General concept*—surgery is the only proven curative therapy. Unfortunately, most patients are not eligible for surgery due to tumour stage or poor liver function.[1,2]
- *Surgical options.*
  - *Surgical resection*—should be offered to suitable patients who have a single lesion and no (or mild) cirrhosis and well-preserved liver function, normal bilirubin, and acceptable hepatic vein pressure gradient (<10mmHg) [B].[1,2]
  - *Liver transplantation*—should be offered to patients with cirrhosis and solitary tumour of <5cm in diameter, or patients with up to three cancer nodules of <3cm in diameter [B].[1,2]
  - *Percutaneous ethanol injection*—safe therapy for patients who cannot tolerate surgical resection, or as a bridge to later transplantation. Most suitable lesions are peripheral smaller nodules (<3cm in diameter) [B].
- *Transarterial chemoembolization*—recommended as a first-line palliative treatment and may have significant effect on survival in some selected patients.[1,2]
- *Systemic or selective intra-arterial chemotherapy*—poor response rate and is not recommended as a standard of care [A]. It should only be offered within a proper trial context.[1,2]
- *Other treatment options*—include radiotherapy, radioimmunotherapy, and chemoembolization.
- *Microwave ablation of HCC*—can be performed by introducing needle electrodes (under appropriate imaging during laparotomy, laparoscopy or percutaneously) into the tumour and delivering multiple pulses of microwave energy. Evidence of efficiency and safety supports its use as one optional technique for carcinoma ablation (within appropriate training and clinical governance setting).[3] Radiofrequency is superior and more predictable than ethanol injection.[1,2] However, evidence is conflicting to support any significant advantages of this procedure over traditional methods, and further work is required.[3]

Further reading

1. Ryder SD; British Society of Gastroenterology (2003). Guidelines for the diagnosis and treatment of hepatocellular carcinoma (HCC) in adults. *Gut* 52 (Suppl 3), iii1–8.
2. American Association for the Study of Liver Diseases (2005). Management of hepatocellular carcinoma. Available from: http://www.guideline.gov/summary/summary.aspx?doc_id=9401.
3. National Institute for Health and Clinical Excellence (2007). Microwave ablation of hepatocellular carcinoma. Available from: http://www.nice.org.uk/nicemedia/pdf/IPG214guidance.pdf.

Part 9

Spleen

Prevention of post-splenectomy sepsis (PSS)*

* The guidelines on this chapter have been sourced and summarized from different
UK, Europe, and international government sources, professional organizations, and
medical specialty societies. Leading guidelines have been listed in the Key guidelines box.

Prevention of post-splenectomy sepsis (PSS)

- British Committee for Standards in Haematology (2002). Update of guidelines for the prevention and treatment of infection in patients with an absent or dysfunctional spleen.
- British National Formulary 57 (2009).

Basic facts
- **Definition of PSS**—fulminant, potentially lethal, infection affecting post-splenectomy patients.[1]
- **Incidence**—PSS affects about 4.4% of splenectomized children under the age of 16y (mortality rate ~2.2%) and ~0.9% of splenectomized adults
  (mortality rate ~0.8%).[3] The risk of late septicaemia in patients undergoing splenectomy increases by 12.6-fold (and 8.6-fold in traumatic cases) compared to the general population.[4]
- **Lifetime risk**—most PSS attacks occur within 2y of splenectomy. About one third of all pneumococcal infections occur after 5y. The risk of subsequent severe infection among survivors of a first episode is more than 6-fold above average, and the risk of a third episode among second-time survivors is more than 2-fold.[1,3,5]
- **Pathogens in PSS**—most commonly are encapsulated organisms, including *Streptococcus pneumoniae* (~60%), *Haemophilus influenzae*, and *Neisseria meningitidis*. The mortality rate ranges from 60% in *Streptococcus pneumoniae* to 30% in the other two.[1,5]

Recommended investigations
- **High index of suspicion**—any fever developing in patients with known splenectomy should be considered as possible PSS attack. Deterioration can occur over few hours if treatment has not been commenced immediately.[1]
- **Clinical presentation**—varies from headache, gastrointestinal symptoms, rigors, and high fever to rapid development of severe sepsis with petechiae, purpura, and meningitis (more common in children).[1]

Recommended treatment (Fig 43.1)

General approach
- Early recognition and following the principles of managing severe sepsis (see Ch. 16) are the mainstay of effective treatment. Prophylactic oral antibiotics should be changed into systemic [C].[1] Consultation with the ICU team and microbiologist is essential.

Prevention.[1,2]
- **Avoid splenectomy**—when possible.

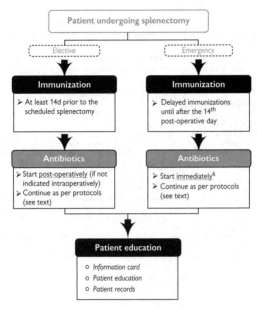

Fig. 43.1 Algorithm for the prevention of post-splenectomy sepsis

- *Immunization.*
  - *Choice of vaccine.*
    - *Pneumococcal immunization*—to all splenectomized patients and to those with functional hyposplenism [B].
    - *Haemophilus influenza type b vaccine*—to all patients not previously immunized [C].
    - *Meningococcal group C conjugate vaccine*—to all patients not previously immunized [C].
  - *Timing*—at least 14d prior to the scheduled splenectomy, where possible.[2] Otherwise, delay immunizations until after the fourteenth post-operative day (to get the best functional antibody response).[1]
    - *Patients on immunosuppressive chemotherapy or radiotherapy*— delayed immunization is recommended for at least 3mo after completion of their treatment.[1]
    - Re-immunization—currently recommended every 5y.[1,6]
- *Antibiotic prophylaxis.*
  - Lifelong prophylactic antibiotics with oral phenoxymethylpenicillin [B] or erythromycin [C] are still recommended.[1] Evidence-based local protocols should be followed where appropriate (e.g. minimum 2y prophylactic antibiotics for adults in general and lifelong for patients with lymphoproliferative disease or sickle cell disease).[6]

- *Patient information.*
  - *Information card*—should be given to all patients to alert caring health care professionals of the high susceptibility for overwhelming infection [C].[1]
  - *Patient education*—should be effective, including advice on the potential risk of overseas travel to epidemic areas [B] and the risk of animal bites [C].[1]
  - *Patient records*—should be clearly labelled as high risk for infection [C].[1]

Further reading

1. Davies JM, Barnes R, Milligan D; British Committee for Standards in Haematology. Working Party of the Haematology/Oncology Task Force (2002). Update of guidelines for the prevention and treatment of infection in patients with an absent or dysfunctional spleen. *Clin Med* 2, 440–3.
2. British National Formulary 57 (2009). BNF 57. Available from: http://www.bnf.org/bnf/bnf/current/3707.htm. Accessed May 2009.
3. Holdsworth RJ, Irving AD, Cuschieri A (1991). Post-splenectomy sepsis and its mortality rate: actual versus perceived risks. *Br J Surg* 78, 1031–8.
4. Cullingford GL, Watkins DN, Watts AD, Mallon DF (1991). Severe late postsplenectomy infection. *Br J Surg* 78, 716–21.
5. Kyaw MH, Holmes EM, Toolis F et al. (2006). Evaluation of severe infection and survival after splenectomy. *Am J Med* 119, 276.
6. Nottingham Antibiotic Guidelines Committee (2006). Adults and children summary for patients with absent or dysfunctinoal spleen. Available from: http://www.nuh.nhs.uk/nch/antibiotics/Full%20Guidelines/Updated%20splenectomy%20guidelines09.2006.pdf.

Part 10

Vascular

Chronic limb ischaemia*

* The guidelines on this chapter have been sourced and summarized from different UK, Europe, and international government sources, professional organizations, and medical specialty societies. Leading guidelines have been listed in the Key guidelines box.

Chronic limb ischaemia

Key guidelines

- Norgren L, Hiatt WR, Dormandy JA et al. (2007). Inter-Society consensus for the management of peripheral arterial disease (TASC II).
- American College of Cardiology/American Heart Association Guidelines (2006). Peripheral Arterial Disease.
- Scottish Intercollegiate Guidelines Network (2006). Diagnosis and management of peripheral arterial disease.

Basic facts

- *Incidence*—common overlooked syndrome in western countries. Affects ~3–10% of the population on objective non-invasive tests, and ~15–20% of those over 70 year of age.[1,2]
- *Risk factors*—see Table 44.1.
- *Anatomical classification*—of chronic limb ischaemia (also called peripheral arterial disease (PAD)) is useful for descriptive as well as planning purposes. Aorto-iliac occlusive segmental disease occurs when the infrarenal aorta, common, and/or external iliacs are affected (also called inflow disease). Femoro-popliteal segmental disease occurs when the common femoral, superficial, profunda, and/or popliteal arteries are affected. Tibial-peroneal segmental disease (run-off or outflow disease) occurs when distal arteries (tibials and/or peroneal arteries) are affected.
- *Clinical presentation*—most patients have limited walking ability and exercise performance (Table 44.2).[1,2] Critical limb ischaemia (CLI) is the presence of ischaemic rest pain, ulceration, or gangrene in objectively proven PAD patients.[2]
- *Physical examination*—should include measuring BP in both arms, examining carotid pulses, abdomen, and legs. Pulse examination should include brachial, radial, ulnar, femoral, popliteal, dorsalis pedis, and posterior tibial pulses. Pulse characteristics and arterial bruits (over subclavian arteries, carotid arteries, abdominal aorta, and femoral arteries) are traditionally examined as well.[1,2]
- *Differential diagnosis*—should be considered and other diseases should be identified in each individual case (Table 44.3).

Recommended investigations

Basic investigations

- *Handheld Doppler examination*—should support the clinical impression [C], especially in suspected critically ischaemic legs [B].[1,2]
  - Handheld Doppler can reliably detects the presence, type, and strength of blood flow signals in peripheral arteries.

Table 44.1 Risk factors for PAD

- *General*—male (OR × 1.1–2.1) and elderly (OR × 2–3 per 10y ageing) patients.

- *Smoking*—the most important risk factor (OR × 3–4). The number of cigarettes smoked correlates strongly with the severity of PAD. Risk declines gradually upon smoking cessation (RR drops from ~3.5 to ~1.5 within 5y).[1]

- *Diabetes*—significant risk factor (OR × 3). Risk of having PAD increases by 26% for every 1% chronic increase in HbA1c.[1]

- *Hypertension*—OR × 2.

- *Dyslipidaemia*—OR × 2. Incidence of symptomatic PAD doubles if fasting cholesterol level were >7mmol/L (270mg/dL).[1]

- *Hyperhomocysteinaemia*—occurs commonly in PAD patients compared to the general population, and is associated with increased risk of PAD (OR × 1–3).

- *Others*—chronic kidney disease (OR × 2) and raised CRP (OR × 2).[1]

Table 44.2 Clinical features of chronic limb ischaemia

- *Intermittent claudication*—fatigue, aching or cramping pain, commonly in the calf, thigh or buttocks, brought on by walking (typically within the same distance), and relieved by rest within 10min. Pain increases significantly by walking uphill or against a wind, and changes with the change in the speed of walking. Pain is reproduced by exercise and does not present on taking the first step. Pain varies slightly from day to day in the same person, and may become prominent if significant changes in general health (severe anaemia, heart failure) occur.[1,2]

- *Ischaemic rest pain*—severe intolerable pain, affects the most distal part of the limbs, commonly awakes the patient up from sleep, and typically relieved by hanging the foot out of bed or even sleeping in a chair.

- *Arterial-type leg ulcers*—are sharp, small, superficial erosions over the bony prominences of the leg (head of metatarsals, malleolus, and heel).

- *Digital gangrene*—are blackened, mummified areas of skin that cannot be mistakable to the observer.

Table 44.3 Differential diagnosis of intermittent claudication

- *Nerve root compression*—sharp, lancinating pain, radiates down the leg posteriorly, starts immediately on commencing exercises (or even without doing any movement), and is not relieved easily with rest. Changing back position may help.

- *Arthritis and inflammatory processes*—aching pain, affects foot and joints predominantly, starts after variable degree of exercises, not relieved quickly on rest. May be relieved by taking certain positions.

- *Others*—spinal stenosis (weakness more than pain, body positions have significant effect), hip arthritis (pain usually localized to hip and gluteal region), and peripheral arthritis.

• *Ankle brachial pressure index (ABPI)*—is a quick and cost-effective method to confirm or exclude the presence of significant lower limb PAD, and is indicated for any patient with suspected chronic limb ischaemia as an objective baseline measurement [B] (Table 44.4).[1,2]

Advanced investigations

● *General approach*—patients with established PAD (based on clinical history and basic investigations), which has no significant effect on their quality of life, require no further advanced investigations and should be managed conservatively (i.e. risk factor optimization etc., see Table 44.6) [A].[1,2] Advanced investigations are indicated for critically ischaemic legs, intermittent claudicants with significant effect on quality of life who have failed the more conservative measures, and where a clear favourable risk-benefit ratio for intervention exists [A].[1,2]

● *Toe brachial index (TBI)*—measures the digital perfusion and requires small cuffs and well-trained investigators. TBI is useful in patients with non-compressible arteries (long-standing diabetes, renal failure, or advanced age) [B].[1,2]

● *Colour flow duplex USS*—is a reliable, non-invasive, and reproducible investigation for PAD patients. In experienced hands, a duplex scan can accurately map the diseased artery and identify the haemodynamic properties of each lesion [A], identify candidates for endovascular interventions [B], and reliably select candidates for surgical bypass [B].[1,2] Duplex scan is recommended for the routine surveillance of the patency of femoro-popliteal/distal bypass grafts [A].[2] The accuracy of duplex scan is highest in outflow (sensitivity of ~85% and specificity of ~95%) and slightly lower in inflow disease (sensitivity of ~89% and specificity of ~90%).[4]

● *MRA*—is a reliable and accurate modality for localizing stenotic lesions and estimating the degree of stenosis [A].[1,2] MRA can identify lesions suitable for endovascular interventions [B] and can reliably select candidates for surgical bypass [B].[1,2]

● *CT angiogram*—can be considered to obtain an accurate map of the arterial tree, especially in more proximal inflow lesions [B].[1,2] CT angiogram can provide high-quality images that are comparable to those from angiogram or MRI scan.

● *Digital subtraction arteriography (DSA)*—remains the gold standard technique for investigating PAD patients and plan for surgical treatment (Table 44.5).

● *Other investigations*—may be useful in selected cases, including leg segmental pressure measurement [B], pulse volume recordings [B], and continuous wave form (CWF) Doppler ultrasound [B].[2]

Table 44.4 Ankle Brachial Pressure Index

- *Technique*—systolic pressure in posterior tibial and/or dorsalis pedis arteries is measured for each leg using a sphygmomanometer cuff and a handheld Doppler. These are compared against the higher brachial pressure of either arm (using handheld Doppler) to formulate the ABPI.

- *Findings.*
  - *Resting ABPI <0.90*—correlates well with a haemodynamically significant arterial stenosis, and is often used as a cut-off point for the definition of PAD,[1] with a sensitivity of ~95% in detecting arteriogram-positive PAD, and specificity of ~100% in identifying healthy persons (when combined to the signal type).
  - *6min walk test*—can provide an objective assessment of functional capacity in selected cases when normal resting ABPI measurements do not correlate with the clinical findings [B].[2]

Table 44.5 DSA—facts and figures

- *Technique*—arterial access is gained using a modified Seldinger technique (floppy guidewire passing through a hollow puncture needle). This is followed by the injection of contrast material to obtain detailed images in different angles.

- *Benefits*—provides detailed map of the arterial system, estimation of arterial inflow and outflow, and allows for therapeutic interventions (angioplasty, stent insertion, coil insertion) via the same access [B].[2]

- *Quality standards*—a full history and complete vascular examination should be performed prior to referral for angiography [C].[2] Iliacs, femorals, and tibials should be visualized [B]. A history of contrast allergy should be documented clearly [B]. Hydration should be provided prior to angiography in patients with renal impairment [B]. Follow-up clinical examination and renal tests are recommended after 2wk [C].[2] Metformin (Glucophage®), an oral agent used in the management of diabetes mellitus, has been associated with the development of severe lactic acidosis following administration of IV contrast media.[10] It is recommended by many experts to stop the metformin therapy pre-procedure, and for at least 48h following the administration of contrast material.

Recommended management

- *Natural history*—in 5 years' time, 70–80% of patients with non-critical ischaemic lower legs will remain stable. Claudication will get worse in 10–20%, and will develop into critical ischaemia (rest pain, ulcer, or gangrene) in 5–10% of cases with a high probability of amputation within 6mo.[1,2] The main causes of morbidity and mortality in symptomatic PAD patients remain in cardiovascular events rather than vascular events. About 20% of symptomatic non-critical PAD patients will sustain a non-fatal MI or stroke, and a further 10–15% will die of cardiovascular (75%) or non-cardiovascular (25%) event.[1] In one year's time, 25% of CLI patients will be dead and 30% will end up with an amputation. Of the remaining pool of patients, less than 50% will have their critical ischaemia resolved satisfactorily.[1]

Intermittent claudication

- *Overall strategy*—patients with intermittent claudication who have no significant life-limiting symptoms should be offered conservative management (control of risk factors, exercises, and consideration for drug therapy) as a first-line treatment [A].[1,2]
- Deteriorating or resistant symptoms require further advanced investigations and consideration for endovascular or surgical revascularization where benefits clearly outweigh risks [A].[1,2]
- *Management of risk factors*—is an essential first step (Table 44.6).
- *Supervised structured exercises*—effective and safe modality and is a recommended option for all patients with intermittent claudication [A].[1,2] An effective programme should be performed in sessions (30–45min each), 3 times a wk or more for 3mo. Each session should contain a proper exercise (treadmill, track walking) that is able to bring the claudication pain on before taking a rest [A].[1,2] Structured exercise can result in increased maximum walking time (mean difference 6.5min), which may sometimes exceed that seen with angioplasty at 6mo (mean difference 3.3min).[8]

Table 44.6 Risk factor modification

- *Smoking cessation*—essential for improving symptoms and reducing cardiovascular risks as well as improving the success rate of any revascularization intervention [B].[2] Smoking cessation is best achieved by advising patients on behavioural modification techniques, frequent follow-ups (1y smoking cessation success rate is ~5% vs 0.1% when no formal follow-up by health care professionals has been arranged), and providing patients with nicotine replacement therapy (1y success rate increases up to ~16%) and/or bupropion (1y success rate ~30%).[2,5]

- *Antiplatelets*—aspirin (75mg od) is recommended to reduce the risk of cardiovascular death [A].[2] Aspirin can significantly reduce the risk of subsequent vascular events (non-fatal MI, non-fatal stroke, and vascular death) by ~22%.[6] Clopidogrel (75mg od) is a safe and effective alternative to aspirin (~5% of aspirin-intolerant patients) in reducing cardiovascular death [B].[2] Oral anticoagulants are NOT indicated for cardiovascular prophylactic purposes [C].[2]

- *Statins (simvastatin 40mg od)*—have been shown to significantly reduce the risk of stroke, MI, or the need for revascularization by ~25%.[7] The 2007 TASC II guidelines provide no graded recommendations pending further analysis of trials.

- *Hypertension*—should be well controlled (140/90 or 130/80 for diabetic and renal insufficiency patients) [A].[2] ACE inhibitors are a reasonable first option [B] and their effect appears to extend to non-hypertensive PAD patients [C].[2]

- *Hyperlipidaemia*—all patients with PAD should have their LDL cholesterol lowered to <100mg/dL (2.6mmol/L) [B].[1,2] In patients with PAD and atherosclerosis in other vital organs, it is advisable to lower the LDL cholesterol to <70mg/dL (1.8mmol/L) [B].[2]

- *Control of diabetes*—aggressive management of blood glucose levels with a HbA1c goal of <7.0% (or as close to 6.0% as possible) is currently recommended to reduce microvascular complications and potentially improve cardiovascular outcomes [C].[1,2] Proper care of the diabetic foot is essential [B].[2]

- *Pharmacotherapy*—is not widely adopted as part of the initial management for intermittent claudication. Level 1 evidence supports the use of cliostazole [A] and naftidrofuryl [A].[1,2,9] Nevertheless, there is currently insufficient data to recommend their use on a routine basis.
- *Endovascular treatment*—should be considered for those who fail the conservative management where claudication is significantly affecting their quality of life [A].[2] Arterial lesions should be of the types that will most likely benefit from endovascular intervention [A].[2]
  - *TASC II classification of PAD lesions*—may be used for descriptive and research purposes. Lesions are classified according to their site (inflow, outflow), length (short, long), number (single, multiple), and exact location (critical, preferred site) into types A to D. Angioplasty results are best in type A and not favourable (if any) in type D.[2]
  - *Stent placement*—should be considered for iliac, femoral, popliteal, or tibial lesions with suboptimal (or failed) angioplasty results [B].[2] The effectiveness of distal stents has not been fully established yet.[2]
  - *Other modalities of treatment (including atherectomy, cutting balloons, thermal devices, and lasers)*—are yet to be established.
- *Surgery*—is rarely required (or justifiable) in pure intermittent claudication. Surgery remains an option in selected patients where intermittent claudication has a significant effect on the mobility, effective conservative management has failed to improve symptoms, and the lesion is likely to benefit from surgical intervention [B].[2]

Critically ischaemic leg

- *Basic treatment*—includes effective pain control (see 📖 Chapter 19, pp.133–140), appropriate management of ulcers and wounds (see 📖 Chapter 9, pp.65–74), and control of infection (see 📖 Chapter 18, pp.123–132).[1]
- *Pharmacological therapy*—includes the use of parenteral prostaglandin E1 or ileoprost for 7–28d (limited efficiency to some patients) [A], and possible use of angiogenic growth factors within a trial context [C].[1,2]
- *In general terms, TASC II recommends endovascular treatment of inflow lesions*—as the preferred initial treatment of choice [B].[1,2] Outflow lesions should be addressed if the inflow lesion correction is not expected to lead to acceptable improvement in symptoms and signs [B].[2]
- *Surgery*—is indicated where endovascular procedure is not expected (or has failed) to achieve adequate inflow and/or outflow results [B].[2]
  - *Examples of inflow procedures*—include aorto-bifemoral bypass procedure iliac endarterectomy, aorto-iliac or aorto-femoral bypass, femoro-femoral cross-over bypass, axillo-femoral bypass, and axillofemoral-femoral bypass graft.[1,2]
  - *Examples of outflow procedures*—include fem-above knee (AK) popliteal vein graft, fem-AK popliteal prosthetic graft, fem-below knee (BK) popliteal vein graft, fem-BK popliteal prosthetic graft, fem-tibial vein graft, fem-tibial prosthetic graft.
  - *Amputation*—should be considered primarily for unsalvageable limbs or where surgical intervention carries a significant risk. Amputation may be the only effective option to manage the pain. The decision to proceed with amputation should take into consideration the ability of the amputation wound to heal, the rehabilitation requirements, and the overall quality of life [C].[1]

Further reading

1. Norgren L, Hiatt WR, Dormandy JA et al. (2007). Inter-Society consensus for the management of peripheral arterial disease (TASC II). *Eur J Vasc Endovasc Surg* 33 (Suppl 1), S1–75.
2. American College of Cardiology/American Heart Association. Guidelines. Peripheral Arterial Disease, 2006. Available from: http://circ.ahajournals.org/cgi/reprint/113/11/e463. Accessed May 2009.
3. Scottish Intercollegiate Guidelines Network (2006). Diagnosis and management of peripheral arterial disease. Available from: http://www.sign.ac.uk/pdf/sign89.pdf.
4. Moneta GL, Yeager RA, Antonovic R et al. (1992). Accuracy of lower extremity arterial duplex mapping. *J Vasc Surg* 15, 275–84.
5. Jorenby DE, Leischow SJ, Nides MA et al. (1999). A controlled trial of sustained-release bupropion, a nicotine patch, or both for smoking cessation. *N Engl J Med* 340, 685–91.
6. Antithrombotic Trialists' Collaboration (2002). Collaborative meta-analysis of randomized trials of antiplatelet therapy for prevention of death, myocardial infarction, and stroke in high risk patients. *BMJ* 324, 71–86.
7. Collins R, Armitage J, Parish S, Sleight P, Peto R; Heart Protection Study Collaborative Group (2004). Effects of cholesterol-lowering with simvastatin on stroke and other major vascular events in 20,536 people with cerebrovascular disease or other high-risk conditions. *Lancet* 363, 757–67.
8. Leng GC, Fowler B, Ernst E (2000). Exercise for intermittent claudication. *Cochrane Database Syst Rev* 2, CD000990.
9. Thompson PD, Zimet R, Forbes WP, Zhang P (2002). Meta-analysis of results from eight randomized, placebo-controlled trials on the effect of cilostazol on patients with intermittent claudication. *Am J Cardiol* 90, 1314–9.
10. McCartney MM, Gilbert FJ, Murchison LE, Pearson D, McHardy K, Murray AD (1999). Metformin and contrast media—a dangerous combination? *Clin Radiol* 54, 29–33.

Carotid artery stenosis*

* The guidelines on this chapter have been sourced and summarized from different UK, Europe, and international government sources, professional organizations, and medical specialty societies. Leading guidelines have been listed in the Key guidelines box.

Carotid artery stenosis

Key guidelines

- Cochrane Database Systematic Reviews. (i) (1999). Carotid endarterectomy for symptomatic carotid stenosis; (ii) (2005). Carotid endarterectomy for asymptomatic carotid stenosis.
- American Academy of Neurology (2005). Carotid endarterectomy—an evidence-based review.
- CREST (2006). Guidelines for investigation and management of transient ischaemic attack.
- National Institute for Health and Clinical Excellence (2006). Carotid artery stent placement for carotid stenosis.
- National Institute for Health and Clinical Excellence (2008). Stroke.
- Scottish Intercollegiate Guidelines Network. (i) (2002). Management of patients with stroke: rehabilitation, prevention and management of complications, and discharge planning; (ii) (2008). Management of patients with stroke or TIA: assessment, investigation, immediate management and secondary prevention.

Basic facts

- *Definitions*—transient ischaemic attack (TIA) is a medical emergency, indicating an unstable brain ischaemia with a high risk of imminent, potentially preventable, stroke.[3] See Table 45.1 for definitions.
- *Incidence*—TIA affects ~66 per 100,000 population every year and precedes ischaemic stroke in 15–25% of patients.[3,11] Stroke is the third most common cause of death in developed countries, affecting ~0.2% of population every year.[3,11]
- *Pathogenesis*—atherosclerotic stenotic lesion of the large extra- or intracranial arteries in ~50% of cases, causing tightness ('low flow' TIA) or artery-to-artery embolism ('embolic' TIA). Other causes of TIA are cardiogenic embolism (20% of TIA cases), small artery disease (25%), and haematologic or non-atheromatous diseases (10%).[3,9]
- *Clinical presentation*—varies widely depending on the area of the brain involved (Table 45.2).

Recommended investigations (Fig 45.1)

- *Basic investigations for TIA/minor stroke*—include basic blood tests (FBC, CRP, U&E, blood sugar, lipid profile, and clotting screen if on warfarin), ECG, and CXR.[3] Echocardiography is indicated if a cardiogenic embolism is suspected (and 24h ambulatory ECG for paroxysmal cardiac arrhythmias if necessary) [C].[3,6]
- *Coagulopathy screening*—is required for cases with no identifiable risk factors.[3] Screening tests include coagulation screen, thrombophilia screen, anti-cardiolipin antibody, and screening for vasculitis auto-antibody and plasma homocysteine.[3]

- *Carotid imaging*—first-line specialist vascular investigation for patients with suspected hemispheric (carotid territory) TIA who are fit for surgery (Fig. 45.1, Table 45.3) **[B]**.[3,6] Carotid stenosis are expressed differently between the European and American trials centres and this should be taken into consideration.[9]

Recommended management

Best medical treatment (Table 45.4)

- *Smoking*—should be completely discontinued (within a lifestyle changing approach) **[A]**.[1,5]
- *High blood pressure and high lipids*—should be well controlled. **[A]**.[1,5,6]
- *Other comorbidities (e.g. cardiac, diabetes)*—should be optimized.

Table 45.1 Definitions

- *Stroke*—a clinical syndrome consisting of 'rapidly developing clinical signs of focal (at times global) disturbance of cerebral function, lasting more than 24h or leading to death with no apparent cause other than that of vascular origin'.[5,17]

- *Transient ischaemic attack (TIA)*—stroke symptoms and signs that resolve within 24h (arbitrary cut-off time).[3,5,8]

Table 45.2 TIA/stroke clinical presentation

- *TIA common presentation*—temporary monocular blindness (amaurosis fugax), difficulty speaking (dysphasia), weakness on one side of the body (hemiparesis), and numbness or tingling (paraesthesia), usually on one side of the body.[3,8]

- *Stroke*—presents with **t**otal **a**nterior **c**irculation **i**nfarction (TACI: extensive sensory, motor, and higher cortical dysfunction), **p**artial **a**nterior **c**irculation **i**nfarction (PACI: more localized and less extensive neural dysfunction), **p**osterior **c**irculation **i**nfarction (POCI: blindness, diplopia, vertigo, ataxia, etc.), and **lac**unar **i**nfarction (LACI: pure motor or sensory dysfunctions).[3,9]

Table 45.3 Carotid duplex scan[9]

- **Technique**—a two-dimensional image (B-mode) of the carotid is obtained using real time USS. A waveform analysis of the blood flow within the artery lumen is then performed and displayed diagrammatically.

- **Diagnostic criteria**—an accurate estimation of the carotid stenosis depends on the judicious and validated use of B-mode images and spectral analysis. The use of peak systolic velocity (PSV) and end diastolic velocity (EDV) are of special use in estimating the degree of narrowing. For example, a PSV value of >125cm/s and EDV value of 140m/s predict a carotid stenosis of >50% with ~89% accuracy (sensitivity of ~96% and specificity of ~85%). A PSV value of >270m/s and EDV value of >110m/s predict a carotid stenosis of >70% with ~93% accuracy (sensitivity of ~96% and specificity of ~91%).

Table 45.4 Best medical management for carotid stenosis

- **BP control is essential**—two RCTs (PROGRESS and HOPE) showed significant risk reduction (RRR × 20–30%) in stroke rate in patients using ACE inhibitors. Nevertheless, no specific recommendation on their routine use has been published.[17,18]

- **Aspirin** (300mg for first 2wk, then long-term antithrombotic treatment)[5]—first-line agent. Significantly reduces the risk of stroke (by about 25–30%).[20] People with a history of dyspepsia should have PPI protection.
  - **Clopidogrel**—is a good alternative or additional treatment to aspirin.[21]

- **Control of other risk factors**—include smoking, hyperlipidaemia, diabetes, and optimization of cardiovascular and respiratory condition.

Surgical treatment
- **Carotid stenosis in symptomatic patients.**
  - *Key trials*—recommendations are mainly based on two international randomized trials.
    - North American Symptomatic Carotid Endarterectomy Trial (NASCET).[13]
    - European Carotid Surgery Trial (ECST).[14]
  - *Current recommendations.*
    - *Severe stenosis*—carotid endarterectomy (CEA) has established safety and effectiveness for recently symptomatic (within previous 6mo) patients with 70–99% internal carotid artery (ICA) stenosis when performed by an experienced surgeon [A].[1,2,6] CEA significantly reduces the risk of disabling stroke (from 28 to 9% (NASCET) or 19 to 11% (ECST); RRR × 45–70%).

- *Moderate stenosis*—CEA may be beneficial for patients with
50–69% symptomatic stenosis, and should be considered for
patients with expected life expectancy of minimum 5y by a
centre/surgeon with reported perioperative stroke/death rate of
<6% for symptomatic patients [A].[1,2,6] CEA moderately reduces
the risk of disabling stroke or death (RRR × 27%).[1]
- *Mild stenosis*—CEA has established harm for symptomatic patients
with <50% stenosis and should not be considered [A].[1,2,6] The
risk of a disabling stroke or death increases by 20%.[1] Best
medical management is recommended [A].[1,2,6]
- *Carotid stenosis in asymptomatic patients.*
  - *Key trials.*
    - Endarterectomy for asymptomatic carotid artery stenosis
(ACAS).[15]
    - Asymptomatic Carotid Stenosis Trial (ACST).[16]
  - *Current recommendations.*
    - *Severe stenosis*—it is reasonable to consider CEA for youngish
patients (age 40–75) with asymptomatic stenosis of 60–99%
(ACST) who has an expected life expectancy of minimum 5y,
where the centre/surgeon has a reported perioperative stroke/
death rate of <3% for asymptomatic patients [A].[1,2] CEA
moderately reduces the risk of disabling stroke or death
(from 11 to 5% (ACAS) or 12 to 6% (ACST) at 5y; RR × 0.71).[1]

Prognosis—the risk of stroke, myocardial infarction, or vascular death after
a TIA event is ~9% per year.[12] Most patients die from heart disease (~40%)
or other disorders (30%) rather than another stroke (25%).[12]

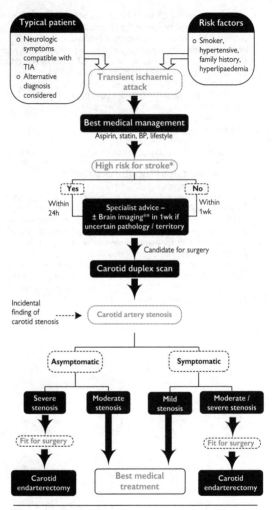

* for example, using the ABCD scoring system: **age** >60 = 1 point; **BP** >140/90 = 1 point; **clinical features** (speech disturbance = 1 point, unilateral weakness = 2 points); **duration** (<60min = 1 point, >60min = 2 points). Score ≥4 is high risk for stroke[5]
** preferably diffusion-weighted MRI[5]

Fig. 45.1 Recommended approach to carotid artery stenosis

Further reading

1. Cina C, Clase C, Haynes RB (1999). Carotid endarterectomy for symptomatic carotid stenosis. *Cochrane Database Syst Rev* 3, CD001081; Chambers BR, Donnan G (2005) Carotid endarterectomy for asymptomatic carotid stenosis. *Cochrane Database Syst Rev* 4, CD001923.

2. Chaturvedi S, Bruno A, Feasby T et al. (2005). Carotid endarterectomy—an evidence-based review: report of the Therapeutics and Technology Assessment Subcommittee of the American Academy of Neurology. *Neurology* 65, 794–801.

3. CREST (2006). Guidelines for investigation and management of transient ischaemic attack. Available from: http://www.crestni.org.uk/tia-guidelines.pdf.

4. National Institute for Health and Clinical Excellence (2006). Carotid artery stent placement for carotid stenosis. Available from: http://www.nice.org.uk/nicemedia/pdf/ip/IPG191guidance.pdf.

5. National Institute for Health and Clinical Excellence (2008). Stroke. Available from: http://www.nice.org.uk/nicemedia/pdf/CG68QuickRefGuide.pdf.

6. Scottish Intercollegiate Guidelines Network (2002). Management of patients with stroke: rehabilitation, prevention and management of complications, and discharge planning. Available from: http://www.sign.ac.uk/pdf/sign64.pdf; Scottish Intercollegiate Guidelines Network (2008) Management of patients with stroke or TIA: assessment, investigation, immediate management and secondary prevention. Available from: http://www.sign.ac.uk/pdf/sign108.pdf.

7. Lip GYH, Kalra L (2008). Stroke prevention. *BMJ Clin Evid* 9, 207.

8. Wikipedia. Stroke. Available from: http://en.wikipedia.org/wiki/Stroke; Wikipedia. Transient ischaemic attack. Available from: http://en.wikipedia.org/wiki/Transient_ischemic_attack.

9. Naylor AR, Gaines PA (2006). Extracranial cerebrovascular disease. In: *Vascular and endovascular surgery*, 3rd ed, Elsevier Saunders, London.

10. Rothwell PM, Giles MF, Flossmann E et al. (2005). A simple score (ABCD) to identify individuals at high early risk of stroke after transient ischaemic attack. *Lancet* 366, 29–36.

11. Rothwell PM, Coull AJ, Silver LE et al. (2005). Population-based study of event rate, incidence, case fatality, and mortality for all acute vascular events in all arterial territories (Oxford Vascular Study). *Lancet* 366, 1773–83.

12. Van Wijk I, Kappelle LJ, van Gijn J et al. (2005). Long-term survival and vascular event risk after transient ischaemic attack or minor ischaemic stroke: a cohort study. *Lancet* 365, 2098–104.

13. North American Symptomatic Carotid Endarterectomy Trial Collaborators (1991). Beneficial effect of carotid endarterectomy in symptomatic patients with high-grade carotid stenosis. *N Engl J Med* 325, 445–53.

14. European Carotid Surgery Trialists' Collaborative Group (1991). MRC European Carotid Surgery Trial: interim results for symptomatic patients with severe (70–99%) or with mild (0–29%) carotid stenosis. *Lancet* 337, 1235–43.

15. Executive Committee for the Asymptomatic Carotid Atherosclerosis Study (1995). Endarterectomy for asymptomatic carotid artery stenosis. *JAMA* 273, 1421–8.

16. Halliday A, Mansfield A, Marro J et al. (2004). Prevention of disabling and fatal strokes by successful carotid endarterectomy in patients with out recent neurological symptoms: randomised trial. *Lancet* 363, 1491–502.

17. Hatano S (1976). Experience from a multicentre stroke register: a preliminary report. *Bull World Health Organ* 54: 541–53.

18. PROGRESS Collaborative Group (2001). Randomized trial of a perindopril-based blood-pressure-lowering regime among 6,105 individuals with previous stroke or transient ischaemic attack. *Lancet* 358, 1033–41.

19. The Heart Outcomes Prevention Evaluation Study Investigators (2000). Effect of an angiotensin-converting enzyme inhibitor, ramipril, on cardiovascular events in high-risk patients. *N Engl J Med* 342, 145–53.

20. Antiplatelet Trialists' Collaboration (1988). Secondary prevention of vascular disease by prolonged antiplatelet treatment. *Br Med J* 296, 320–31.

21. CAPRIE Steering Committee (1996). A randomized blinded trial of clopidogrel versus aspirin in patients at risk of ischaemic event (CAPRIE). *Lancet* 348, 1329–39.

Abdominal aortic aneurysm (AAA)*

---

* The guidelines on this chapter have been sourced and summarized from different UK, Europe, and international government sources, professional organizations, and medical specialty societies. Leading guidelines have been listed in the Key guidelines box.

Abdominal aortic aneurysm (AAA)

Key guidelines
- ACC/AHA practice guidelines (2006). Management of patients with peripheral arterial disease (lower extremity, renal, mesenteric, and abdominal aortic)
- Vascular Society of Great Britain and Ireland (2004). Screening for abdominal aortic aneurysm.
- National Institute for Health and Clinical Excellence (2006). Stent-graft placement in abdominal aortic aneurysm.

Basic facts
- **Definition**—abnormal, persistent, localized dilatation of the aorta. An anteroposterior aortic diameter of ≥3cm (1.5 times the diameter measured at the level of the renal arteries) is considered aneurysmal, based on epidemiologic information of normal sizes of aorta in healthy adults adjusted to age and gender.[1]
- **Prevalence**—about 7–8% of the male population over the age of 65.[1,2] Males are affected five times more than females.
- **Pathogenesis**—appears to be multifactorial (Table 46.1). The combination of aortic wall degenerative changes (associated with abnormal elastolytic and proteolytic activities), chronic inflammatory process (correlated with raised CRP and interleukin (IL)-6), and the haemodynamic forces progressively applied on the aortic wall play a major role in the formation and development of AAA.[1,2,8] Most cases are associated with, but not necessarily caused by, atherosclerotic changes. Most (95%) are infrarenal aneurysms.
- **Clinical presentation**—the majority are asymptomatic until they rupture. Usually detected incidentally during investigations for other reasons (Table 46.2). About 15–25% of patients have multiple aneurysms (e.g. popliteal and iliac).[1] Only 30% of AAA <4cm can be detected clinically, rising to 75% when AAA reaches 5cm or more.[9]
- **Natural history**—only 10% of untreated AAA patients (depending on the aneurysm size) would be alive in 8 years' time (compared to 65% of non-AAA age-matching population).[2,11] Ruptured AAA accounts for ~30–50% of death in this group (Table 46.3).[2,11]

Recommended investigations
- **USS**—highly reliable for detecting AAA (accuracy ~97–100%) **[B]**.[1,3,9,10] USS is less reliable in screening iliac aneurysms and obese patients.
- **Abdominal contrast spiral CT scan/MRI/CT angiography**—should be used selectively (e.g. excluding other causes of abdominal pain, thorough assessment of aorta and iliacs, planning for open or endovascular aortic procedures).[1,10]
- **Screening recommendations for AAA**—see Table 46.4.

Table 46.1 Risk factors for AAA

- *Ageing process*—significant increase in prevalence with advancing age (~1.5% for men aged 45–55y, rising to 12.5% for men aged 75–85y).[1,6,7] Screening (abdominal physical examination and one-time USS) should be offered to male patients at age 65, (and to those aged 65–75y who have never smoked as per US recommendations [B]).[1,2,21]

- *Genetic*—higher risk (×4–10) in patients with affected first-degree relative.[1,2] Risk rises to 20 times if a sister is affected.[3] Screening (abdominal physical examination and USS) should be offered to first-degree male relatives of AAA patients [B].[1] Proper advice on stopping smoking (including smoking cessation interventions) should be offered to patients with a family history of aneurysms [B].[1]

- *Smoking*—major risk factor (OR × 5.6) for the formation, growth, and rupture of AAA.[6] Proper smoking cessation interventions (e.g. behavioural modification and nicotine replacement) should be offered to AAA patients [C].[1]

- *Atherosclerosis*—more common in AAA patients (MI, carotid stenosis, peripheral arterial disease)[1], and vice versa.

- *Hypertension*—relatively small effect (OR × 1.2).[8]

Table 46.2 Symptoms of AAA

- *Asymptomatic*—detected incidentally or on rupture

- *Symptomatic*—worsening abdominal or back pain (steady hypogastric gnawing pain for hours or days) and tender aneurysm are usually associated with recent expansion or inflammatory process and high risk for rupture.[1] Distal embolization can also occur.

- *Ruptured aneurysm*—presents (if patient survives long enough to get medical attention) with abdominal or back pain, hypotension, and/or a pulsatile abdominal mass.

Table 46.3 Estimated risk of AAA rupture*[2,11]

Size (cm)	Risk of rupture per year (%)
<3	~0
3–5	~0.5–1.0
5–6	~3.5
6–7	~9
7–8	~24

* Based on a meta-analysis of 13 studies

Recommended management

Best medical treatment
- **Smoking**—should be completely discontinued [C].[1]
- **High BP and high lipids**—should be well controlled [C].[1]
  - **β-blockers**—may be considered for AAA patients who are being followed non-operatively [B].[1,14,15,16] Patients undergoing AAA repair have been recommended to considered β-blockers in the perioperative period (if no contraindications exist) [A].[1,14,15,16]
  - **POISE trial**—is the largest trial to date. A total of 8,351 patients with or at risk of atherosclerotic disease undergoing non-cardiac surgery (42 % vascular surgery) were randomly assigned to either fixed dose metoprolol or placebo given 2–4h before surgery and repeated 0–6h after surgery. POISE results as well as two other meta-analyses confirmed that β-blockers decreases the risk of MI (RR = 0.73), but increases the risk of death (RR = 1.29) due to other causes (mainly stroke).[22]

Follow-up surveillance for small aneurysms
- **Asymptomatic AAA (3.0–5.5cm)**—should be managed conservatively (watchful waiting) to balance the risks of rupture (Table 46.4) with the risk of operation (Table 46.5) [A].[1] Monitoring with regular USS (or CT scan) is recommended 6–12 monthly (depending on the initial size and expansion rate of the aneurysm [A].[1]

Surgical treatment
- **General approach**—factors to be considered include the size and rate of growth of the aneurysm, perioperative expected risk (see 📖 Chapter 6, pp.31–44), quality of life issues, and patient's wishes and expectations.
- **Aneurysm key trials**—include the UK Small Aneurysm trial and VA Aneurysm Detection and Management (ADAM) Trial (US).[17,18,19] EVAR 1 and 2 trials (see Table 46.5) and their updates are key cornerstones for the current recommendations of AAA repair.[23,24]
- **Large-sized infrarenal asymptomatic AAA (>5.5cm)**—would benefit from elective repair (endovascular or open) in fit (good or average) and willing patients [B].[1] Elective repair for screen-detected AAA can offer an extra 9y of life to over 3,000 men per year in the UK (Table 46.4).[2]
- **Symptomatic AAA**—requires surgical repair (endovascular or open) regardless of the size in fit and suitable candidates [C].[1] Aneurysms increasing by ≥ 0.5cm in diameter per year should also be considered for repair.
- **Surgical options**—include open and endovascular surgical repair (Table 46.5 and 📖 Beyond the guidelines, p.354). EVAR patients should undergo immediate and long-term surveillance to detect endoleaks, displacement, and any need for further intervention [B].[1]

Table 46.4 Screening recommendations for AAA

- *Key trial*—the Multicentre Aneurysm Screening Study (MASS) trial: 4 centres (7,000 men); screening (and treatment) vs control group. The screening arm had AAA-related mortality reduction by 42%; emergency ruptured AAA mortality reduction by 70%; reduced disruption to elective work; and better management of risk factors and ICU/HDU beds.[2,12,13]

- *Cost-effectiveness*—estimated at ~£28,500 per QALY (quality adjusted life year) after 4y, and at ~£10,000 per QALY after 10y (cost-effective NHS screening programme should be less than £30,000 per QALY).[2]

- *Estimated increase in workload*—one extra AAA repair per month for a general hospital serving ~400,000 population.[2]

- *Current recommendations*—screening (abdominal physical examination and one-time USS) should be offered to male patients at the age of 65 (Table 46.1) [B].[1] This should be repeated in appropriate intervals to detect progression.

Table 46.5 Surgical treatment of AAA

- *Elective open repair.*
  - *Surgical technique*—involves full laparotomy, assessment of the aneurysm, full control of proximal, distal and collateral ends, and placement of appropriate aortic bypass graft.
  - *Risks*—recorded in-hospital mortality rate is 2–8% depending on the surgeon and the centre.[1,19] Operative non-fatal morbidity (CVA, MI, renal failure, ischaemic bowel, ischaemic legs) differs between centres as well (5% on average). Graft infection and impotence can also occur.

- *Elective endovascular aneurysm repair (EVAR).*
  - *Surgical technique*—collaboration of vascular surgeons and interventional radiologists. Bilateral groin access allows wires, catheters, and graft delivery systems to be delivered into the aorta and the bypass graft to be deployed under X-ray guidance.
  - *Risks*—recorded in-hospital mortality rate is <3%.[1] Operative non-fatal morbidity (CVA, MI, renal failure, ischaemic bowel, ischaemic legs) is ~3% on average. Graft infection and endoleak (persistent flow into aneurysm sac after deployment of graft) can also occur.

- *Laparoscopic repair of AAA*—can be performed using a hand-assisted or total laparoscopic surgery. Current evidence on safety and efficacy supports the use of this procedure by well-trained surgeons in appropriate clinical governance setting and multidisciplinary patient selection.[20]

Beyond the guidelines and the future

All patients with AAAs should now be offered EVAR. The EVAR l trial has shown a 3% reduction in aneurysm-related mortality at 30d, and this reduction continues out to 4y. The trial did show EVAR was more expensive than open surgery. However, these costs are now even less due to no ICU stay and shorter hospital stay for EVAR patients, using ultrasound for long-term monitoring and improvements in stent graft technology reducing the incidence of significant endoleak. In the future, the majority of aortic aneurysms will be treated by EVAR, as there are now endovascular options for the more complex aneurysm such as juxta-renal and thoraco-abdominal aneurysms.

Major centres in the UK, Europe, and North America are now embarking on stent-graft repair of ruptured AAAs. In practice, this is difficult to achieve due to the manpower and stock of devices required. However, it is likely that there will soon be a randomized controlled trial of EVAR vs open repair for ruptured aortic aneurysms.

With the increasing skill base and technology required, it is likely that all aortic aneurysms in the future will be treated in major vascular units with very few, if any, being treated in district general hospitals.

Mr Mark McCarthy

Further reading

1. Hirsch AT, Haskal ZJ, Hertzer NR *et al.* (2006). ACC/AHA 2005 Practice guidelines for the management of patients with peripheral arterial disease (lower extremity, renal, mesenteric, and abdominal aortic): a collaborative report from the American Association for Vascular Surgery/Society for Vascular Surgery, Society for Cardiovascular Angiography and Interventions, Society for Vascular Medicine and Biology, Society of Interventional Radiology, and the ACC/AHA Task Force on Practice Guidelines (Writing Committee to develop guidelines for the management of patients with peripheral arterial disease): endorsed by the American Association of Cardiovascular and Pulmonary Rehabilitation; National Heart, Lung, and Blood Institute; Society for Vascular Nursing; TransAtlantic Inter-Society Consensus; and Vascular Disease Foundation. *Circulation* 113, e463–654.
2. Vascular Society of Great Britain and Ireland (2004). Screening for abdominal aortic aneurysm. Available from: http://www.vascularsociety.org.uk/Docs/3208_A5Booklet1.pdf.
3. National Institute for Health and Clinical Excellence (2006). Stent-graft placement in abdominal aortic aneurysm. Available from: http://www.nice.org.uk/nicemedia/pdf/ip/IPG163guidance.pdf.
4. Finnish Guidelines. AAA. http://www.guideline.gov/summary/summary.aspx?ss=15&doc_id=7377&nbr=4359. Available from: http://www.guideline.gov/summary/summary.aspx?doc_id=12786&nbr=006588&string=AAA. Accessed May 2009.
5. Lederle FA, Johnson GR, Wilson SE *et al.* (2000). The aneurysm detection and management study screening program: validation cohort and final results. Aneurysm Detection and Management Veterans Affairs Cooperative Study Investigators. *Arch Intern Med* 160, 1425–30.
6. Powell JT, Greenhalgh RM (2003). Clinical practice. Small abdominal aortic aneurysms. *N Engl J Med* 348, 1895–901.
7. Scott RA, Ashton HA, Kay DN (1991). Abdominal aortic aneurysm in 4,237 screened patients: prevalence, development and management over 6 years. *Br J Surg* 78, 1122–5.
8. Lederle FA, Johnson GR, Wilson SE *et al.* (1997). Prevalence and associations of abdominal aortic aneurysm detected through screening. Aneurysm Detection and Management (ADAM) Veterans Affairs Cooperative Study Group. *Ann Intern Med* 126, 441–9.

9. Lederle FA Simel DL (1999). The rational clinical examination: does this patient have abdominal aortic aneurysm? *JAMA* 281, 77–82.

10. Lederle FA, Wilson SE, Johnson GR et al. (1995). Variability in measurement of abdominal aortic aneurysms. Abdominal Aortic Aneurysm Detection and Management Veterans Administration Cooperative Study Group. *J Vasc Surg* 21, 945–52.

11. Law MR, Morris J, Wald NJ (1994). Screening for abdominal aortic aneurysms. *J Med Screen* 1, 110–5.

12. Ashton HA, Buxton MJ, Day NE et al. (2002). The Multicentre Aneurysm Screening Study (MASS) into the effect of abdominal aortic aneurysm screening on mortality in men: a randomized controlled trial. *Lancet* 360, 1531–9.

13. Fleming C, Whitlock EP, Beil TL, Lederle FA (2005). Screening for abdominal aortic aneurysm: a best-evidence systematic review for the U.S. Preventive Services Task Force. *Ann Intern Med* 142, 203–11.

14. Propanolol Aneurysm Trial Investigators (2002). Propranolol for small abdominal aortic aneurysms: results of a randomized trial. *J Vasc Surg* 35, 72–9.

15. POISE Study Group, Devereaux PJ, Yang H et al. (2008). Effects of extended-release metoprolol succinate in patients undergoing non-cardiac surgery (POISE trial): a randomized controlled trial. *Lancet* 371, 1839–47.

16. Devereaux PJ, Beattie WS, Choi PT et al. (2005). How strong is the evidence for the use of perioperative beta blockers in non-cardiac surgery? Systematic review and meta-analysis of randomized controlled trials. *BMJ* 331, 313–21.

17. The UK Small Aneurysm Trial Participants (1998). Mortality results for randomized controlled trial of early elective surgery or ultrasonographic surveillance for small abdominal aortic aneurysms. *Lancet* 352, 1649–55.

18. Lederle FA, Wilson SE, Johnson GR et al. (2002). Immediate repair compared with surveillance of small abdominal aortic aneurysms. *N Engl J Med* 346, 1437–44.

19. Lederle FA, Kane RL, MacDonald R, Wilt TJ (2007). Systematic review: repair of unruptured abdominal aortic aneurysm. *Ann Intern Med* 146, 735–41.

20. National Institute for Health and Clinical Excellence (2007). Laparoscopic repair of abdominal aortic aneurysm. Available from: http://www.nice.org.uk/nicemedia/pdf/IPG229Guidance.pdf.

21. National Screening Committee (2009). Abdominal aortic aneurysm. Available from: http://www.library.nhs.uk/screening/ViewResource.aspx?resID=60457.

22. Fleisher LA, Poldermans D (2008). Perioperative beta blockade: where do we go from here? *Lancet* 371, 1813–4.

23. EVAR trial participants (2005). Endovascular aneurysm repair versus open repair in patients with abdominal aortic aneurysm (EVAR trial 1): randomized controlled trial. *Lancet* 365, 2179–86.

24. EVAR trial participants (2005). Endovascular aneurysm repair and outcome in patients unfit for open repair of abdominal aortic aneurysm (EVAR trial 2): randomized controlled trial. *Lancet* 365, 2187–92.

Chronic venous
insufficiency (CVI)*

* The guidelines on this chapter have been sourced and summarized from different UK,
Europe, and international government sources, professional organizations, and medical
specialty societies. Leading guidelines have been listed in the Key guidelines box.

Chronic venous insufficiency (CVI)

Key guidelines

- BMJ Clinical Evidence (2007). Varicose veins.
- National Institute for Health and Clinical Excellence (2001). Referral advice: a guide to appropriate referral from general to specialist services.
- Cochrane Database of Systematic Reviews (2004). Surgery versus sclerotherapy for the treatment of varicose veins.
- National Institute for Health and Clinical Excellence (2007). Ultrasound-guided foam sclerotherapy for varicose veins.
- National Institute for Health and Clinical Excellence (2004). Endovenous laser treatment of long saphenous vein.

Basic facts

- *Definitions*—CVI is the impairment of venous return in the lower limbs, presenting with a broad clinical spectrum, including varicose veins, skin changes, and venous ulceration (Table 47.1).
- *Incidence*—CVI affects ~2–9% of the population.[11] Varicose veins affect ~40% of men and 16% of women aged 18–64y.[1,10] Telangiectases and reticular veins occur in ~80–85% of both genders.[1,10] Ankle oedema is present in ~7% of men and 16% women.[1,10] Venous leg ulcers (active or healed) occur in ~1% of the population.[1,10]
- *Impact on health resources*—tremendous. Most venous leg ulcers require an average of 1y to heal satisfactorily, 20% require >2y, and 66% of patients complain of episodes of ulceration for >5y.[10] The cost of care for chronic venous disease accounts for ~1–3% of the total health care budget in developed countries.[10]
- *Pathophysiology*—not fully understood (Table 47.2).
  - Risk factors for venous insufficiency include multiple pregnancies (RR × 1.2 after two pregnancies), age, obesity in women (RR × 1.3), and a history of phlebitis or venous thrombosis.[1,10,12–14]
- *Clinical presentation*—ranges from cosmetically upsetting, but otherwise asymptomatic, ectatic veins to severe skin changes, oedema, and ulcerations (Table 47.1).
- *Classification*—the Clinical, Etiologic, Anatomic, and Pathophysiologic (CEAP) classification was developed in 1994 by an international consensus conference and is widely accepted (Table 47.3).[8,15]

Recommended investigations

- *General approach*—the diagnosis of venous insufficiency and incompetent valve system is mainly based on thorough clinical history, detailed physical examination, and appropriate use of invasive and non-invasive investigations. The widespread use of the non-invasive Doppler and duplex scan has reduced the need for more time-consuming clinical tests such as Trendelenburg (selective occlusion) test.[9]

Table 47.1 Clinical presentation of varicose veins

- *Aching pain and heaviness*—fullness feeling, leg cramps during night, aching discomfort, or leg heaviness. Discomfort may be made worse upon standing, during menstrual cycle, and with the progression of pregnancy. Pain may interfere with normal daily activities and makes ambulation difficult.

- *Dilated veins*—vary in size and palpability.
  - Telangiectases are tiny (<1mm), bluish, ecstatic, non-palpable venules located intradermally.
  - Reticular veins presents as small, tiny (<3mm), dilated, non-palpable veins located subdermally.
  - Varicose veins are larger (>3mm), dilated, palpable veins located subcutaneously.

- *Leg and ankle oedema*—usually associated with varicose veins at an early stage. Oedema is made worse with prolonged standing positions and improves significantly (at the initial stages of the disease) with leg elevation and walking. Oedema becomes persistent as the disease progresses.

- *Skin changes*—occur at a later stage; reddish brown colour skin changes on the medial aspects of leg and ankle. Lipodermatosclerosis (heavily pigmented skin with extensively fibrotic, and impeding lymphatic and venous flow) results from the fibrosing panniculitis of subcutaneous tissue.

- *Venous ulcer*—usually located on the medial shin over a perforating vein, or along the line of long or short saphenous veins. The ulcer is typically tender, varies in diameter, is shallow with sloping edges, and usually has irregular, but not undermined edges.

Table 47.2 Pathophysiology of CVI

- In most cases, CVI results from an obstruction to venous flow, dysfunction of venous valves, and/or failure of the venous pump.[1,10] This results in an abnormal direction of the venous blood flow from the deep to the superficial system, with resultant local tissue anoxia, inflammation, white cell trapping, and occasionally, necrosis. The resulting 'subcutaneous fibrosing panniculitis' obstructs further the proximal lymphatic and venous flow.[1,10]

- *Handheld Doppler*—can detect the presence of reflux in the saphenofemoral junction (SFJ), long saphenous vein, saphenopopliteal junction (SPJ), and occasionally, perforating veins.[9] Reported accuracy is ~75%.[16] Limitations include the inability to identify the specific veins and it is operator-dependent.

- *Duplex scanning*—(B-mode USS combined with wave Doppler scan) is the investigation of choice for CVI.[8,9,17,18] Duplex scan can accurately delineate venous anatomy, including areas of venous reflux disease. Reported accuracy is ~95% when compared to traditional venography.[17,18] The impact of duplex scanning on long-term recurrence rate has not been properly validated.

- *Other investigations*—may occasionally be required, including venography and functional calf volume measurements. A full description of available investigations for CVI with their benefits and limitations can be found in Nicolaides's review article.[9]

Recommended treatment

- *General approach.*
  - *The main treatment goal in CVI*—is to improve the venous and lymphatic back flow. This in turn would improve the oxygen transport to the skin and subcutaneous tissues, and reduce the inflammatory process, which will allow for the reduction of oedema, elimination of fibrosing panniculitis of the subcutaneous tissue, and eventually healing of the venous ulcers, if present.
  - Venous and lymphatic back flow can be improved using general (leg elevation, etc.), pharmacologic (e.g. injection sclerotherapy), and operative measures (e.g. treatment of incompetent varicose veins, reconstruction of deep veins). The local treatment of chronic ulcers can be found in Ch. 9.
- *General measures*—include elevation of the legs above the heart level at rest, regular exercises (sensible option, but lack evidence), avoidance of long standing, and management of confounding factors such as obesity [G].[1,19]
- *Graduated compression stockings*—is the primary effective management of CVI. Stockings that apply the highest pressure around the ankle (~30–40mmHg) and decreases proximally has been validated in a Cochrane systematic review to significantly increase the healing rate of leg ulcers, especially when multi-component systems (three or four layers bandages) that contain an elastic bandage were used.[1,20] Caution should be taken when applied in patients with concurrent arterial disease. The reported healing rate is ~93% in a mean duration of 5.3mo.[21] Surgical correction of superficial venous reflux in addition to compression bandaging has been shown in ESCHAR trial **NOT** to be superior to compression bandaging alone in improving the ulcer healing, but was able to reduce the recurrence of ulcers at 4y and resulted in a greater proportion of ulcer-free time.[25]

Table 47.3 CEAP classification

Classification	Description/definition
C: Clinical (subdivided into A for asymptomatic, S for symptomatic)	
0	No venous disease
1	Telangectiases
2	Varicose veins
3	Oedema
4	Lipodermatosclerosis or hyperpigmentation
5	Healed ulcer
6	Active ulcer
E: aEtiologic	
Congenital	Present since birth
Primary	Undetermined aetiology
Secondary	Associated with post-thrombotic, traumatic
A: Anatomic distribution (alone or in combination)	
Superficial	Great and short saphenous veins
Deep	Cava, iliac, gonadal, femoral, profunda, popliteal, tibial, and muscular veins
Perforator	Thigh and leg perforating veins
P: Pathophysiological	
Reflux	Axial and perforating veins
Obstruction	Acute and chronic
Combination of both	Valvular dysfunction and thrombus

Table 47.4 Injection sclerotherapy—technique and side effects

- *Technique*—following marking the varicosities while patient is standing, a small (25–30G) needle is used to inject a small amount (0.25–0.50mL) of an appropriate sclerosing agent slowly into the lumen of the vein. Compression stockings are then applied for few weeks and the patient is asked to walk for half an hour.

- *Contraindications*—include allergy to the agent in use, peripheral vascular disease, immobility, and acute thrombophlebitis.

- *Complications*—are rare, including thrombosis, ulceration, and anaphylactic reactions.

Table 47.5 Ultrasound-guided foam sclerotherapy[4]

- *Technique*—a variation of the traditional liquid sclerotherapy. Under ultrasound guidance, a sclerosant foam is injected into the vein and compression stockings are applied.

- *Safety*—no major safety concerns according to current available evidence. Transient side effects in a small proportion of patients have been noticed. Possible adverse effects include skin pigmentation (~30% of cases), skin necrosis (~1.5%), local neurological injury (<1%), transient visual disturbance (0–6%), and rare cases of stroke, MI, epilepsy, and DVT.

- *Efficiency*—successful vein occlusion occurs in >85% of cases. Compared to surgery, no significant difference was noticed. Recurrence rate ranged from 1–15%.

- *Terms of use*—special arrangements should be undertaken for clinical governance, patient consent, audit, and review of all outcome results by a dedicated team.

Table 47.6 Endovenous laser therapy (EVLT)[5,24]

- *Technique*—following injection of a local anaesthesia, a catheter is placed into the long saphenous vein under ultrasound guidance. The laser fibre is passed through to just below (distal) the SFJ. Further local anaesthesia is injected, then energy from a diode laser is delivered while slowly withdrawing the laser fibre.

- *Safety*—no major safety concerns were reported according to current available evidence. Possible complications include minor skin burns (~0.5%) and temporary paraesthesia (~2%).

- *Efficiency*—appears to be more effective in the short term, and at least as effective overall as the comparative procedure of junction ligation and vein stripping for the treatment of varicose veins.[24]

- *Terms of use*—special arrangements should be undertaken for clinical governance, patient consent, audit, and review of all outcome results by a dedicated team.

- **Injection sclerotherapy for varicose veins**—has been shown in a recent Cochrane review to have significant effect (improved symptoms and cosmetic appearance) when used for recurrent varicose veins following surgery and thread veins (such as telangectiasia or spider veins).[1,22] Compared to surgery, injection sclerotherapy appears to have superior results in the short term, but inferior results after 5y, although the evidence is weak.[1,23] Table 47.4 summarizes the technique, contraindications, and possible side effects.
  - *Ultrasound-guided foam sclerotherapy*—current evidence on the safety and efficacy of this treatment for varicose veins appears adequate to support its use within the appropriate setting (Table 47.5).[4]
- **Endovascular treatment of varicose veins.**
  - *Endovenous laser therapy (EVLT)*—current evidence on the safety and efficacy of this treatment for incompetent long saphenous vein appears adequate to support its use within the appropriate setting (Table 47.6).[5,24]
  - *Radiofrequency ablation of varicose veins*—this technique involves accessing the long saphenous vein (puncture or small incision) and heating the wall of the diseased vein using a bipolar generator and specially designed catheters. By manually withdrawing the catheter at 2.5–3cm/min, the vein wall temperature can be maintained at 85°C. Current evidence on the safety and efficacy of this treatment for incompetent long saphenous vein appears adequate to support its use as an alternative to open surgery within the appropriate setting.[6]
- **Open surgery for varicose veins.**
  - *Technique*—ligation of the SFJ, stripping of the long saphenous vein, and avulsion of the remaining varicosities is the traditional varicose vein operation, and one of the commonest sources of litigation in the UK.
  - *Benefits*—a Cochrane systematic review should that open surgery has significantly reduced the risk of varicose vein recurrence and improved cosmetic appearance when compared with injection sclerotherapy alone.[23]
  - *Standards of surgery*—include adequate preoperative investigation and marking, adequate and thorough patient consultation, using day surgery as a norm (see 📖 Chapter 4, pp.21–6), and appropriate stripping and avulsion techniques.

Further reading

1. Tisi P (2007). Varicose veins. *BMJ Clin Evid* 10, 212.
2. National Institute for Health and Clinical Excellence (2001). Referral advice: a guide to appropriate referral from general to specialist services. Available from: http://www.nice.org.uk/nicemedia/pdf/Referraladvice.pdf.
3. Rigby KA, Palfreyman SJ, Beverley C, Michaels JA (2004). Surgery versus sclerotherapy for the treatment of varicose veins. *Cochrane Database Syst Rev* 4, CD004980.
4. National Institute for Health and Clinical Excellence (2007). Ultrasound-guided foam sclerotherapy for varicose veins. Available from: http://www.nice.org.uk/Guidance/IPG217.
5. National Institute for Health and Clinical Excellence (2004). Endovenous laser treatment of long saphenous vein. Available from: http://www.nice.org.uk/Guidance/IPG52.
6. National Institute for Health and Clinical Excellence (2003). Radiofrequency ablation of varicose veins. Available from: http://www.nice.org.uk/Guidance/IPG8.

7. National Institute for Health and Clinical Excellence (2004). Transilluminated powered phlebectomy for varicose veins. Available from: http://www.nice.org.uk/Guidance/IPG37.

8. Eberhardt RT, Raffetto JD (2005). Chronic venous insufficiency. *Circulation* 111, 2398–409.

9. Nicolaides AN (2000). Investigation of chronic venous insufficiency: a consensus statement. *Circulation* 102, e126–63.

10. Bergan JJ, Schmid–Schönbein GW, Smith PD, Nicolaides AN, Boisseau MR, Eklof B (2006). Chronic venous disease. *N Engl J Med* 355, 488–98.

11. Evans CJ, Fowkes FG, Ruckley CV, Lee AJ (1999). Prevalence of varicose veins and chronic venous insufficiency in men and women in the general population: Edinburgh Vein Study. *J Epidemiol Community Health* 53, 149–53.

12. Criqui MH, Denenberg JO, Bergan J, Langer RD, Fronek A (2007). Risk factors for chronic venous disease: the San Diego Population Study. *J Vasc Surg* 46, 331–7.

13. Scott TE, LaMorte WW, Gorin DR, Menzoian JO (1995). Risk factors for chronic venous insufficiency: a dual case-control study. *J Vasc Surg* 22, 622–8.

14. Chiesa R, Marone EM, Limoni C, Volonte M, Petrini O (2007). Chronic venous disorders: correlation between visible signs, symptoms, and presence of functional disease. *J Vasc Surg* 46, 322–30.

15. Porter JM, Moneta GL (1995). Reporting standards in venous disease: An update. *J Vasc Surg* 21, 635–45.

16. Campbell WB, Niblett PG, Ridler BM, Peters AS, Thompson JF (1997). Handheld Doppler as a screening test in primary varicose veins. *Br J Surg* 84, 1541–3.

17. Khaira, HS, Parnell, A (1995). Colour flow duplex in the assessment of varicose veins. *Clin Radiol* 50, 583–6.

18. Smith JJ, Brown L, Greenhalgh RM, Davies AH (2002). Randomized trial of preoperative colour duplex marking in primary varicose vein surgery: outcome is not improved. *Eur J Vasc Endovasc Surg* 23, 336–43.

19. The Alexander House Group (1992). Consensus paper on venous leg ulcer. *J Dermatol Surg Oncol* 18, 592–602.

20. Cullum N, Nelson EA, Fletcher AW, Sheldon TA (2002). Compression for venous leg ulcers. *Cochrane Database Syst Rev* 2, CD000265.

21. Mayberry JC, Moneta GL, Taylor LM Jr, Porter JM (1991). Fifteen year results of ambulatory compression therapy for chronic venous ulcers. *Surgery* 109, 575–81.

22. Tisi PV, Beverley C, Rees A (2006). Injection sclerotherapy for varicose veins. *Cochrane Database Syst Rev* 4, CD001732.

23. Rigby KA, Palfreyman SJ, Beverley C, Michaels JA (2004). Surgery versus sclerotherapy for the treatment of varicose veins. *Cochrane Database Syst Rev* 4, CD004980.

24. Medical Services Advisory Committee (2008). Endovenous laser treatment for varicose veins (ELT), MSAC application 1113. Available from: http://www.msac.gov.au/internet/msac/publishing.nsf/Content/app1113-1.

25. Gohel MS, Barwell JR, Taylor M *et al.* (2007). Long-term results of compression therapy alone versus compression plus surgery in chronic venous ulceration (ESCHAR): randomized controlled trial. *BMJ* 335, 83.

Part 11

Breast

Breast cancer*

* The guidelines on this chapter have been sourced and summarized from different UK, Europe, and international government sources, professional organizations, and medical specialty societies. Leading guidelines have been listed in the Key guidelines box.

Breast cancer

Breast cancer

Key guidelines
- Cancer Research UK (2008). Breast cancer.
- Association of Breast Surgery (2005). Guidelines for the management of symptomatic breast disease.
- Scottish Intercollegiate Guidelines Network (2005). Management of breast cancer in women.
- National Institute for Health and Clinical Excellence (2002). Improving outcomes in breast cancer—manual update.

Basic facts
- *Incidence*—the commonest cancer affecting women and commonest cause of cancer death in women worldwide. Over 50% increase in incidence since 1980 (more than 1% each year). In 2004, about 44,500 new cases were diagnosed in the UK, 80% occurred in women aged over 50. Rare in men (less than 1% of all cancer cases).[1,6] Incidence is highest in industrialized world (North America and Northern Europe) and lowest in Asia and Africa.[1]
- *Risk factors*—most related to the effect of exposure to oestrogen (Table 48.1).
- *Clinical presentation*—ranges from a highly suspicious breast lesion to a completely asymptomatic screen-detected cancer (Table 48.2). The estimated doubling time of breast cancer is 100–300d with frequent exceptions.[16] A 1cm^3 tumour usually requires ~30 doublings (≥7y) to become palpable clinically.[16,19] Palpability depends also on the volume of breast, location of cancer, surrounding stromal reaction, and experience of the examiner.[18] Breast screening detects many cancers at the pre-clinical stage (about 20–35% of all breast cancer cases in the UK).[4]

Recommended investigations
- *Urgent referral to breast unit*—for all patients with a breast lump if age ≥30, skin ulceration, nodules or distortion, nipple eczema, retraction or unilateral discharge.[4] Less urgent referrals should be reserved for low suspicious cases (asymmetric nodularity, bilateral nipple discharge, etc).[4]
- *Triple assessment*—the mainstay of diagnosis [B].[2,4,38] This includes clinical examination, breast imaging (two-view mammography, digital mammography, and ultrasound), and histology confirmation (core biopsy or fine needle aspiration (FNA)).[6]
  - *Accuracy*—depends on the quality of each constituent test. Reported sensitivity is ≥99% if all investigations concur.[36] False negative rates are low, but higher in younger patients.[1]
  - *Quality standards*—bilateral mammography prior to any definitive treatment is essential in any patient with early breast cancer [B].[38] Mastectomy should not be performed on the basis of an FNA alone wherever possible [B].[4] Core biopsy also has the advantage of making the assessment of hormone receptor status possible.

Table 48.1 Risk factors for breast cancer

- *Patient age*—rare under the age of 30 (estimated risk is 1 in 1,900). Steady increase up to the age of 50 (estimated risk is 1 in 50). Most cases (8 out of 10) diagnosed in the 50–64 age group (estimated risk at age 70 is 1 in 15). The incidence curve flattens after the age of 75 to 80 with a slight decrease thereafter.[1]

- *Socioeconomic status*—more common in higher socioeconomic status females (up to 2-fold).[1,7] More common in North America and Northern Europe. Possibly caused by the special modern reproductive lifestyle (parity, age at first live birth, etc.).[1,7]

- *Reproductive history*—more common in women with early age of menarche (each year menarche is delayed after age 12 reduces the risk by 3–7%), in women with late childbearing (risk increases by 3% for each year of delay), in nulliparous women (risk increases by 30% in nulliparous vs parous women), in women with no history of breastfeeding (each year of breastfeeding reduces the risk by 4.3%), and in women with delayed menopause (risk increases by 3% for each year delay in menopause).[1,8–9]

- *Personal and family history of breast cancer*—personal history increases the risk of a second primary breast cancer by 2–6 times.[1,10] A positive family history of breast cancer in one first-degree relative (mother or sister) increases the risk of breast cancer by two. Two or more affected relatives increase the risk further. Note that over 85% of women with a close relative who had a breast cancer will never develop the disease.[1,11]

- *Other risk factors*—current or recent use of oral contraceptives (RR × 1.25)[12] and use of HRT (RR × 1.66), especially for oestrogen-progestagen combinations and for long users. High BMI increases the risk in post-menopausal women (30% increased risk for BMI >28 compared to BMI <21).[1,13,14] Vigorous exercises for a few hours per week reduces the risk by 30–40%.[1] Alcohol consumption increases the risk by 7% for each daily alcoholic drink consumption.[1,15] No proven link of tobacco to the risk of breast cancer.[1] Other factors include mammographic density and exposure to ionizing radiation.

Table 48.2 Breast cancer—clinical features

- *Local features*—include breast lump (often hard, painless, can be immobile, fixed to surrounding tissues, to overlying skin, or to the underlying pectoral muscle), nipple discharge (usually unifocal, bloodstained, or clear), and skin changes (skin distortion, puckering, and peau d'orange sign).

- *Regional features*—include axillary and supraclavicular lymphadenopathy.

- *Distant features*—include hepatomegaly, ascites, and ovarian mass.

- *Mammographic abnormalities*—detected in most cancers.[20] The overall sensitivity and specificity is 80–85% (therefore, it cannot be the only diagnostic test for symptomatic breast patients).[2,3]
  - *Most common findings*—suggestive of cancer are clustered microcalcifications and spiculated masses. Microcalcifications (calcium shadows measuring between 0.1 and 1mm in diameter, taking various shapes and sizes, and grouping as a cluster of more than 4–5/cm^3) are found in about 60% of mammographically-detected cancers. Spiculated masses are found in about a third of non-calcified breast cancer.[37] Other suspicious findings include linear branching microcalcifications and granular calcifications.
  - *Summary of findings*—is best performed using the Royal College of Radiologists scoring system (Table 48.3), indicating the likelihood of a normal, benign, or malignant diagnosis.[21]
- *USS*—complements the clinical examination and mammography, especially in undetermined cases (palpable masses with normal mammogram, breast masses in dense breasts, young ages, etc.).[2,4] Sensitivity, specificity, and negative predictive values when adding USS in such cases are around 97, 95, and 99%, respectively.[22,23] Very beneficial in predicting (and downstaging) cancer size, and in guiding real-time FNA, core biopsy, or wire insertion in small or non-palpable lesions.[4] Pretreatment assessment of axilla with USS and ultrasound-guided FNA is recommended as per local protocols.
- *Other imaging modalities (such as MRI scan[39])*—should be used in specific occasions after discussion at the MDT meeting. MRI scan is specifically useful for evaluating undetermined cases where a discrepancy between clinical and radiological assessments exists, in increased breast density, and as part of the assessment of the size of invasive lobular carcinoma if conservative surgery is planned.
- *Breast biopsy*—is essential prior to any definitive treatment. Breast biopsy can be obtained by using FNA cytology (FNAc), core biopsy, or occasionally open surgical biopsy.
  - *FNAc*—should be performed by a trained person to achieve accurate results. The rate of false negative results in experienced hands ranges from 0–32%.[40] FNA findings should be reported as in Table 48.3.
  - *Core biopsy*—is more adequate than FNAc for proper sampling and is able to distinguish invasive from *in situ* cancers in most cases. Findings should be reported using a standardized reporting system (Table 48.3).
  - *Other methods*—can occasionally be used for sampling purposes in certain cases, including open biopsy and stereotactic biopsy.

Recommended initial staging (Fig. 48.1)

- *MDT discussion*—essential prior to any definitive treatment [C*].[3,4] Main issues affecting treatment should be discussed, agreed, and documented (Table 48.4). Joint treatment recommendations should be documented and communicated to the patient as and when appropriate (see below).

- *Basic investigations*—should include baseline blood tests (FBC, LFTs, etc.) for all patients, and CXR for patients with no clinical suspicion of metastatic disease. Other staging tests (liver imaging or bone scan) are not required for early operable breast cancer [C],[1,2] and only minimal investigations for asymptomatic patients with early breast cancer should be performed [A].[38] Agreed local protocols in well-established breast units should be followed.
- *Metastatic cancer*—should be suspected in locally advanced cancers, aggressive histologic and cellular cancer type (large tumours, poor differentiation, etc.), and abnormal LFTs. Further staging with CT and bone radionuclide scan should be considered in such cases.[3]
- *PET scan*—should only be used to make a new diagnosis of metastasis where imaging is suspicious, but not diagnostic.
- *Breaking bad news*—an essential step to ensure adequate compliance. Should be done in a professional and effective way (Table 48.5). The role of cancer care nurse is essential.[2]

Table 48.3 Recommended reporting standards in breast cancer[2]

- **Clinical findings**—P1: normal. P2: benign. P3: probably benign. P4: probably malignant. P5: malignant.
- **USS**—U1: normal. U2: benign. U3: probably benign. U4: probably malignant. U5: malignant.
- **Mammography**—R1: normal. R2: benign. R3: probably benign. R4: probably malignant. R5: malignant.
- **FNAc**—C1: inadequate. C2: benign. C3: atypia probably benign. C4: suspicious of malignancy. C5: malignant.
- **Core biopsy**—B1: unsatisfactory/normal tissue only. B2: benign. B3: lesions of uncertain malignant potential. B4: suspicion of malignancy. B5a: *in situ* malignancy. B5b: invasive malignancy. B5c: malignant, *in situ*/invasive status not assessable.

Table 48.4 Points to discuss at MDT meeting

- **Surgeon's assessment**—includes clinical findings, patient's personal circumstances and attitude to treatment options, technical challenges (including breast/cancer relative sizes), and any other relevant findings.
- **Radiologist's assessment**—includes the extent of breast involvement, existence of any other concomitant cancers, need for further imaging or histologic confirmation, axillary lymph gland involvement (with FNA if possible), and preoperative requirement for localization of cancer.
- **Pathologist's assessment**—includes confirmation and histologic features of cancer, biological markers (including oestrogen receptors (ERs), progesterone receptors (PRs), and human epidermal growth factor receptor-2 (HER-2)), lymphovascular invasion, genomics, Nottingham Prognostic Index (NPI), and any other relevant issues.
- **Breast care nurse contribution**—is essential.

Table 48.5 Points to discuss with the patient in the result clinic

- Confirmation of diagnosis, available treatment options (including immediate reconstruction even if that treatment is not available in that unit), expected perioperative period experience, contact details and sources for further information (including patient support groups).
- Discussion should be documented and communicated to other members of the team (GP, oncologists, breast care nurses, etc.).

Recommended management (Fig. 48.1)

Lobular carcinoma in situ (LCIS)

- **Biological features**—very slow-growing tumour, indolent biologic behaviour, and very low probability of progression to invasive disease.[31] Typically positive to ERs and has no overexpression of *HER2/neu* oncogene.
- **Risk of invasive cancer**—not considered pre-malignant, but high and very powerful risk marker to invasive cancer. 20–30% of patients develop invasive cancer of various types in both biopsied and opposite sides (RR is 2–18 times higher than average population).[2, 26,31]
- **Management**—see Table 48.6.

Ductal carcinoma in situ (DCIS)

- **Biological features**—malignant precursor of invasive cancer.[2]
- **Management**—see Table 48.7.

Operable (early stage) breast cancer

- **In general**—HRT should be stopped. Surgical excision is the treatment of choice irrespective of age [A].[2,4] Locally invasive cancers may require neoadjuvant therapy before considering surgery.
- **Surgical options**—should be based on the individual patient needs following a thorough informed consent on benefits and risks of each option [A].[2,4] Breast-conserving surgery (BCS) is suitable for the majority if deemed acceptable by the patient (Table 48.8). BCS should preserve cosmetically acceptable breast without sacrificing survival. Mastectomy (following proper staging of the axilla) is the option if BCS is contraindicated or not suitable [A].[3,5]
- **Axillary surgery**—management of regional lymph nodes should be determined according to the biologic features of the tumour.
  - All invasive operable breast cancer patients should undergo axillary surgery for staging and/or treatment purposes [A].[3,4] Axillary imaging has become a common practice in many cancer centres prior to commencing axillary surgery.[41] Axillary surgery can take one or more of the following types of procedures:
    - Sentinel lymph node biopsy (SLNB)—(a preferable option) is performed by selectively removing the first draining node/s following appropriate radio colloid mapping/Methylene blue labelling.
    - Axillary node sampling (ANS).
    - Axillary node clearance (ANC)—provided there is a definitive evidence of lymph node involvement. Macro- or micrometastases found following SLNB requires proceeding to ANC. Patients with isolated tumour cells in the lymph nodes can be treated as lymph node negative.[41]

Table 48.6 Management of LCIS

- Optimal management is controversial. A policy of close surveillance (regular physical examination and annual or biennial mammography) is safe and acceptable [C].[2,4,27]
- LCIS found coincidentally in biopsy for other lesions does not require further excision (even if margins contain LCIS).[2,28,29]
- Prophylactic tamoxifen or raloxifene reduces the risk of invasive cancer by 38%. Its use should follow locally agreed protocols.[30]
- Prophylactic bilateral mastectomy is an option in individual cases, but is not generally recommended.

Table 48.7 Management of DCIS

- *Surgical resection is recommended.* In general terms, mastectomy should be considered for DCIS >4cm or multifocal disease. Otherwise, wide local excision with appropriate free margins.
- Decisions should be based on the lesion/breast size ratio, pathological features of DCIS, age, fitness to surgery or radiotherapy, and patient preferences.[1,2,6] Tamoxifen not advised for those who have had breast-conserving surgery.[41]
- Axillary surgery is not required.[1]
- Radiotherapy may be necessary.[1]

Table 48.8 Management of early stage breast cancer—BCS benefits, risks, and contraindications

- *Benefits and risks of BCS*—10y outcome (cancer-related death, local and regional recurrence) is similar to that for mastectomy,[32] good, long-term local control, and very acceptable cosmetic results (compared to mastectomy). BCS requires radiotherapy to reduce the possibility of recurrence in the breast. Radiation-related side effects are a possibility. BCS may also require further surgery to clear margins.
- *Contraindications*—include mismatched tumour size to breast size (e.g. 4cm cancer can be treated with BCS in a large breast, and 3cm cancer requires mastectomy in a small breast), multifocal lesion or extensive microcalcifications on mammography, and inability to tolerate radiotherapy [C].[4]

Breast reconstruction
- Should be discussed and offered (preferably during the initial operation) to all patients undergoing mastectomy [C].[2,3,4]

Surgical treatment of locoregional recurrence
- Depends on the type of primary surgery and should be managed within the multidisciplinary setting.[2]
  - *Recurrence in previously conservatively managed breast*—requires mastectomy (or conservative re-excision if safe and appropriate) and re-staging to exclude distant metastasis.
  - *Recurrence in mastectomy patients*—should be managed with excision of recurrence (in solitary, confined, recurrent tumour) or as per the MDT decision.
  - *Recurrence in regional lymph nodes*—should be managed with completion of axillary clearance or radiotherapy following local MDT recommendations.

Adjuvant systemic therapy
- ***Adjuvant! Online***—has been used widely by many MDT teams and centres to guide discussions and decision-making.[41]
- ***Radiotherapy***—40Gy in 15 fractions can significantly reduce the risk of local or regional recurrence following breast conservative surgery (RR × 3.3) and selected cases of mastectomy, and is a recommended practice following MDT discussion [A].[4,41] Post-mastectomy radiotherapy to chest wall is also indicated if the cancer's features are deemed high risk of recurrence, including those with 4 or more involved lymph nodes.[41] Those with fewer lymph nodes involved should be entered into the SUPREMO trial.[41] Radiotherapy to the nodal areas are indicated only if axillary node dissection is not possible or incomplete and to supraclavicular nodes if heavy lymph node involvement.[41]
- ***Adjuvant chemotherapy***—should be based on a sound risk-benefit judgement [A].[4] It should start within 6wk of surgery. Docetaxel, and not paclitaxel, offered to node-positive patients with early breast cancer.[41]
- ***Neoadjuvant chemotherapy***—should be offered for large, but early, breast cancers if the patient's preference is for breast-conserving surgery [A].[4,41]
- ***Endocrine therapy***—is indicated for oestrogen-positive cancers. Tamoxifen is suitable for pre-menopausal women. Aromatase inhibitors (AI) are suitable for post-menopausal women, especially if tamoxifen has relative contraindications (e.g. high risk of thromboembolism).[41] Patients starting on an AI should have baseline DEXA assessment of bone mineral density.[41]
- Post-menopausal ER-positive patients not considered low risk should have initial adjuvant treatment with an AI (exemestane or anastrozole). Those on tamoxifen for 2–3y and those treated for 5y should be considered for transfer to letrozole.[41]
- ***Biological therapy***—trastuzumab (Herceptin®) should be given 3-weekly for 1y or until disease recurrence as adjuvant treatment for HER-2-positive patients following surgery, chemotherapy, or radiotherapy when appropriate. Requires cardiac function assessment pre-treatment and 3-monthly during treatment.[41]

Follow-up

- Patients to have a written care plan with a copy to the GP. The need for clinical follow-up is debated, but the patient with early breast cancer should, after completion of radiotherapy and systemic adjuvant therapies, be given the options, and this includes primary, secondary, or shared care.[4,41]
- *Annual mammography*—until a minimum age of 70 and this includes those treated for DCIS.[41]
- *Lymphoedema*—patients must have access to specialized support.
- *Menopausal symptoms*—selective serotonin uptake inhibitors (paroxetine, fluoxetine) are useful for patients with hot flushes, but not if they are on tamoxifen. Clonidine, venlafaxine, and gabapentin should only be used if the patients understand the side effects.[41]

Management of advanced disease[41]

- Careful assessment of each individual patient's needs and circumstances, and close integration with the different clinicians involved in the management to avoid mixed messages.
- *Hormone therapy*—If ER-positive, the first-line therapy is hormone treatment unless life-threatening in which case chemotherapy followed with hormone therapy. Offer ovarian suppression to pre- and perimenopausal patients who have previously been treated with tamoxifen. Treat male ER-positive patients with tamoxifen.
- *Chemotherapy*—use sequential single agent chemotherapy in the majority of patients, starting with anthracyclines, progressing to docetaxel as a single agent, second-line vinorelbine, or capecitabine, thirdly vinorelbine or capecitabine depending on what was used previously. Gemcitabine with paclitaxel have been used and paclitaxel in combination with trastuzumab can be offered to HER-2-positive patients scoring 3+.
- *Bone secondaries*—offer bisphosphonates to patients with bone secondaries and localized radiotherapy 8Gy to painful bone secondaries. Orthopaedic surgeons should be involved if there is a risk of long bone fracture.
- *Brain secondaries*—surgery in rare circumstances. Whole brain radiotherapy more often indicated.

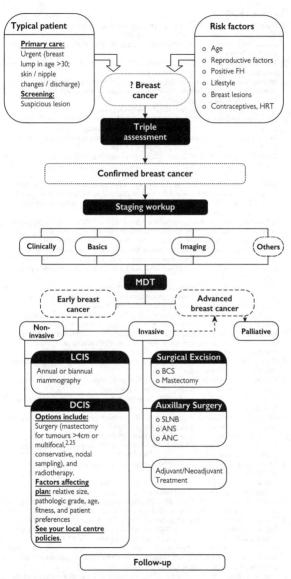

Fig. 48.1 Recommended approach to patients with breast cancer

Further reading

1. Cancer Research UK (2008). Breast cancer at a glance. Available from: http://info. cancerresearchuk.org/cancerandresearch/cancers/breast/.
2. Association of Breast Surgery (2005). Surgical guidelines for the management of breast cancer. *Eur J Surg Oncol* 35 (Suppl 1), 1–22.
3. Scottish Intercollegiate Guidelines Network (2005). Management of breast cancer in women. Available from: http://www.sign.ac.uk/pdf/sign84.pdf.
4. National Institute for Health and Clinical Excellence (2002). Improving outcomes in breast cancer—manual update. Available from: http://www.nice.org.uk/nicemedia/pdf/Improving_ outcomes_breastcancer_manual.pdf.
5. Breast Cancer Care. Available from: http://www.breastcancercare.org.uk/.
6. BMJ Clinical Evidence. Breast Cancer. 2008. Available from: http://www.clinical evidence.bmj.com/ceweb/conditions/woh/0102/0102.jsp. Accessed May 2009.
7. Kelsey JL, Fischer DB, Holford TR et al. (1981). Exogenous oestrogens and other factors in the epidemiology of breast cancer. *J Natl Cancer Inst* 67, 327–33.
8. Clavel-Chapelon F; E3N–EPICGroup (2002). Differential effects of reproductive factors on the risk of pre- and postmenopausal breast cancer. Results from a large cohort of French women. *Br J Cancer* 86, 723–7.
9. Ewertz M, Duffy SW, Adami HO et al. (1990). Age at first birth, parity and risk of breast cancer: a meta-analysis of 8 studies from the Nordic countries. *Int J Cancer* 46, 597–603.
10. Chen Y, Thompson W, Semenciw R, Mao Y (1999). Epidemiology of contralateral breast cancer. *Cancer Epidemiol Biomarkers Prev* 8, 855–61.
11. Collaborative Group on Hormonal Factors in Breast Cancer (2001). Familial breast cancer: collaborative reanalysis of individual data from 52 epidemiological studies including 58,209 women with breast cancer and 101,986 women without the disease. *Lancet* 358, 1389–99.
12. Collaborative Group on Hormonal Factors in Breast Cancer (1996). Breast cancer and hormonal contraceptives: collaborative reanalysis of individual data on 53,297 women with breast cancer and 100,239 women without breast cancer from 54 epidemiological studies. *Lancet* 347, 1713–27.
13. Key T, Appleby P, Barnes I, Reeves G; Endogenous Hormones and Breast Cancer Collaborative Group (2002). Endogenous sex hormones and breast cancer in postmenopausal women: reanalysis of nine prospective studies. *J Natl Cancer Inst* 94, 606–16.
14. Van den Brandt PA, Spiegelman D, Yaun SS (2000). Pooled analysis of prospective cohort studies on height, weight, and breast cancer risk. *Am J Epidemiol* 152, 514–27.
15. Hamajima N, Hirose K, Tajima K (2002). Alcohol, tobacco and breast cancer—collaborative reanalysis of individual data from 53 epidemiological studies, including 58,515 women with breast cancer and 95,067 women without the disease. *Br J Cancer* 87, 1234–45.
16. Greenall MJ, Wood WC (2001). Cancer of the breast. In: *Oxford Textbook of Surgery*, 2nd ed. Oxford University Press, Oxford.
17. Morrow M , Khan S (2006). Breast disease. In: *Greenfield's surgery: scientific principles and practice*, 2nd ed, Lippincott Williams & Wilkins, Philadelphia.
18. Querci della Rovere G, Warren R (2001). Detection of breast cancer. Mammography should be available. *BMJ* 322, 792–3.
19. Mittra I, Baum M, Thornton M, Houghton J (2000). Is clinical breast examination an acceptable alternative to mammographic screening? *BMJ* 321, 1071–3.
20. Smart CR, Hartmann WH, Beahrs OH, Garfinkel L (1993). Insights into breast cancer screening of younger women. Evidence from the 14-year follow-up of the Breast Cancer Detection Demonstration Project. *Cancer* 72, 1449–56.
21. The Royal College of Radiologists (1990). Quality assurance guidelines for radiologists. NHSBSP Publications, Oxford.
22. Flobbe K, Bosch AM, Kessels AG et al. (2003). The additional diagnostic value of ultrasonography in the diagnosis of breast cancer. *Arch Intern Med* 163, 1194–9.
23. Soo MS, Rosen EL, Baker JA, Vo TT, Boyd BA (2001). Negative predictive value of sonography with mammography in patients with palpable breast lesions. *AJR Am J Roentgenol* 177, 1167–70.
24. Tilanus-Linthorst MM, Obdeijn IM, Bartels KC (2005). MARIBS study. *Lancet* 365, 1769–78.
25. Saslow D, Boetes C, Burke W et al. (2007). American Cancer Society guidelines for breast screening with MRI as an adjunct to mammography. *CA Cancer J Clin* 57, 75–89.
26. Fisher ER, Land SR, Fisher B, Mamounas E, Gilarski L, Wolmark N (2004). Pathologic findings from the National Surgical Adjuvant Breast and Bowel Project: twelve-year observations concerning lobular carcinoma in situ. *Cancer* 100, 238–44.
27. Bradley SJ, Weaver DW, Bouwman DL (1990). Alternatives in the surgical management of *in situ* breast cancer. A meta-analysis of outcome. *Am Surg* 56, 428–32.

28. Abner AL, Connolly JL, Recht A et al. (2000). The relation between the presence and extent of lobular carcinoma *in situ* and the risk of local recurrence for patients with infiltrating carcinoma of the breast treated with conservative surgery and radiation therapy. *Cancer* 88, 1072–7.

29. Stolier AJ, Barre G, Bolton JS, Fuhrman GM, Looney S (2004). Breast conservation therapy for invasive lobular carcinoma: the impact of lobular carcinoma *in situ* in the surgical specimen on local recurrence and axillary node status. *Am Surg* 70, 818–21.

30. Cuzick J, Powles T, Veronesi U et al. (2003). Overview of the main outcomes in breast-cancer prevention trials. *Lancet* 361, 296–300.

31. Gump FE (1990). Lobular carcinoma *in situ*. Pathology and treatment. *Surg Clin North Am* 70, 873–83.

32. Morris A D, Morris RD, Wilson JF et al. (1997). Breast-conserving therapy vs mastectomy in early-stage breast cancer: a meta-analysis of 10-year survival. *Cancer J Sci Am* 3, 6–12.

33. Al-Ghazal SK, Blamey RW (1999). Cosmetic assessment of breast-conserving surgery for primary breast cancer. *Breast* 8, 162–8.

34. Wazer DE, DiPetrillo T, Schmidt–Ullrich R, Weld L et al. (1992). Factors influencing cosmetic outcome and complication risk after conservative surgery and radiotherapy for early-stage breast carcinoma. *J Clin Oncol* 10, 356–63.

35. Liljegren G, Holmberg L, Westman G (1993). The cosmetic outcome in early breast cancer treated with sector resection with or without radiotherapy. Uppsala–Orebro Breast Cancer Study Group. *Eur J Cancer* 29A, 2083–9.

36. Eltahir A, Jibril JA, Squair J et al. (1999). The accuracy of 'one-stop' diagnosis for 1,110 patients presenting to a symptomatic breast clinic. *J R Coll Surg Edinb* 44, 226–30.

37. Costantini M, Belli P, Lombardi R, Franceschini G, Mulè A, Bonomo L (2006). Characterization of solid breast masses: use of the sonographic breast imaging reporting and data system lexicon. *J Ultrasound Med* 25, 649–59.

38. The Royal College of Radiologists' Clinical Oncology Information Network (1999). Guidelines on the non-surgical management of breast cancer. *Clin Oncol (R Coll Radiol)* 11, S90–133.

39. Peters NH, Borel Rinkes IH, Zuithoff NP, Mali WP, Moons KG, Peeters PH (2008). Meta-analysis of MR imaging in the diagnosis of breast lesions. *Radiology* 246, 116–24.

40. Ljung BM, Drejet A, Chiampi N et al. (2001). Diagnostic accuracy of fine-needle aspiration biopsy is determined by physician training in sampling technique. *Cancer* 93, 263–8.

41. National Institute for Health and Clinical Excellence (2009). Breast cancer (early and locally advanced): diagnosis and treatment. Available from: http://www.nice.org.uk/guidance/CG80.

Benign breast diseases

Benign breast diseases

Key guidelines

- Association of Breast Surgery @ BASO, Royal College of Surgeons of England (2005). Guidelines for the management of symptomatic breast disease.
- Vaidyanathan L, Barnard K, Elnicki DM (2002). Benign breast disease: when to treat, when to reassure, when to refer.
- American Society of Breast Surgeons.
- Review: benign breast diseases. (US)
- Santen RJ, Mansel R (2005). Benign breast disorders.
- BMJ Clinical Evidence. 2008.
- University of Michigan Health System (2007). Common breast problems.

Fibroadenoma

Basic facts

- *Incidence*—the most common benign lesion affecting women younger than 30. Fibroadenomas are found in 2–23% of women in their mid-20s.[4]
- *Pathogenesis*—abnormal excessive response of lobules and stroma of the breast to hormonal stimuli, with the resultant development of a single or multiple, palpable, rubbery, encapsulated mass lesions. Underlying and acquired genetic changes may have a role, including the possible loss of heterozygosity as a result of deletions of small segments of DNA.[4]
- *Clinical presentation*—well-defined, extremely mobile, solitary or multiple breast lumps. May increase in size during pregnancy or with oestrogen therapy, and regress after menopause.

Recommended approach

- *In general*—the approach should typically follow the triple assessment approach [B].[1,2] This applies especially to women over the age of 35 with dominant lumps.[4]
- *Natural history*—spontaneous resolution (or decrease in size) in ~35% of patients, persistent size with minimal changes in ~50%, and growing in size in ~10% within 2y of follow-up.[8]
- *Risk of cancer*—related to the histologic type of fibroadenomas and the presence of a family history of breast cancer.[4,7,8]
  - *Simple fibroadenoma with negative family history*—is unlikely to increase the risk of cancer (based on follow-up data for >25y).
  - *Complex fibroadenomas with proliferative changes.*
  - *Type of lesions*—fibroadenomas with cysts >3mm, sclerosing adenosis, epithelial calcifications, or papillary apocrine changes.
  - *Risk of cancer*—small but definite increased risk (estimated RR 1.5–2.0).[4] The presence of atypia increases the relative risk to 3.0.
  - *Positive family history*—increases the risk of subsequent breast cancer, even in the non-proliferative cases. The estimated RR is 1.6.

Treatment options

- **General approach**—surgical excision of small, simple fibroadenomas is not required on an oncological basis because of the extremely low malignancy potential. Disadvantages of surgical excision include the incision site scar, dimpling of breast, damaging the breast's ductal system, and inducing mammographical changes (increased focal density, architectural distortion, skin thickening) that might interfere with the detection of cancer in the future.
- **Indications for surgery**—lesions that are large enough to cause physical deformity, discomfort, or significant emotional distress to patients.
- **Conservative management**—safe and acceptable. Patients are followed up as appropriate. Repeated ultrasonography is required if no histological confirmation has been performed during the 'triple' assessment.
- **Newer methods of management.**
  - Ultrasound-guided percutaneous excision with a vacuum-assisted core biopsy device.
  - Cryoablation.

Fibrocystic breast change

- **Definition**—increased exhibition of cysts or fibrous tissue in an otherwise normal breast. Considered as normal phase of the spectrum of histologic features of normal breast. Fibrocystic disease is a term used when fibrocystic changes are associated with pain, lumpiness, or nipple discharge.
- **Incidence**—presents in up to 50–60% of healthy women.[4]
- **Pathogenesis**—results from an abnormal excessive response of lobules and stroma of the breast to hormonal stimuli, with consequent blockage or dilatation of ducts. The stromal oedema, ductal dilatation, and associated inflammation may result in breast pain. Underlying and acquired genetic changes may also be involved.[4]
- **Clinical presentation**—varies between different age groups. The most common type in women in their 20s is hyperplasia, characterized by upper outer quadrant and axillary tail induration and pain. Women in their 30s are commonly affected by adenosis, characterized by the development of multiple breast nodules 2–10mm in size. Women in their 30s and 40s present usually with solitary or multiple cysts, commonly associated with green to brownish nipple discharge.
- **Diagnosis**—should typically follow the triple assessment approach [B].[1,3] This applies especially to women over the age of 35 with dominant lumps.[4]
- **Natural history**—spontaneous resolution in about two thirds of patients within 2y or no regression in ~12% within five years' time.[4,7,8]
- **Risk of cancer**—related to the histologic type associated with fibrocystic changes. Non-proliferative changes have slightly increased risk of cancer (RR × 1.27). The risk is more significant in lesions with proliferative changes with or without atypia (RR of 4.24 and 1.88, respectively). Family history is an independent risk factor. A positive family history increases the relative risk to about 1.5.[7]
- **Treatment options**—usually aimed at relieving the pain and reassuring the patient following triple assessment.

- *Simple reassurance*—that there is no evidence of cancer can provide adequate relief for ~85% of patients.
- *Diet and lifestyle changes*—have not been clearly demonstrated to provide significant symptom relief.
  - *Low-fat (15% calories), high-carbohydrate diet*—may reduce the severity of self-reported premenstrual breast swelling and tenderness at 6mo when compared with general diet.
  - *Caffeine reduction*—have long been recommended, but the evidence is weak to support any association with fibrocystic disease. Caffeine reduction cannot be recommended as a treatment or preventative measure according to currently available evidence.[5] Nevertheless, placebo effect might result in pain relief in some patients.
  - *Smoking cessation*—may be associated with improved symptoms, although this may also result from placebo effect. Smoking cessation is generally recommended for other health benefits.
  - *Vitamin E*—no evidence to suggest any significant effect on improving breast pain.[5]
  - *Evening primrose oil (EPO)*—has no significant effect in reducing the severity or frequency of pain compared to placebo at 6mo (average 12–15% reduction in pain for EPO and placebo). The Committee for Safety of Medicines in the UK has withdrawn the prescription licence from EPO due to the lack of efficacy, but EPO is still available to purchase over the counter.
- *Medical management.*
  - *Topical NSAIDs*—effective therapy in relieving breast pain (general expert consensus).[5] Topical NSAIDs can reduce the pain by 6 scores on average (measured on visual analogue scale from 0 = no pain to 10 = intolerable pain) compared to placebo (average reduction of pain is 1.2).[5] No adverse effects have been noticed with topical NSAIDs usage.
  - *Diuretics*—no evidence on any beneficial effect in women with breast pain and are not indicated or licensed for this purpose.
  - *Danazol*—androgenic steroid and has significant effect in achieving a 50% reduction in breast pain after 6mo of therapy. Possible side effects include weight gain, menorrhagia, deepening of voice, and muscle cramps. Reducing the dose of danazol to 100mg daily after achieving a good symptomatic relief and restricting treatment to 2wk preceding menstruation can significantly reduce the risk of significant side effects.
  - *Tamoxifen*—can reduce breast pain in over 50% of women with severe mastalgia over 3–6mo.[5] Tamoxifen dose of 10mg provides equivalent breast pain relief compared to 20mg. Possible serious side effects include venous thromboembolism. Tamoxifen is not currently licensed for general physicians to treat breast pain in the UK or US. Its use is restricted to supervised cases for no more than 6mo at a time.
  - *Other medications*—Simple pain killers, toremifene, gestrinone, and gonadorelin analogues may reduce the breast pain.
  - *Other options*—Pain management strategies, eg. hyprotherapy and acupuncture.

Further reading

1. Association of Breast Surgery @ BASO, Royal College of Surgeons of England (2005). Guidelines for the management of symptomatic breast disease. *Eur J Surg Oncol* 31 (Suppl 1), 1–21.
2. Vaidyanathan L, Barnard K, Elnicki DM (2002). Benign breast disease: when to treat, when to reassure, when to refer. *Cleve Clin J Med* 69, 425–32.
3. American Society of Breast Surgeons. Available from: http://breastsurgeons.org/statements/Management_of_Fibroadenomas_of_the_Breast_4-29-08.pdf. Accessed May 2009
4. Santen RJ, Mansel R (2005). Benign breast disorders. *N Engl J Med* 353, 275–85.
5. BMJ ClinicalEvidence. 2008. Available from: http://clinicalevidence.bmj.com/ceweb/conditions/woh/0812.jsp. Accessed May 2009.
6. University of Michigan Health System (2007). Common breast problems. Guidelines. (US) Available from: http://www.guidelines.gov/summary/summary.aspx?doc_id=12015&nbr=006199&string=breast+AND+pain. Accessed May 2009.
7. Hartmann LC, Sellers TA, Frost MH et al. (2005). Benign breast disease and the risk of breast cancer. *N Engl J Med* 353, 229–37.
8. Dixon JM (1991). Cystic disease and fibroadenoma of the breast: natural history and relation to breast cancer risk. *Br Med Bull* 47, 258–71.

Endocrine

Thyroid nodules and cancer*

* The guidelines on this chapter have been sourced and summarized from different
UK, Europe, and international government sources, professional organizations, and
medical specialty societies. Leading guidelines have been listed in the Key guidelines box.

Thyroid nodules

Key guidelines

- British Association of Endocrine Surgeons (2003). Guidelines for the surgical management of endocrine disease.
- British Thyroid Association (2006). UK guidelines for the use of thyroid function tests.
- American Association of Clinical Endocrinologists and Associazione Medici Endocrinologi (2006). Medical guidelines for clinical practice for the diagnosis and management of thyroid nodules.
- European Thyroid Association.

Basic facts

- *Incidence*—very common. Clinically apparent thyroid nodules present in ~3–7% of women (<1% of men).[8] True prevalence on ultrasound surveys or autopsy studies range from 37% to 57% of the population.[8,9]
- *Risks of malignancy*—about 5% of all thyroid nodules, independent of their size.
- *Histologic classification*—four main types (Table 50.1).
- *Clinical presentation*—often discovered incidentally by patient, examining physician, or through imaging tests performed for other reasons. The absence of symptoms does not rule out the presence of malignancy [C].[3] Clinical history should include the onset and rate of growth, the presence of any compression symptoms (e.g. dysphagia, hoarseness), and any relevant medical or family history.
  - *Past medical history*—any previous disease or therapy involving the neck (history of head and neck irradiation during childhood), and any recent pregnancy.[3]
  - *Family history*—the presence of benign or malignant thyroid diseases, familial adenomatous polyposis, Gardner's syndrome, and Cowden's disease.
  - *ALARM factors*—Table 50.2.

Recommended investigations

- *Blood tests*—all patients with thyroid nodule should have measurement of serum TSH concentration, using third generation high sensitive assay techniques, if available [B].[1,3]
  - Free thyroxine (T4) and free triiodothyronine (T3) should be measured if the TSH level is low (<0.5μIU/mL) [C].[1,3]
  - Free T4 and thyroid peroxidase antibody (TPOAb) should be measured if the TSH level is high (>5.0μIU/mL) [C].[1,3]
  - There is no indication for routine measurement of thyroglobulin and no clear benefits of measuring serum calcitonin without any evidence of medullary thyroid cancer (MTC) on FNA or relevant family history [C].[3]
- *FNA*—safe, reliable and simple 'office' procedure (Table 50.3). FNA is recommended in the UK and Europe for all patients with solitary thyroid nodule or dominant nodule in multinodular goitre.[1,4] FNA is performed in the US based on the results of thyroid USS [B].[3]

Table 50.1 Histologic classification of thyroid nodules

- **Simple, non-proliferative nodules**—colloid, simple, or haemorrhagic. Cystic lesions account for 20% of thyroid nodules.[7]
- **Adenomas**—colloid adenomas, multinodular goitre, and follicular adenomas.
- **Thyroiditis-related nodules**—Hashimoto's thyroiditis.
- **Malignant nodules**—papillary, follicular, medullary, anaplastic, lymphoma, and metastatic.

Table 50.2 ALARM factors in thyroid nodules

- Any previous history of head and neck irradiation.
- Family history of thyroid cancer (MTC or MEN type 2).
- Patients younger than 20 (×2 risk) or older than 70, males (×2 risk).
- Suspicious nodule features—growing nodule with firm or hard consistency and fixed nodules.
- Any signs of invasion—cervical adenopathy, persistent hoarseness, dysphagia, and dyspnoea.

Table 50.3 Fine needle aspiration

- **Technique**—with the patient supine, a 23–27G needle is inserted into the nodule without applying suction. Once in the nodule, suction is applied and the needle is moved within the nodule. In a few seconds, the aspirate appears in the needle hub, suction is released, and the needle withdrawn. The smears should be prepared by filling the syringe (after removing the needle) with air, attaching the needle, and placing the material onto multiple slides.
- **Accuracy**—sensitivity, specificity, and positive predictive value of FNA are excellent when performed by an experienced person (83, 92, and 75%, respectively).[3] False negative rate (patients with negative FNA whose nodule have malignant or microfollicular histology) is ~5%. False positive rate (patient with FNA showing malignant, suspicious, or indeterminate cytology, who has a benign macrofollicular adenoma) is ~5%.[3] Follicular cytology cannot usually distinguish between adenoma and carcinoma as diagnosis depends on capsule invasion.
- **Results**—most (70%) are benign (negative), 5% are malignant (positive), 10% are suspicious (indeterminate), and 10–20% are non-diagnostic (unsatisfactory).[3]
- **Side effects**—can cause slight discomfort and minor haematoma. No significant side effect or seeding effect has been reported.

- *USS*—indicated in the UK and Europe for selected patients with atypical solitary thyroid nodule, multinodular goitre, or as part of the evaluation of neck lymphadenopathy.[1,4] Recommended in the US in all palpable thyroid nodules and multinodular goitres [C].[3]
  - *Other indications*—include high-risk patients (positive family history, MEN type 2, and external radiation) and patients with suspicious adenopathy in the neck region. USS is not indicated as a screening tool for the general population [C].[3]
  - *Findings and accuracy*—see Table 50.4.
- *Radionuclide scanning*—indicated in patients with TSH level below the lower limits of the normal range (thyrotoxic). Thyroid FNA is not indicated in such cases [B].[1,3] Also indicated in exploring suspected ectopic thyroid tissue, suspected retrosternal goitre, and in iodine-deficient areas (US recommendations) [B, C].[3]
- *Other diagnostic tests*—CT scan, MRI, laryngoscopy, and CXR.[1]

Recommended management

- *FNA-positive or suspicious thyroid nodules (papillary, medullary or follicular carcinoma)*—surgical resection is recommended (see thyroid cancer below) [B].[1,3]
- *FNA-negative 'benign' nodule/s.*
  - *Conservative management (wait and watch)*—if no other indications for surgical resection exist.[1,3]
    - *Thyroid cysts*—may be cured by aspiration to dryness.[3,7] Recurrence is common, and may require surgical resection[7] or consideration of percutaneous ethanol injection (PEI) if experience is available [B].[3] PEI has a low recurrence rate (2–5% over 1y) and can avoid surgical resection where malignancy has been excluded.[3]
    - *Levothyroxine (LT4) suppression therapy*—is not indicated in most cases although the issue remains controversial.[3,7] LT4 therapy has a clear beneficial effect in iodine deficiency areas (effective reduction of nodule volume),[3] young people diagnosed with 'benign' small thyroid nodule, and in non-functioning nodular goitres [C].[3] Long-term use is usually required [B], and accurate monitoring to ensure incomplete suppression of thyroid function is essential [C].[3]
  - *Surgical resection* is indicated in certain cases (Table 50.5).[1,3]
    - *Post-operative follow-up.*[1]
    - *Calcium check*—within the first 24h of surgery and subsequently if required.
    - *Calcium replacement*—consider if corrected calcium falls below 2mmol/L (IV calcium gluconate if below 1.8mmol/L) or if the patient is symptomatic. Ensure that calcium levels are stable without IV calcium before discharge.

Table 50.4 Thyroid USS—findings and accuracy

- *Findings*—suspicious features of a thyroid nodule include hypoechoic nodules over 10mm with irregular margins, chaotic intranodular vascular spots, a shape that is 'more tall than wide', and microcalcifications. The suggestion of extracapsular growth or metastatic lymph nodes requires immediate cytological evaluation [B].[3]

- *Accuracy*—the presence of more than one feature of malignancy on USS increases the diagnostic accuracy to ~90%.[3] USS can detect other small nodules in over 50% of patients with a clinical 'solitary' thyroid nodule. Histologic sampling should be performed on suspicious lesions, which might not be the largest or most clinically dominant nodule [C].[3]

Table 50.5 Surgical resection for 'benign' thyroid nodule[1,3]

- *Indications.*
  - Clinical suspicion of malignancy.
  - Associated pressure signs or symptoms.
  - Cosmetic, discomfort, or anxiety reasons.
  - Growth of nodule/s, especially in retrosternal goitres.

- *Recommended approach.*
  - Solitary benign nodule—lobectomy and/or isthmusectomy.
  - Bilateral nodules/multinodular goitre—total/near total thyroidectomy.

- *Post-operative complications*—permanent hypoparathyroidism or recurrent laryngeal nerve injury should not exceed 1%.[2]

- *Intra-operative nerve monitoring during thyroid surgery (IONM)*—is used as an adjunct to conventional thyroid surgery by placing electrodes close to the vocal cords.[10] The procedure has no major safety issues, and is more efficient when used in thyroid re-operation and in operating on giant thyroid nodules.[10]

Table 50.6 Radioiodine for 'benign' thyroid nodule

- *Indications.*
  - Small hyperactive goitres (<100mL) or autonomous nodules.
  - High risk for surgery.

- *Not recommended.*
  - Compressive symptoms.
  - Large nodules that require high dose of radiation.
  - Immediate resolution of thyrotoxicosis is required.

- *T4 replacement*—should commence prior to being discharged from hospital for all total/near total thyroidectomies.
- *TSH levels*—should be checked at follow-up.
- *Radioiodine therapy for benign disease*—is indicated as in Table 50.6.

Further reading

1. British Association of Endocrine Surgeons (2003). Guidelines for the surgical management of endocrine disease. Available from: http://www.baes.info/Pages/BAETS%20Guidelines.pdf.
2. British Thyroid Association (2006). UK guidelines for the use of thyroid function tests. Available from: http://www.british-thyroid-association.org/info-for-patients/Docs/TFT_guideline_final_version_July_2006.pdf.
3. Gharib H, Papini E, Valcavi R et al. (2006). American Association of Clinical Endocrinologists and Associazione Medici Endocrinologi medical guidelines for clinical practice for the diagnosis and management of thyroid nodules. *Endocr Pract* 12, 63–102.
4. European Thyroid Association. http://www.hotthyroidology.com/ebook/file_info/download1.php?file=_ebook_ht_2008-2009.pdf. Accessed May 2009.
5. Hegedüs L (2004). Clinical practice. The thyroid nodule. *N Engl J Med* 351, 1764–71.
6. Anderson CE, McLaren KM (2003). Best practice in thyroid pathology. *J Clin Pathol* 56, 401–5.
7. Jones MK (2001). Management of nodular thyroid disease. The challenge remains identifying which palpable nodules are malignant. *BMJ* 323, 293–4.
8. Wass J, Shalet S, eds (2002). *Oxford Textbook of Endocrinology and Diabetes*. Oxford University Press, Oxford.
9. Reiners C, Wegscheider K, Schicha H et al. Prevalence of thyroid disorders in the working population of Germany: ultrasonography screening in 96,278 unselected employees. *Thyroid* 14, 926–32.
10. National Institute for Health and Clinical Excellence (2008). Intraoperative nerve monitoring during thyroid surgery. Available from: http://www.nice.org.uk/nicemedia/pdf/IPG255Guidance.pdf.

Thyroid cancer

Key guidelines

- British Association of Endocrine Surgeons (2003). Guidelines for the surgical management of endocrine disease.
- British Thyroid Association (2006). UK guidelines for the use of thyroid function tests.
- American Association of Clinical Endocrinologists and Associazione Medici Endocrinologi (2006). Medical guidelines for clinical practice for the diagnosis and management of thyroid nodules.
- European Thyroid Association.

Basic facts

- *Incidence*—uncommon (top 20 most common cancers for females in the UK). Affects ~2.5 per 100,000 females and 1.4 per 100,000 males. The male to female ratio is 1:3. Incidence has been rising slightly in the UK for females.[9]
- Worldwide incidence varies considerably. The highest incidence in Europe was reported in Malta (7 times the lowest ranking EU country) and highest rates in the world occur in Northern America (~8 per 100,000 females).[9]

Differentiated thyroid cancer

- *Types*—papillary and follicular thyroid cancers. Biologically different cancers, but often treated similarly.
- *Diagnosis*—may be made preoperatively (suspicious thyroid nodule), intra-operatively (frozen section), or post-operatively (definitive histology).
- *Preoperative staging*—thyroid function tests, CXR, and laryngoscopy are recommended prior to surgery.[1] Staging scintigraphy is not a recommended practice in the UK prior to the first operation.[1] Evaluation of level 2, 3, and 4 lymph nodes using USS is recommended for all thyroid cancer patients in the US [D].[3] CT or MRI scans are indicated in patients with extensive or recurrent disease.[1]
- *Surgery*—is indicated in almost all cases [B].[3]
  - *Total lobectomy*—is safe and appropriate in early thyroid cancers (cancers <1cm in diameter, no evidence of lymph node involvement (clinically or on USS), no evidence of diseased contralateral lobe, and no distant metastasis).[1,3]
  - *Total or near total thyroidectomy*—is recommended for more advanced cancers (tumours >1cm, multifocal, familial thyroid cancer, tumour capsular invasion, and/or involved lymph nodes (clinically or on USS), Hurthle cell tumours).[1,3]
  - *Lymph nodes*—central compartment lymph node (level 6) dissection is recommended for all grossly involved lymph nodes (or routinely as per the American Thyroid Association guidelines).[3,11] All suspicious lymph nodes (clinically or on USS) should be removed and sent for histology.[1,3] Modified or radical lymph node dissection can be considered (but not in all cases)[1] in the presence of histologically confirmed regional metastatic cancer following multidisciplinary meeting discussion.[1,3]

- Post-operative management—as for benign lesions except that:
  - *Triiodothyronine 20µg tds*—should be commenced post-operatively because of its short half-life prior to a pre-ablation scan if the patient has had a total thyroidectomy. Any residual thyroid tissue is destroyed by radioiodine (see adjuvant treatment). Long-term TSH suppression using T4 is recommended for thyroid cancers[1]
  - *Surveillance*—to check for TSH suppression and thyroglobulin estimation is recommended for frankly invasive lesions.[1] Note that thyroglobulin is not of value as a preoperative test as it is produced by normal as well as malignant tissue but is an important monitoring tool after a total thyroidectomy
- *Staging*—using the TNM pathological classification is recommended.[1]
- *Adjuvant therapy*—using radioiodine ablation is recommended for the ablation of residual thyroid tissue and treatment of residual or metastatic thyroid cancer. External beam radiotherapy may be indicated in certain cases (metastatic cancers refractory to radioiodine).
- *Recurrent disease*—should be considered for further surgery, radioiodine, or external radiotherapy.[1]
- *Prognosis*—the overall 5y survival rates in England and Wales, corrected for age and sex, is ~80%, being best in younger ages (~98% survival rate for patients younger than 40) and worst in the elderly (~45% at the age of 70–79).[12]

Anaplastic thyroid cancer

- *Diagnosis*—additional diagnostic tests include immunocytochemistry (to differentiate from other types of cancers) and CT/MRI scan for all patients.[1]
- *Treatment*—usually palliative. External radiotherapy may be helpful for symptom relief. Limited resection may occasionally be considered to relieve compression signs and for tumour size over 5cm.[1]
- *Prognosis*—very poor (85% mortality rate in 1y).[1]

Medullary thyroid cancer

- *Incidence*—rare. Occurs as sporadic cancer or as part of familial predisposition (sporadic familial or MEN type 2a or 2b).[1]
- *Diagnosis*—additional diagnostic investigations include a detailed thorough history and appropriate tests to exclude phaeochromocytoma. Other additional investigations include USS for all patients (or CT/MRI), basal calcitonin levels, and genetic screening in suspected familial cases.[1]
- *Treatment*—total thyroidectomy and central compartment (tracheal and paratracheal) lymphadenectomy are recommended for all patients.[1] Neck dissection and hyperparathyroidism should be planned and treated during the first operation based on preoperative investigations. Prophylactic thyroidectomy has a role in familial cases.[1]
- *Prognosis*—the 5y and 10y disease-free survival rates range from 75–95% and 50–65%, respectively.[12]

Thyroid lymphoma
- *Type*—almost always non-Hodgkin's.
- *Diagnosis*—additional diagnostic tests include immunocytochemistry (to differentiate from other types of cancers) using core biopsy (recommended to be performed in theatre).[1]
- *Treatment*—prompt referral to oncologists. Steroids may be very efficient in relieving compression symptoms.[1]
- *Prognosis*—good for early stage lymphomas (50–85% 5y survival rate) and poor for advanced stage lymphomas (15–35% 5y survival rate).[1]

Further reading

1. British Association of Endocrine Surgeons (2003). Guidelines for the surgical management of endocrine disease. Available from: http://www.baes.info/Pages/BAETS%20Guidelines.pdf.
2. British Thyroid Association (2006). UK guidelines for the use of thyroid function tests. Available from: http://www.british-thyroid-association.org/info-for-patients/Docs/TFT_guideline_final_version_July_2006.pdf.
3. Gharib H, Papini E, Valcavi R et al. (2006). American Association of Clinical Endocrinologists and Associazione Medici Endocrinologi medical guidelines for clinical practice for the diagnosis and management of thyroid nodules. Endocr Pract 12, 63–102.
4. European Thyroid Association. Available from: http://www.hotthyroidology.com/ebook/file_info/download1.php?file=_ebook_ht_2008-2009. pdf. Accessed May 2009.
5. Hegedüs L (2004). Clinical practice. The thyroid nodule. N Engl J Med 351, 1764–71.
6. Anderson CE, McLaren KM (2003). Best practice in thyroid pathology. J Clin Pathol 56, 401–5.
7. Jones MK (2001). Management of nodular thyroid disease. The challenge remains identifying which palpable nodules are malignant. BMJ 323, 293–4.
8. Wass J, Shalet S, eds (2002). Oxford Textbook of Endocrinology and Diabetes. Oxford University Press, Oxford.
9. Cancer Research UK. Available from: http://info.cancerresearchuk.org/cancerstats/types/thyroid/?a=5441. Accessed May 2009.
10. National Comprehensive Cancer Network (2009). NCCN clinical practice guidelines in oncology. Available from: http://www.nccn.org/professionals/physician_gls/f_guidelines.asp.
11. de Groot JW, Plukker JT, Wolffenbuttel BH, Wiggers T, Sluiter WJ, Links TP (2006). Determinants of life expectancy in medullary thyroid cancer: age does not matter. Clin Endocrinol (Oxf) 65, 729–36.
12. Cancer Research UK (2008). Thyroid cancer survival statistics. Available from: http://info.cancerresearchuk.org/cancerstats/types/thyroid/survival/.

Surgery for hyperparathyroidism*

* The guidelines on this chapter have been sourced and summarized from different UK, Europe, and international government sources, professional organizations, and medical specialty societies. Leading guidelines have been listed in the Key guidelines box.

Surgery for hyperparathyroidism

Key guidelines

- British Association of Endocrine Surgeons (2003). Guidelines for the surgical management of endocrine disease.
- The American Association of Clinical Endocrinologists and the American Association of Endocrine Surgeons (2005). Diagnosis and management of primary hyperparathyroidism.
- National Institute for Health and Clinical Excellence (2007). Thoracoscopic excision of mediastinal parathyroid tumours.

Basic facts

- *Definition*—hyperparathyroidism (HPT) is the abnormal excessive production of parathyroid hormone (PTH) from the parathyroid gland(s), often with resultant hypercalcaemia (Table 51.1).
- *Incidence*—HPT affects ~1% of adult population.[2] Incidence increases after the age of 55, and women are more commonly affected (3× men).[2]
- *Pathogenesis*—HPT results from solitary parathyroid adenoma (85%) or multiple hyperfunctioning parathyroid glands (including parathyroid hyperplasia, multiple adenomas, and polyclonal hyperfunction) (Table 51.2).[1,7,8] Hyperfunctioning parathyroid carcinoma accounts for ~1% of cases.[1,2,7,8]
- *Clinical presentation*—over 80% of primary hyperparathyroidism (PHP) in Western countries are found incidentally by routine biochemical tests.[2,10] Symptoms and signs result usually from the combined effect of increased PTH secretion and hypercalcaemia (Table 51.3).
  - A thorough clinical history usually shows subtle neurobehavioural symptoms (fatigue, weakness, anorexia, mild depression, and mild cognitive or neuromuscular dysfunction) in up to 50% of cases.[7]
  - Symptoms and signs have been immortalized historically by Walter St Goar in the mnemonic 'bones (bone pain and fractures), stones (renal or ureteric stones), abdominal groans (pancreatitis, constipation, and peptic ulcer), and psychiatric moans (depression and cognitive or neuromuscular dysfunction)'.

Recommended investigations (Fig. 51.1)

- *Diagnosis*—can be established by demonstrating persistent hypercalcaemia (or serum calcium at the high normal levels) in the presence of elevated (or inappropriately normal) PTH concentrations and elevated urinary calcium excretion.[1,2]
- *Other laboratory tests*—include measurement of 24h urinary calcium excretion and 25-hydroxyvitamin D for undetermined cases.[1]
- *Differential diagnosis*—should always be reviewed (Table 51.4). The surgeon has the ultimate responsibility to check that other causes of hypercalcaemia have been excluded.[1]

Table 51.1 Hyperparathyroidism—definitions and classification

- *Primary hyperparathyroidism (PHP)*—the autonomous overproduction of PTH from the parathyroid gland(s), often with resultant hypercalcaemia.[2]

- *Secondary hyperparathyroidism*—the excessive secretion of PTH in response to hypocalcaemia with associated hypertrophy of the parathyroid glands. Most commonly associated with chronic renal failure.

- *Tertiary hyperparathyroidism*—the excessive autonomous calcium-insensitive secretion of PTH after a long period of secondary HPT.

Table 51.2 Parathyroid tumours—molecular biology

- *Activation of oncogenes*—cyclin D1/PRAD1 for sporadic tumours and RET gene for familial tumours.[8,9,14]

- *Deactivation of tumour suppression genes*—MEN1 gene for sporadic and familial tumours and HRPT2 gene in familial tumours.[8,9,14]

- *Confirmed risk factors.*
  - *History of irradiation to the head and neck (external radiation or atomic bomb)*—dose-dependent effect. High radiation dose (≥12Gy) increases the risk by >50%; low doses (1Gy) increase the risk by 5–10 times (<1% at 35y).[12,13]
  - *MEN type 1 or 2 syndromes*—PHP is the most common component of MEN1 and represents the initial manifestation of the syndrome in most patients. About 1–2% of all cases of PHP are due to MEN1.[14] MEN2A syndrome is associated with a predisposition to medullary thyroid cancer (90%), phaeochromocytoma (40–50%), and primary parathyroid hyperplasia (10–20%).[14] Parathyroid hyperplasia is not a feature of MEN2B syndrome.[14]

Table 51.3 Clinical manifestations

- *Effect on bone metabolism*—loss of bone mineral density (measured by the dual energy X-ray absorptiometry (DEXA) test), increase in fracture risk (×2–3), distributed variably between cortical sites (mainly long bones), and trabecular sites (mainly vertebrae).[4] Osteitis fibrosa cystica, brown tumours, and subperiosteal bone resorption on the radial aspect of the middle phalanges are found only in patients with prolonged, severe disease.[10]

- *Nephrolithiasis*—occurs in ~15–20% of patients. Only ~5% of patients with nephrolithiasis will have HPT.[10,11]

Recommended treatment (Fig. 51.1)

- **Natural history**—the progress of HPT is usually slow in most patients, if at all. Nevertheless, about 25–60% of untreated asymptomatic patients will develop symptomatic disease during a 10y period.[2,7]
- **Surgical resection**—the treatment of choice for all symptomatic and asymptomatic patients who are fit for surgery.[1,2,6]
  - *Recommendations for asymptomatic patients*—controversial since the recommendations from the NIH consensus conference (2002).[15] Nevertheless, more recent evidence has shown clear benefits of surgical resection as well as significantly reduced risks of operative intervention (see below).[1,2,6] Surgery has become the currently recommended approach for all asymptomatic patients who are fit for anaesthesia and surgery by most authorities.[1,2,6]
  - *Benefits of early surgical intervention*—include reduced mortality from cardiovascular diseases, improved physical and neuropsychological well-being, decreased risk of kidney stones, improved bone mineral density, and possible decrease of fracture risk.[1,2,6] Surgical intervention is possibly more cost-effective than any single hospital admission for a complication of HPT.[16]
  - *Recommendations for technical aspects*—see Table 51.5.
  - *Thoracoscopic excision of mediastinal parathyroid tumours*—should only be performed within a proper trial and clinical governance setting.[3]
  - *Post-operatively*—check serum calcium within the first 24h (and thereafter, if abnormal). Serum calcium should be checked in 1y for solitary adenoma patients.[1]
  - *Re-operative parathyroid surgery*—should be managed within a multidisciplinary setting by a specialist centre with appropriate facilities.[1]
- **Medical management**—has little contribution to the curative management plan.[2] Good hydration, furosemide, oestrogen replacement in post-menopausal women, and bisphosphonate therapy have all some supportive role.[2]
  - *Cinacalcet (an agent which increases the sensitivity of calcium-sensing receptors to extracellular calcium ions, and therefore, inhibits the release of PTH)*—has enough evidence to support its recommendation for the treatment of refractory secondary HPT in patients with end-stage renal disease where surgical excision is contraindicated.[20] Pooled analysis of three largest RCTs (n = 1,136) showed that Cinacalcet can reach the target mean PTH levels in ~40% of patients (compared to 5% of patients receiving placebo, p <0.001).[20]

Table 51.4 Differential diagnosis of hypercalcaemia

- **With associated elevated PTH**—primary HPT (sporadic), familial (MEN I and IIA, familial hypercalcaemic hypocalciuria), tertiary HPT (chronic renal failure).

- **With no associated PTH.**
  - **Malignancy-related.**
  - **Medications**—e.g. vitamin D intoxication, thiazide, diuretics, lithium, excessive vitamin A.
  - **Miscellaneous**—chronic granulomatous disease , hyperthyroidism, phaeochromocytoma, acromegaly, immobilization, parenteral nutrition, milk alkali syndrome.

Table 51.5 Surgical exploration—technical aspects

- **Preoperative localization**—only required if a 'focused' limited neck exploration is to be performed.[1] No current consensus exists on the specific indications or cost-effectiveness of each localization strategy.
  - There is no substitute for an experienced surgeon with meticulous dissection and haemostasis.[1]
  - Current options include: (1) the 99mTc-sestamibi scanning with the use of a single photon emission CT scan,[4] (2) intra-operative measurement of circulating PTH,[5] (3) high resolution USS examination, and (4) intra-operative direct PTH measurement (which can effectively avoid the need for frozen section and confirm cure).[1,2,6]
  - Some surgeons use handheld gamma detection devices for radioguided parathyroidectomy.[2] The combination of 99mTc-sestamibi scanning with USS has a reported combined sensitivity of 94%.[17]

- **Unilateral parathyroid exploration**—can be performed using a collar incision or minimally invasive-type incision. The cure rate following such approach can reach up to 99%.[6,18]

- **Focused parathyroidectomy (FP)**—can be performed using a small lateral neck incision.[6] This can be performed under local or regional anaesthesia and is suitable for day case surgery.[6]
  - **Efficiency and risks**—FP can achieve 100% cure rate (defined as normocalcaemia) when combined with intra-operative PTH (iPTH) measurement.[6,19] The overall complication rate is ~1.2% (compared to 3% for open bilateral exploration), the operating time is ~30min (compared to >60min for open bilateral exploration), and the post-operative stay before discharge (in the day case surgery setting) is 2h.[6,19]

- **Thoracoscopic excision of mediastinal parathyroid tumours**—has limited evidence on safety and efficacy, and should ONLY and STRICTLY be used by well-trained surgeons within appropriate clinical governance setting.

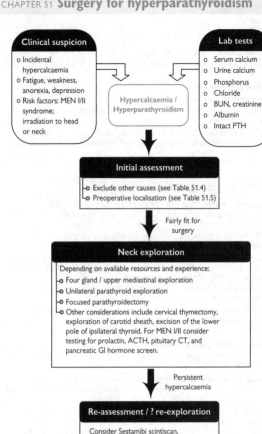

Fig. 51.1 Suggested approach to primary hyperparathyroidism

Further reading

1. British Association of Endocrine Surgeons (2003). Guidelines for the surgical management of endocrine disease. Available from: http://www.baes.info/Pages/BAETS%20Guidelines.pdf.
2. AACE/AAES Task Force on primary hyperparathyroidism (2005). The American Association of Clinical Endocrinologists and the American Association of Endocrine Surgeons position statement on the diagnosis and management of primary hyperparathyroidism. Endocr Pract 11, 49–54.
3. National Institute for Health and Clinical Excellence (2007) Thoracoscopic excision of mediastinal parathyroid tumours. Available from: http://www.nice.org.uk/nicemedia/pdf/IPG247Guidance.pdf.
4. The Society of Nuclear Medicine (2004). Procedure guideline for parathyroid scintigraphy. Available from: http://interactive.snm.org/docs/Parathyroid_v3.0.pdf.
5. National Academy of Clinical Biochemistry (2006). Intraoperative parathyroid hormone. Laboratory medicine practice guidelines: evidence-based practice for point-of-care testing. Available from: http://guidelines.gov/summary/summary.aspx?doc_id=10820&nbr=005645&string=parathyroid.
6. Wishart GC (2006). Recent advances in the diagnosis and management of primary hyperparathyroidism (pHPT). Available from: http://www.endocrinology.org/education/resource/summerschool/2006/ss06/ss06_wis.htm.
7. Marx SJ (2000). Hyperparathyroid and hypoparathyroid disorders. N Engl J Med 343, 1863–75.
8. Ruda JM, Hollenbeak CS, Stack BC Jr (2005). A systematic review of the diagnosis and treatment of primary hyperparathyroidism from 1995 to 2003. Otolaryngol Head Neck Surg 132, 359–72.
9. Hendy GN (2000). Molecular mechanisms of primary hyperparathyroidism. Rev Endocr Metab Disord 1, 297–305.
10. Silverberg SJ, Bilezikian JP (1996). Evaluation and management of primary hyperparathyroidism. J Clin Endocrinol Metab 81, 2036–40.
11. Parks J, Coe F, Favus M (1980). Hyperparathyroidism in nephrolithiasis. Arch Intern Med 140, 1479–81.
12. Tisell LE, Hansson G, Lindberg S, Rangnhult I (1977). Hyperparathyroidism in persons treated with X-rays for tuberculous cervical adenitis. Cancer 40, 846–54.
13. Schneider AB, Gierlowski TC, Shore–Freedman E, Stovall M, Ron E, Lubin J (1995). Dose-response relationships for radiation-induced hyperparathyroidism. J Clin Endocrinol Metab 80, 254–7.
14. Brandi ML, Gagel RF, Angeli A et al. (2001). Guidelines for diagnosis and therapy of MEN type 1 and type 2. J Clin Endocrinol Metab 86, 5658–71.
15. Bilezikian JP, Potts JT Jr (2002). Asymptomatic primary hyperparathyroidism: new issues and new questions—bridging the past with the future. J Bone Miner Res 17 (Suppl 2), N57–67.
16. Sejean K, Calmus S, Durand Zaleski I et al. (2005). Surgery versus medical follow-up in patients with asymptomatic primary hyperparathyroidism: a decision analysis. Eur J Endocrin 153, 915–27.
17. Lumachi F, Ermani M, Basso S, Zucchetta P, Borsato N, Favia G (2001). Localization of parathyroid tumours in the minimally invasive era: which technique should be chosen? Population-based analysis of 253 patients undergoing parathyroidectomy and factors affecting parathyroid gland detection. Endocr Relat Cancer 8, 63–9.
18. Sidhu S, Neill AK, Russell CF (2003). Long-term outcome of unilateral parathyroid exploration for primary hyperparathyroidism due to presumed solitary adenoma. World J Surg 27, 339–42.
19. Gurnell EM, Thomas SK, McFarlane I et al. (2004). Focused parathyroid surgery with intraoperative parathyroid hormone measurement, as a day case procedure. Br J Surg 91, 78–82.
20. National Institute for Health and Clinical Excellence (2007). Cinacalcet for the treatment of secondary hyperparathyroidism in patients with end-stage renal disease on maintenance dialysis therapy. Available from: http://www.nice.org.uk/nicemedia/pdf/TA117guidance.pdf.

Index